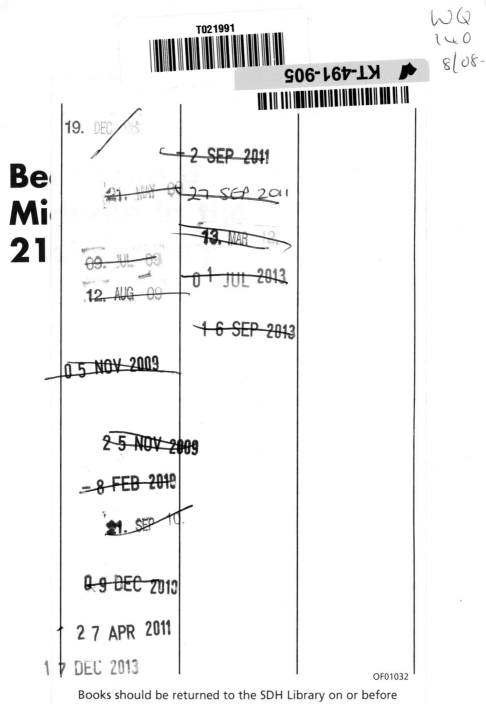

Becoming a Midwife in the 21st Century

Edited by:
Ian Peate
Cathy Hamilton

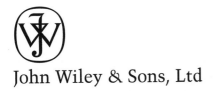

John Wiley & Sons, Ltd

Other Wiley Editorial Offices

Library of Congress Cataloging-in-Publication Data
Becoming a midwife in the 21st century / edited by Ian Peate, Cathy Hamilton.
        p.   ;   cm.
    Includes bibliographical references and index.
    ISBN   978-0-470-06559-4 (alk. paper)
1. Midwifery–Study and teaching.   I. Peate, Ian.   II. Hamilton, Cathy,
1962-   III. Title: Becoming a midwife in the twenty-first century.
    [DNLM: 1.   Home Childbirth–nursing.   2.   Nurse Midwives–organization &
administration.   3.   Nurse Midwives–standards.   4.   Perinatal Care–methods.
5.   Quality Assurance, Health Care. WQ 160 B398 2007]
    RG950.B43 2007
    618.2'0233–dc22

                                                         2007031343

British Library Cataloguing in Publication Data
A catalogue record for this book is available from the British Library

ISBN: 978-0-470-06559-4

Typeset by SNP Best-set Typesetter Ltd., Hong Kong
Printed and bound in Singapore by Markono Print Media Pte Ltd

This book is dedicated to women, their families and to midwives, because they matter.

Contents

List of Contributors

Laura Abbott BA, BSc(Hons), RGN, DipN(Lond), RM, PGCert (supervision) is an Independent Midwife. She is a Supervisor of Midwives for the East of England Local Supervisory Authority and is linked with the team of Supervisors at East and North Herts NHS Trust. Laura has written for midwifery and nursing journals. She also occasionally teaches at The University of Hertfordshire on the pre and post registration midwifery courses and has been a guest speaker at conferences around the UK. Laura has just completed her MSc in Advancing Practice (Midwifery).

Meryl Dimock RGN, RM is a Clinical Facilitator at Watford General Hospital. She is a Labour Ward Co-ordinator and she has trained as an ALSO instructor and a Supervisor of Midwives.

Lyn Dolby BSc(Hons), RGN, RM, DPSM, PG Cert is Senior Midwifery Lecturer at the University of Hertfordshire. After working in ENT and Commando surgery Lyn undertook midwifery training and then worked as a midwife until she joined the Royal Berkshire Hospital as an autonomous rural Community Midwife. She began working in midwifery education at Nottingham University and then joined the University of Hertfordshire in 1996.

Caroline Duncombe BSc(Hons), MSc, RGN, RM, DipHE Midwifery, PGCert is Midwife, Supervisor of Midwives. She is currently an instructor on the ALSO (Advanced Life Saving in Obstetrics) Course and works as a Community Midwife and in the antenatal clinic. Her interests include supporting women with medical complications through their pregnancy and birth.

Tandy Deane-Gray MA, BSc, PGCEA, ADM, RM, RGN is a Senior Lecturer Midwifery at the University of Hertfordshire. She has worked in Midwifery Education since 1988 and her key interests have continued to be midwifery, parenting and communication. She has developed her interest in the psychology and mental health of parents by becoming a psychotherapist.

Sarah Green RM, DipHE Midwifery has been a registered midwife for 11 years. She has worked at West Herts NHS Trust since 1998 and is currently working as a teenage pregnancy midwife with a special interest in high risk pregnancy, especially pre-eclampsia and eclampsia.

Cathy Hamilton BSc(Hons), MSc, RGN, RM, PGDip, PGCert is a Senior Midwifery Lecturer at the University of Hertfordshire and Supervisor of Midwives. In 2004 Cathy undertook the preparation for supervisors programme and has joined the team supervisors of midwives at West Herts NHS Trust.

Eileen Huish DCR(R) is practice Lead for the pre-registration Interprofessional Education at the University of Hertfordshire. Eileen's role is to support and facilitate interprofessional learning in practice and she is currently studying for an MA in Learning and Teaching in Higher Education. Eileen actively supported the Creating an Interprofessional Workforce (CIPW) initiative and chaired the CIPW Practice Learning Working Group. She has recently been appointed co-editor of the Centre of the Advancement of Interprofessional Education (CAIPE) Education Bulletin.

Annabel Jay BA(Hons), MA, FHEA, DipHE, RM, PGDip(HE) is a Senior Lecturer in Midwifery and is currently the admissions tutor for the pre-registration midwifery programme at the University of Hertfordshire and has recently undertaken research into the Objective Structural Clinical Examination (OSCE). Annabel continues to lead parent education classes at an NHS Trust.

Chris Lawrence MSc(Dist), BSc(Hons), RM, RN, PGCEA, Cert Coaching is a Principal Lecturer Midwifery. Chris gained qualifications as an orthopaedic nurse and then as a registered general nurse before undertaking her midwifery training. After studying advanced nursing and midwifery courses and gaining a post graduate diploma in the education of adults she has been in midwifery education for the last 25 years. Her particular interest in organisational development was enhanced by studying this field at Masters level, and is now directed through providing performance coaching and action learning for senior managers in both the nursing and midwifery professions.

Sally Luck MA(Health Law), BSc, RN, RM has been a practising midwife for more than 25 years. She completed a masters degree in Health Law in 2003 and has been working in Clinical Governance and Risk Management for the past two years at Barnet and Chase Farm NHS Trust. She works closely with the Maternity service covering all aspects of risk and governance to help achieve best practice in Maternity care.

Kath Mannion BSc Midwifery, MSc Midwifery, RM, RN, ADM is LSA Midwifery Officer for the North East Strategic Health Authority. Kath's current appointment includes investigating cases of alleged sub-optimal practice by midwives and determining the appropriate supervisory action. She is an Advanced Life Support in Obstetrics (ALSO) Advisory Faculty and serves as a trustee on the executive team within that organisation. She regularly teaches on ALSO Provider and Instructor Courses throughout the UK and Ireland.

Marianne Mead PhD qualified as a nurse in 1974 and as a midwife in 1975. She is now a member of the Executive Board of the European Midwives Association and a member of the ICM French speaking Research Group. She is also a member of the Editorial Board of Evidence-based Midwifery (UK), British Journal of Midwifery (UK) and Les Dossiers de l'Obstetrique (France). Additionally she is a journal referee for Evidence-based Midwifery, Midwifery and Primary Health Care Research and Development.

Chandra Mehta RN, RM is a Supervisor of Midwives. Since 1997, Chandra's clinical role has been based at a stand alone birth centre in Edgware, working as a G grade midwife. Chandra is also a Supervisor of Midwives, qualified in 2004, and has implemented and continues to facilitate the record keeping workshops in the trust for all staff. She is currently undertaking a master's degree at the University of Hertfordshire, Hatfield.

Lisa Nash BSc (Hons), MBA (Herts), RM, PGDip, Dip HE Midwifery is Senior Lecturer in Midwifery at the University of Hertfordshire. Lisa's key areas of interest include health education and promotion, sexual health and management issues. She is currently a senior lecturer within the School of Nursing and Midwifery.

Ian Peate BEd (Hons), MA (Lond), EN(G), RGN DipN (Lond), RNT, LLM is Associate Head of School of Nursing and Midwifery at the University of Hertfordshire. Ian's key areas of interest are nursing practice and theory, sexual health and HIV/AIDS. His portfolio centres on recruitment and marketing and professional academic development with the School of Nursing and Midwifery.

Cathy Rogers MA, RN, RMN, RM, ADM, PGCEA, Supervisor of Midwives qualified as a midwife in 1984 and she has worked in all areas of midwifery practice. She is currently employed as a consultant midwife at Barnet and Chase Farm NHS Trust where she is responsible for leading midwifery led services. She is also an honorary lecturer at the University of Hertfordshire and is specifically involved in the development and the delivery of the postgraduate course for the preparation of supervisors of midwives.

Nada Schiavone RN, RM, MBA, HSM currently works in a risk management role in the Clinical Governance Department at Barnet and Chase Farm Trust. Nada is a registered nurse and midwife and has held a range of challenging roles in nursing and midwifery, including Head of Risk Management and Assistant Director of Nursing prior to her appointment. She has a personal interest in clinical governance and risk.

Celia Wildeman SCM, DipNS, ADM, PGDC, PGDSPCF, Supervisor of Midwives is Senior Lecturer in the Department of Nursing and Midwifery at the University of Hertfordshire. Her special interest include women's sexual health, teenage pregnancy, domestic violence and abuse, equal opportunities and cultural diversity.

Carole Yearley MSc, RN, RM, ADM, PGCEA, PGCERT Supervisor of Midwives is a Principal Lecturer, Midwifery. She is part of the team of Supervisors of Midwives at Barnet Enfield and Haringey Strategic Health Authority and currently is the Programme Tutor for the Post Graduate Certificate in the Supervision of Midwives at the University of Hertfordshire.

Acknowledgements

We would like to thank all of our colleagues for their help, support, comments and suggestions. We thank Anthony Peate who produced the illustrations.

Cathy would like to thank her children Lucy and Elizabeth for their patience, her mother Shirley Richardson for her helpful suggestions, and her partner Gary Martin for his continued support and encouragement.

Ian would like to thank his sister Sharon Brent and his partner Jussi Lahtinen for their support and encouragement.

Introduction

Ian Peate and Cathy Hamilton

This text is primarily intended for midwifery students, health care assistants, associated practitioners, those undertaking SNVQ/NVQ level of study or anyone who intends to undertake a programme of study leading to registration as a midwife. Throughout the text the terms midwife, student and midwifery are used. These terms and the principles applied to this book can be transferred to a number of health care workers at various levels and in various settings in order to develop their skills for caring for women and their families through childbirth.

The unique role and function of the midwife

Midwives provide individual care to women and their families, encouraging them to participate in and determine how they want their pregnancy to progress. Midwives work with women during and after their pregnancy in a variety of settings, for example, in the women's own homes, midwifery-led units and hospitals. Midwife means 'with woman' and this highlights the empowering/partnership role of the midwife – the midwife works with the woman rather than telling her what to do.

The support the midwife offers is determined by assessing the woman's individual needs and working in partnership with her and other health care workers. The midwife is usually the lead health care professional involved in caring for pregnant women. There will be occasions when you will need to work on your own as a midwife and times when you will be working as a member of the wider team. It is important that midwives work collaboratively with other health care professionals, including obstetricians, paediatricians, specialist community public health nurses and paramedics, in order to ensure a high quality of care for women and their families.

According to Medforth et al. (2006) the definition of a midwife was first officially formulated in 1972. This followed discussions and debates among various organisations and committees and is as follows:

> 'A midwife is a person who, having been regularly admitted to a midwifery educational programme, duly recognised in the country in which it is located, has successfully completed the prescribed course of studies in midwifery and has acquired the requisite qualifications to be registered and/or legally licensed to practise midwifery.'

The midwife is the senior professional attending over 75 per cent of births in the UK; she provides total care to mother and baby from early pregnancy onwards, throughout childbirth and until the baby is 28 days old (Medforth et al. 2006). The role of the midwife is thus multifaceted.

The midwife's role in public health

Another important aspect of that role is within the context of public health. Public health can be defined as improving the health of the population, as opposed to treating the diseases of individuals. This is particularly appropriate in midwifery as you will be caring for healthy individuals going through the physiological process of childbirth. Public health functions (DH 2004) include:

- Health surveillance, monitoring and analysis
- Investigation of disease outbreaks, epidemics and risk to health
- Establishing, designing and empowering communities
- Creating and sustaining cross-government and inter-sectoral partnerships to improve health and reduce inequalities
- Ensuring compliance with regulations and laws to protect and promote health
- Developing and maintaining a well-educated and trained, multidisciplinary public health workforce
- Ensuring the effective performance of NHS services to meet goals in improving health, preventing disease and reducing inequalities
- Research, development, evaluation and innovation
- Quality assuring the public health function

Public heath activities can take place with individuals, their families or communities, on a national or international level. The midwife is ideally placed to influence and enact public health policy when working with women and their families as well as being able to develop a population perspective within midwifery.

All the chapters in this text are concerned with midwifery practice, and as such are rooted in public health. Midwives make a substantial contribution to public health by promoting the long-term well-being of women, their babies and their families. They provide information and advice regarding screening and testing, sexual health, nutrition, exercise and healthy lifestyles. The midwife promotes breastfeeding, offering support and advice, as well as providing guidance to women and their families in relation to immunisation (RCM 2001). Public health in midwifery is not new; midwives have always provided care that has a public health focus. Public health is at the heart of all aspects of midwifery practice.

Terminology

There are number of terms that can be used to describe women who use maternity services. 'Patient', 'woman' and 'client' are used throughout this text and refer to all groups and individuals who have direct or indirect contact with health care workers and in particular registered midwives, nurses and specialist community public health nurses.

Patient is the term commonly used within the NHS. It is acknowledged that not everyone approves of the passive concept associated with it or the way in which it can emphasise a medical focus. However, the term is used in this text in the knowledge that it is widely understood. The other two commonly used terms – woman and client – are also used to reflect changes in the way midwives and other care providers are considering their relationships with users of maternity services. The term client emphasises the professional nature of the relationship that the midwife has with the women she cares for. The term consumer is taken from the marketplace and highlights the concept of service-users as consumers of products such as medications or care services. Client and consumer have their roots in health care provision during the 1980s and 1990s, when – particularly in the health service – market forces and consumerism were in vogue. Another term used is expert. Experts are said to be on an equal footing with expert care providers (for example, midwives and obstetricians). They are often patients who live with long-term health conditions.

Table I.1   Number of midwives on the midwives' section of the professional register

Number of midwives	
Male	163
Female	42 718
Total	42 881

Source: NMC 2006

There are 42 881 midwives on the midwives' section of the professional register (see Table I.1). The majority of midwives in the UK are women. And whilst it is acknowledged that the number of men entering the midwifery profession is increasing, for the sake of brevity this text uses the pronoun she.

The Nursing and Midwifery Council and Quality Assurance (Education)

The primary aim of the Nursing and Midwifery Council (NMC), an organisation established by Parliament, is to protect the public by ensuring that midwives and nurses provide a high standard of care to their patients and clients.

The NMC is the regulatory body responsible for promoting best practice amongst the midwives and nurses registered with them. The key role of the NMC is central to ensuring that women receive the best possible care. It is the responsibility of the NMC to set and monitor standards in training (Nursing and Midwifery Order 2001). The NMC has produced a framework for quality assurance of education programmes. This framework relates to all programmes that lead to registration or to the recording of a qualification on the professional register.

The programme you have embarked on, or are going to embark on, must meet certain standards. These include the standards set by your educational institution – for example, your university's policies and procedures relating to quality assurance and external influences. The NMC and the Quality Assurance Agency (QAA) standards must be satisfied before a programme of study can be validated and deemed fit for purpose (Quality Assurance Agency for Higher Education 2000). Other external factors that must be given due consideration are the European Directives. Two European Directives – 77/453/EEC and 89/595/EEC – and their implications are discussed.

The Nursing and Midwifery Order 2001 provides the NMC with powers in relation to quality assurance and, as a result of this, the production of a framework that education providers (for example, universities) that offer, or intend to offer, NMC-approved programmes leading to registration or recording on the register have to adhere to. There are many provisions in place in the UK that ensure the quality of education programmes.

The NMC has to be satisfied that its standards for granting a licence to practise are being met as required and in association with the law. They do so by setting standards to maintain public confidence, as well as to protect the public. By appointing representatives they can be satisfied that they are represented during the quality assurance process in relation to the approval, re-approval and annual monitoring activities associated with programmes of study.

Each programme of study for pre-registration midwifery must demonstrate explicitly and robustly that it has included the rules and standards of the NMC so that those who complete a recognised programme of study are eligible for registration. The Standards of Proficiency for Pre-registration Midwifery Education (NMC 2004a) are examples of standards that must be achieved prior to registration.

Midwives Rules and Standards

The Nursing and Midwifery Order 2001 demands that the NMC sets rules and standards for midwifery and Local Supervising Authorities (LSAs) for the function of statutory supervision of midwives. *The Midwives Rules and Standards* (NMC 2004c) replace those produced in 1998. The current *Rules and Standards* came into force on 1 August 2004 (see Table I.2).

Becoming a proficient midwife

Those who wish to study to become a midwife, and then go on to register with the NMC and afterwards practise as a midwife, must undertake a three-year (or equivalent) programme of study. The programme must by law comprise 2300 hours of practice and another 2300 hours of theory.

The title registered midwife is protected in law. This means it can only be used by a person who is registered with the NMC and her name must appear on the national register. There are three parts to the professional register:

Table 1.2 The 16 midwifery rules

Rule	Description
1	Citation and commencement
2	Interpretation
3	Notification of intention to practise
4	Notification by LSA
5	Suspension from practice by LSA
6	Responsibility and sphere of practice
7	Administration of medicines
8	Clinical trials
9	Records
10	Inspection of premises and equipment
11	Eligibility for appointment as a Supervisor of Midwives
12	The supervision of midwives
13	The local supervising authority midwifery officer
14	Exercise local supervising authority of its function
15	Publication of local supervising authority procedures
16	Annual report

Source: NMC 2004c

- Nurses
- Midwives
- Specialist community public health nurses

The student who wishes to undertake midwifery education must meet the NMC's requirements for age of entry. Those entering a programme of pre-registration midwifery education must be no less than 17 years and 6 months of age on the first day of the commencement of the programme. However, in certain exceptional circumstances and related to specific programmes the NMC may agree to an earlier age, but this will never be less than 17 years. Currently this requirement is index review.

As well as satisfying the NMC's age requirement, general entry requirements must also be met. Educational requirements are set by each educational institution; and there must also be evidence of literacy and numeracy. How these requirements are set is the prerogative of the educational institution; however, the NMC must agree to and permit these requirements. Those wishing to practise in Wales must also be able to demonstrate proficiency in the use of the Welsh language where this is required. On entry, during and on completion of their programme all applicants must demonstrate that they have good health and good character sufficient for safe and effective practice. It is the responsibility of educational institutions to have procedures in place to ensure assessment of health and character. Any convictions or cautions related to criminal offences that the applicant has must be declared. There are several ways in which this can be achieved, for example, self-disclosure, and/or criminal record checks conducted by accredited organisations.

Completion of the programme and achievement of the proficiencies mean that the student will graduate with both a professional qualification (Registered Midwife (RM)) and an academic qualification at degree or enhanced diploma level. The good character and good health declaration is made on an approved form provided by the NMC. This must be supported by the registered midwife whose name has been notified to the NMC, who is responsible for directing the educational programme at the university, or his/her designated registered midwife substitute. This midwife is known as the Lead Midwife for Education (LME).

Once registered with the NMC the midwife is accountable for her actions or omissions and is bound by the tenets enshrined in the *Code of Professional Conduct* (NMC 2004b). Legal requirements, such as participating in continuing professional development and the maintaining a personal professional portfolio, must be addressed. This text provides you with insight into how to become a proficient midwife.

There are 15 standards associated with pre-registration midwifery. These range from the appointment of the LME to standards of proficiency (see Table I.3). This text will address the standards of proficiency for entry to the register for midwives.

Currently, no texts are available that describe in the same detail as this text does the standards of education required to achieve the NMC standards of proficiency (standard 15) as demanded by the NMC.

The proficiencies

The format of the text draws upon that used by the NMC in their publication *Standards of Proficiency for Pre–Registration Midwifery Education* (NMC 2004a). Standard 15 concerns the standards of education and is divided into four domains.

Domain I   Effective Midwifery Practice
Domain II   Professional and Ethical Practice
Domain III   Developing the Individual Midwife and Others
Domain IV   Achieving Quality Care through Evaluation and Research

Table 1.3   Summary of the standards for pre-registration midwifery

Standard 1	Appointment of the LME
Standard 2	Development, delivery and management of midwifery programmes of education
Standard 3	Signing the supporting declaration for good health and good character
Standard 4	Age of entry
Standard 5	General requirements for admission to approved pre-registration of education and entry to the register: 5.1. Literacy and numeracy 5.2. Good health and good character
Standard 6	Interruption in pre-registration midwifery programmes of education
Standard 7	Admission with advanced standing
Standard 8	Transfer between approved education institutions
Standard 9	Academic standard of programme
Standard 10	Length of programme
Standard 11	Student support
Standard 12	Balance between clinical practice and theory
Standard 13	Supernumerary status
Standard 14	Assessment strategy
Standard 15	Standards of education to achieve NMC standards of proficiency

Source: NMC 2004a

Case notes and activities

Most of the chapters provides the reader with case notes to consider and activities to carry out. They are included to encourage and motivate you, as well as for you to assess your learning and progress. It is also anticipated that they will enable you to link theoretical concepts with what is occurring in the clinical setting. You are encouraged to delve deeper and seek other sources – both human and material – to help with your responses.

In Chapters 2 and 3 you will find useful snippets of midwifery knowledge, gathered and honed as a result of many years midwifery practice, called midwifery wisdom.

The aim of this text is to encourage, inspire and stimulate you, as well as instilling in you the desire, confidence and competence to become a registered midwife. What is required from you is an interest in women and their families through all stages of pregnancy. Becoming a member of the midwifery profession places many demands on you, the key demand being the desire to care with compassion and understanding for the women and families you will have the privilege to work with.

References

Department of Health (2004) *Standards for Better Health*. London: DH.

Medforth, J., Battersby, S., Evans, M. et al. (2006) *Oxford Handbook of Midwifery*. Oxford: Oxford University Press.

Nursing and Midwifery Council (2004a) *The Standards of Proficiency for Pre-registration Midwifery Education*. London: NMC.

Nursing and Midwifery Council (2004b) *The NMC Code of Professional Conduct: Standards for Conduct, Performance and Ethics*. London: NMC.

Nursing and Midwifery Council (2004c) *Midwives Rules and Standards*. London: NMC.

Nursing and Midwifery Council (2006) *Statistical Analysis of the Register: 1 April to 31 March 2006*. London: NMC.

Quality Assurance Agency for Higher Education (2000) *Code of Practice for the Assurance of Academic Quality and Standards in Higher Education*. Gloucester: QAA.

Royal College of Midwives (2001) *The Midwives' Role in Public Health*. Position Paper 24. London: RCM.

Effective Communication

Tandy Deane-Gray

Introduction

The purpose of this chapter is to relate and understand how the development of communication from infancy can influence and inform your skills as adults in order to enhance your work-based experience to meet needs of the clients in your care. The chapter encourages you to draw from the lessons of optimal parent–infant relationships, including sensitive responsiveness, which underpins effective communication, as well as providing an outline of communication issues for practice. This is a condensed chapter on communication skills for midwives, and is designed to stimulate the reader to seek the original sources for expansion of the concepts.

Midwives are in a unique position to observe how humans learn to communicate. When time is taken to observe infants it is apparent that babies are 'pre-programmed' to interact with adults (Stern 1985). This is due to their preference for the sound, sight and movement of adults rather than other comparable stimuli. They are especially attracted to their mother. This is probably a biological instinct, as humans depend on their mother and other adults to care for them to ensure survival.

MacFarlane (1977) highlighted the ability of babies and dispelled many myths about infants, such as the belief that they cannot see. Not only can they see – and focus well at about 30 cm – but they like to look at the contrast and contours found in the human face. They turn to sound, particularly their mother's voice; and will turn to the smell of their mother's breast pad in preference to another woman's. So they develop recognition of their mother very quickly through their senses, and communicate their needs through behaviours (RCM 1999).

Babies also mimic the behaviours of adults, most noticeably by facial expression. If you smile, open you mouth wide or stick out your tongue, the baby will watch carefully and then copy. This is quite remarkable – how do they know that they even have a mouth? This can be observed in the first hour after birth and it is this response to adults that makes the baby a social and communicative being, as they will demonstrate taking turns in their non-verbal responses and vocalisations (Murray and Andrews 2000), provided the adult is sensitive to them.

It is not surprising that adults are attracted to baby features. We find certain attributes of the human infant 'cuddly': a relatively large head with big eyes, a receding chin and large forehead, round body outline and relatively short limbs, small size and high-pitch vocalisation (Eibl-Eibesfeldt 1996). These features normally stimulate caretaking responses and are perceived as loveable.

Care-taking and our sensitivity to infants is normally based on how we were cared for as infants. If we formed a good enough attachment to our parents and they were in tune with our needs, if they were 'baby-centred', then we become secure adults (Steele 2002). Every time babies are changed in a loving way or sympathetically responded to when lonely, tired, hungry or frightened, they take in the experience of being loved in the quality of care received. For a baby, physical discomfort is the same as mental discomfort, and vice versa (Stern 1985).

How do mothers respond sensitively to the specific emotional needs of their infant? Sadly not all of them do. 'Insensitive mothers' base their responses on their own needs and wishes, or general ideas about infants' needs. What is sensitive from an adult's point of view may not be perceived as such by the infant.

As the WAVE (Worldwide Alternatives to Violence) report (Wave Trust 2005, section 3) summarises, it is the parental attunement to the needs of infants, which midwives have a role in fostering, that leads to loved individuals who do not become anti-social. Sinclair (2007) suggests that through our early relationships and communication from conception to 3 years of age, we develop our emotional brain and our capacity for forming relationships occurs. Fundamentally, human beings at any age respond and feel understood when an attuned sensitive other interacts with them. As a professional, if you respond to the client in your care as a sensitive parent would, your communication with her can be improved.

Sensitive responsiveness is one of the key constructs of attachment theory (Bowlby 1973). The early infant–mother relationship has far-reaching consequences for the developing child's later social and mental health. It is the underpinning theory in national agendas and frameworks interventions (e.g. DH 2004; Wave Trust 2005; DfES 2006; Sinclair 2007), and recommended for effective practice in the promotion of family health and parenting skills, which are now a priority politically and professionally.

The concept of sensitive responsiveness includes the ability of parents to perceive and respond to infants' signals accurately, because they are able to see things from the baby's point of view (Paavola 2006). This has been refined by many researchers.

Mothers who are sensitively responsive demonstrate the following (the key concept is in italics):

- They are observers who *listen* and see their strengths and help them with their difficulties
- They have warm and responsive interactions with caretakers. The mother's task is to respond *empathically* – to mind read. Babies have no control or bad intent, but they learn they can self-regulate through maternal containment. They then learn to self-soothe, for example, by sucking
- They offer structure and routine, which is flexible and age-appropriate, and set *boundaries*. They provide psychological and physical holding. Holding also relieves anxiety – they feel held together
- They maintain interest by providing things to look at and do through play and touch, but *in tune*, e.g. they recognise a yawn means 'leave me to sleep'
- Vocalisation is reinforced by response-dialogue. Hearing and *being heard* – respond to parent's voice, familiarity gives sense of security; and babies need to hear talking to develop speech

(Paavola 2006, drawn from DH 2004; Wave Trust 2005; DfES 2006; Ponsford 2006).

Sensitive responsiveness can be facilitated, and when mothers' sensitivity and responsiveness are enhanced, this results in a dramatic increase in secure attachments with fussy infants (Steele 2002).

Our infant–parent attachment patterns are largely acquired, rather than determined by genetic or biological make-up (Steele 2002), so with support we can improve our ability to relate to others. For midwives this means relating to clients and colleagues, but also facilitating parent–infant relationships. This can be done by praising the sensitivity you observe in parents and helping them see and

Table 1.1   Helping parents know their baby

Ask them to tell you about their baby:
- What does he/she like?
- What does he/she like to hear, look at, feel and smell in particular?
- How does he/she get your attention?
- How does he/she tell you they are content?
- What does he/she like when going to sleep? What do you notice about their sleep or their crying?

understand their baby. Using the questions in Table 1.1 might enable parents to realise that they can understand their baby.

The basic method of improving our relationships are those that mothers ideally use with their infants. This is primarily non-verbal, which is not surprising as over 65 per cent of our communication is non-verbal (Pease 1987). Observe bodily and facial cues, and be in touch with what that person might be feeling. This is truly listening and being with another person, and because we are listening and empathising, we provide a safe environment. This is something midwives demonstrate by holding women physically, which seems to help contain the labouring women in their pain, and at birth by encouraging skin-to-skin contact giving the baby a safe framework after being contained in the womb. But we also provide holding psychologically, by being with women and trying to understand what the experience is like for them. This is demonstrating empathy. When we reflect back what the client says and feels by our actions, whether by touch or words, the client feels held and heard.

Humans become socialised and learn that they should not do certain things: they should not upset others; they should stop arguing. We learn to hide our feelings and disguise what we really mean, which in turn leads to a lack of communication.

Dissatisfaction with midwifery care and in family life is often due to lack of communication. Our early skills in relation to communication become set in patterns, and the stamped foot of a toddler's temper tantrum can still be apparent in the adult. Nichols (1995) summarises the four early stages of development of self described by Stern (1985), which helps inform us of how we adopt patterns of acting and reacting which become unconscious responses in adult life. Interesting as these stages are between the ages of 0 and 18 months, this partly explains why, when we are anxious, we become inarticulate because we have reverted to a pre-verbal developmental stage.

Effective communication can be hard to achieve. Sometimes it seems that no matter how carefully we phrase what we say, the listener either does not understand or misunderstands us. In verbal communication we often add emphasis through body language or intonation. We may adopt a defensive or threatening posture to reinforce our message and, of course, we may raise or lower our voice. These techniques are used spontaneously, having developed through our socialisation in childhood.

Some common problems in communication

Bolton (1979) suggests there are six peculiarities or common problems in human communication. These are mainly to do with understanding and listening:

1. Lack of clarity as words can have different meanings
2. Failure to understand because a message is 'coded'
3. Failure to receive the message as another agenda is clouding the issue
4. Being distracted and not hearing the message
5. Not understanding because the message is distorted by perception or other filters
6. Not handling emotions during a conversation

The first problem is poor understanding, often due to an unclear message or ambiguous words, because words may have different meanings for different people. As Ralston (1998) points out, terms such as incompetent cervix or inadequate pelvis are open to a very different interpretation to the non-professional listener. But even straightforward terms such as mayonnaise, when it is not differentiated into 'home-made' (using raw eggs, which should be avoided in pregnancy) and a commercial product, can lead to women misunderstanding the information they are given (Stapleton et al. 2002).

When the message is 'coded' the real meaning is masked; for example, when the client asks you to put her flowers in water, it could be a message to keep her company. It can also often be observed that clients present with one agenda, but really have a different problem – for example, they present with backache, but are really concerned that the pregnancy is normal. Midwives also miss conversational codes for more information from clients (Kirkham et al. 2002a). 'I don't know' and 'What would you do?' are both tactics women use to elicit more information, tactics which unfortunately are not very successful.

The way a message is spoken can also conceal a message within the message. Most speech has both an obvious and a hidden meaning

(Kagan et al. 1989). For example 'What did you say?' has the obvious meaning 'Please say that again', but the hidden meaning could be, 'You're so boring, I wasn't really listening'. However, if we say what we really mean we can hurt another's feelings. So we try to look and act professionally and this creates barriers to communication, because our message is not clear. Indeed, as professionals there are times when we are acutely aware of appropriate interactions and the need to adopt a professional face. For example, it is inappropriate to look cheerful or go into a long explanation of care during a life-threatening emergency (Mapp and Hudson 2005).

Clients also do not hear, or take in, what we say when they are distracted by the environment or physical symptoms. The disruption of a child needing attention during a conversation is an example. A client who is in pain or focused on their child, for example, may miss the information you are giving. However, midwives often miss non-verbal cues and carry on their own conversations neglecting the woman. The woman may interpret this as an 'I've started so I'll finish' attitude, while the midwife thinks 'I know I have given her the information', even if the client 'could not hear'. It is interesting to observe that mothers will say 'Look at me when I am talking to you' when addressing their children, thus ensuring the non-verbal feedback needed, which tells us we are being heard (Yearwood-Grazette 1978). Midwives should ensure that they respond to non-verbal cues with their clients, particularly eye contact.

Midwives and clients can filter information, because of perceptions, emotions or simple hearing what they wish to hear. For example, if you say 'You can go home after the paediatrician has discharged the baby', the client may hear only 'You can go home' and so phones her partner to collect her. Midwives too filter information by avoiding discussion. They emphasise physical tasks and this sends the message that discussion, particularly about how the woman feels, is less important. Indeed, discussions are often avoided by filling time asking for urine samples, ignoring possible anxiety even when the last pregnancy was a stillbirth, for example (Kirkham et al. 2002a). In essence, filters become blocks to communication.

Another block to communication is 'don't worry', a term that is used to reassure (Stapleton et al. 2002). However, paradoxically it causes anxiety as the client is denied the opportunity to express how she is really feeling (Stapleton et al. 2002). The words 'don't worry' should be avoided (Mapp and Hudson 2005). A smile or touch is more helpful and reassuring (Mapp and Hudson 2005).

It is not just what we say and do, it is also how we listen. It is rare for midwives to explore topics such as what foods a client eats to invite discussion (Stapleton et al. 2002), yet this would enable the client to say what she knows. However, the midwife would then need to listen for any relevant missing information. This is hard, so instead there is a tendency to tell clients what to do – things they often already know, such as the advantages and disadvantages of breastfeeding – but not what the client wants to know, e.g. 'what does breastfeeding feel like?' (Stapleton et al. 2002). Kirkham (1993) suggests:

Kirkham 1993

> 'Good care must involve sensitive communication. Good communi-cation is concerned with the exchange of information, ideas or feelings so that both parties understand more and have appropriate expecta-tions. Just to impart our instructions cannot be called good care.'

Finally, people who have difficulty with emotional issues may deny their emotions or become blinded by them (Bolton 1979) because anxiety and fear or any high levels of emotional arousal lock the brain into one-dimensional thinking (Griffin and Tyrrell 2004). Our emotions affect our physiology and hijack the brain's capacity for rational thought. This inhibits our ability to rationalise or enter-tain different perspectives, because traumatic and distressing expe-riences – whether big or small – cause imbalances in the nervous system which create a block or incomplete information-processing. This is why it is difficult to take in medical or other information or advice when we are upset, frightened, angry or in pain. This dys-functional information is then stored in its unprocessed state in both the mind (neural networks) and the body (cellular memory) (Pert 1997). During emergencies poor communication can compound stress, so careful, sensitive communication that is congruent (i.e. the non-verbal matches the verbal) is what is required (Mapp and Hudson 2005).

Non-emergency situations can also involve high emotional arousal. Emotional arousal as a consequence of a power struggle will evoke a defensive response. As the thinking part of the brain becomes inhibited when the client feels conflict or stress, learning and taking in information cannot be effective (Griffin and Tyrrell 2004). When a midwife says, 'I want to tell you about breastfeeding', the emo-tional arousal from the client may come from the unspoken – 'Who are you to tell me how to bring up my family!' It would be more useful to reduce the emotional arousal and reframe or present the information another way, for example, 'It's good you have decided on your method of feeding. I would like to hear more about how you are going to feed your baby.' As Nichols (1995) points out, 'It isn't exuberance or any other emotion that conveys loving apprecia-tion; it's being noticed, understood and taken seriously.'

Midwives may find that employing open questions is time-consuming. However, when information becomes blocked, misunderstanding is increased and this eventually leads to spending more time sorting out the problem later. Midwives also limit their emotional effort and may stereotype in order to increase control over work situations (Kirkham et al. 2002b), although if they were to increase their sensitive responsiveness, clients would be able to get the information they need, understand and feel understood.

Midwives need to give their clients emotional care, particularly those in labour, but this is draining. Many midwives realise they do not have time for their own emotional feelings so they 'pull down the shutters' in order to appear calm. It is this that can give the impression of aloofness, whereas others are perceived as naturally friendly (John and Parsons 2006). As John and Parsons (2006) suggest, support mechanisms need to be developed and implemented in order to reduce stress in practice. According to Nichols (1995):

> 'If you see a parent with blunted emotions ignoring a bright-eyed baby, you're witnessing the beginning of a long, sad process by which unresponsive parents wither the enthusiasm of their children like unwatered flowers.'

Thus far the problems and the ways midwives have been seen to communicate have been discussed. To be more effective in communication our sensitive responsiveness needs to be developed. The scope of this chapter can only scratch the surface in this respect as communication skills need to be developed experientially as our patterns of communicating are often learnt from childhood. Having said that there are areas individuals can develop, which will also improve their professional practice. This particularly includes listening and empathy. Some pointers will be outlined here, but learning these skills needs to be gained through experience in order for long-term change in practice to take place.

Listening

Listening skills are essential. Listening is an active process requiring the individual's full attention as you need to listen and fully hear what is actually being communicated, not just what is being said. Listening involves the mind, senses and emotions to pick up what is not said. Also required is the development of self-awareness, the awareness of when we fail to listen and attend, which, if addressed, is likely to have a positive effect on future communication. Good communication minimises misunderstanding; poor communication can lead to complaints (Sidgewick 2006).

Part of the process of communication is receiving messages. Obviously, verbal messages are heard, but the receiver needs to be actively listening. Passive listening includes encouraging fillers such as 'umm', 'uh huh', as well as non-verbal nods and eye contact (Balzer-Riley 1996). Passive listening implies understanding, but active listening removes the guesswork as it ensures messages are received properly (Balzer-Riley 1996).

Listening skills vary depending on what we are doing. Sometimes passive attentive listening is sufficient. However, if we require more information, or if our clients are giving an emotional account, then a more active approach is helpful (Kagan et al. 1989). Attending is listening to what is really being said. This may also require the skill of appropriate questioning (questioning skills are addressed later). If we focus on our questions, then we go back and forth between what is being said and our reply, and we may not really hear what is being said (Rowan 1993). It cannot be emphasised enough that listening is one of the most important communication skills.

Guidelines for Listening

- Listen without interruption as far as possible; minimise questions
- Remember what is being said, as if you are going to be tested on it. Listen to what is not being said, particularly feelings
- Observe the client's body language as well as your own – is she giving you any clues?
- Have an empathic stance – what would it be like if you were in the client's situation?
- Try not to rush in with explanations and answers. The client generally has the answer
- Look like you have time, or make it clear how much time you have, and give your full attention

(Adapted from Jacobs 2000.)

Unfortunately, because much of midwifery requires information from the client we focus on questions rather than listening. Questions are so much part of conversation they seem almost to have replaced the ability to listen or respond in any other way, because we are already forming the next question. In order to enable clients to talk and midwives to listen and talk less, it is generally useful to begin with open questions. Open questions usually begin with words such as would, could, tell me, seem to be, I think, I feel, or I wonder. Questions that begin how, what, where and particularly *why* can leave the client feeling they are under interrogation, whereas an open question allows them to describe their experience.

Activity

One of our tasks is to ask personal questions. Some of us find these easier to ask than others. However, you still have to ask them. So think about the following – could they be rephrased into more open questions?

- When was the first day of your last menstrual period?
- Have you had you bowels open?
- When did you last have sex?
- Can I see your sanitary towel?
- How are your breasts?

The following are part of the activities for daily living which may be used on admission forms. How would you phrase the questioning order to gain the information you need? How could you broach the question on issues such as:

- Expressing sexuality
- Death
- Safer sex
- Termination of pregnancy
- Alcohol consumption
- Domestic violence
- Mental health

When trying to establish legal responsibility for a child, how will you ask this when the child's surname is different from the mother's and the 'next of kin' – who is the 'father'?

Listening to what is not being said

In ordinary listening we are often interested in the content or subject. We generally try to relate this to our own experience (this is sympathy), thinking of interesting replies to carry the conversation on. In contrast, in a therapeutic relationship we are listening not only to the content, but also to the message within the message. This may be about the client's emotions, so if our own thoughts, experiences and emotions arise, we should put them aside because it is the client's experience that is the focus (Rowan 1993).

Jacobs (2000) recommends that we listen to the 'bass line' of a conversation, as if it were a piece of music. This invites us to listen to what is not being openly said, but possibly being felt by the client.

Activity

Tom, a young father-to-be, is talking about his dissatisfaction with his partner's maternity care. Whether or not he is justified, what can Tom's bass line tell you? Imagine how you might feel in his position.

What is Tom's bass line saying? He is young, so possibly has little experience of the world, and the transition to parenthood is not without stress, partly due to the unknown. He may be unsure of himself, so any threat might elicit a defensive/hostile response. Tom may be feeling helpless and powerless as he feels he can do little for his new family. He may be concerned for his partner or their baby. These are all possibilities, so what are the feelings he could be expressing – anxiety, anger, frustration?

Activity

Tom is talking about his dissatisfaction with his partner's maternity care.

Tom: Excuse me, you said you would give my wife some more of those tablets to get her started in labour, we have been waiting for hours.

Think how you would answer. The labour ward has been busy and you were told not to induce Tom's partner. You also have been frantically trying to discharge clients in order to give beds to the women waiting to clear the delivery ward. The paediatrician has not discharged the babies and the consultant wants to do a round with you.

Midwife: I am sorry, we are busy and have not had time.
Tom: You seem to be making time for everyone else who has babies already.
Midwife: Well the delivery ward does not have space for you anyway.
Tom: Then why were we dragged in here at 7 am?
Midwife: Well, it's one of those things. We do not know what the work-load will be like.

Now think how you could answer differently.

The midwife has been polite, but she is defensive, and her answers sound like excuses to Tom. The midwife feels stressed and is having trouble coping with her workload. Her factual response does not demonstrate any understanding or concern for Tom and his partner. Concern and understanding will be demonstrated by letting Tom know you have heard him. Giving full attention is difficult in this case. I am sure you have heard a conversation like this while the midwife is on the phone and writing up some notes. Pushing the mute button on the phone, putting the pen down and giving good eye contact may have been the midwife's first reaction and would go a long way to contributing to Tom's perception that she really was listening. Furthermore, reflecting back or summarising what was said might ensure the midwife understands and Tom would feel heard.

Case Notes

Tom: Excuse me, you said you would give my wife some more of those tablets to get her started in labour, we have been waiting for hours.

Here are some possible replies that are more likely to help Tom feel heard and understood.

- Yes I did. You have been waiting a long time.
- Yes I did. I am sorry you have been waiting so long, it must be very frustrating for you.
- You have been waiting a long time, and it's disappointing when you expected the induction to have begun by now.

Not only are some of Tom's words being used to help him feel heard, but also the midwife has listened to the 'bass line' and is tentatively reflecting possible feelings. The midwife may be stressed and she might have started the conversation by using factual replies as that is an old habit, but she could recover or repair the communication by demonstrating empathy.

Tom: Excuse me, you said you would give my wife some more of those tablets to get her started in labour, we have been waiting for hours.
Midwife: I am sorry, we are busy and have not had time.
Tom: You seem to be making time for everyone else who has babies already.
Midwife: You seem concerned that there is no time for you and your wife. You feel anxious because it seems like the induction is never going to happen.

Empathy

Jacobs (2000) suggests that if you listen to yourself and how you might feel in a given situation, this will be a way of understanding – the first step towards empathy. Empathy involves the capacity to recognise the bodily feelings of another and is related to our imitative capacities. We associate the bodily movements and facial expressions we see in another with the feelings and corresponding movements or expressions in ourself.

Mothers help babies regulate their emotions in this way. You may have observed a distressed baby being cuddled gently by its mother whose facial expression is as pained as the infant's. Her tone of voice and touch mirror the infant's state – 'Oh dear! There there' gradually soothing into a calmer state with soft voice and holding: 'I know. Mummy is here, you can cope' (Gerhardt 2004). Humans also seem to make the same immediate connection between tone of voice and other vocal expressions and inner emotion. Thus, empathy is a synonym for communicated understanding (Balzer-Riley 1996). It is mentally putting yourself in the shoes of another so that you can understand how they are feeling in an accepting way without judgement or evaluation (Balzer-Riley 1996).

A midwife needs to be empathic and also has to understand the woman and provide the care and support needed while watching the process of labour and any deviation that might cause concerns (Ralston 1998). The midwife who gets this right is truly 'with woman'. By being empathic she is unlikely to have a different perception from the patient's.

Midwives also convey compassion, understanding and empathy through touch. Not being touched is related to emotional deprivation, yet midwives have been observed to touch the fetal heart monitor and not the woman in labour, thus distancing themselves from the intimacy of the relationship (Yearwood-Grazette 1978). Sensitive touch can help relax a person in pain, but the midwife needs to recognise when this becomes intrusive (Ralston 1998), just as a mother does who is sensitive and does not ignore or over-stimulate her baby (RCM 1999).

To be empathic requires you to listen and identify the emotion. As in the mother–infant relationship we tune in non-verbally, noting behaviours. Sometimes we pick up the feeling in our own body – our stomach may be in knots. If these factors are taken into account along with what we imagine it must be like, then we can identify the emotion. However, we also need to communicate this to our client.

Jacobs (2000) cautions that we should choose our words carefully when describing others' emotions. Clients may not feel that you understand them if you suggest they are furious when they are just feeling mildly irritated, and vice versa. However, if you truly are sincere and congruent (your words match your behaviours and emotions), then you will find that people will simply correct you when they respond. Nevertheless, it is important to recognise accurately the shades of emotion which might be present in a particular interaction.

Empathy can be expressed as a phrase, a word or even sensitive touch. But first the emotion needs to be identified (Tschudin 1985). For example, a friend tells you they are happy to be pregnant. You already have the information that she is pleased to be pregnant, hence the one emotion you could respond with empathetically is 'happy'. A phrase that might reflect a similar feeling is: 'You look like you're on cloud nine.' Often we congratulate people on their achievements, so you could say, 'You must be delighted with your achievement'. Or you can simply state 'You feel happy because you are pregnant'. These responses may not feel right to you, but remember it is how you say them that shows you are trying to understand. In responding empathetically the client is aware that you have heard and are trying to understand.

Developing empathetic understanding is about staying with the client's experience and not being judgemental or giving advice. One of the difficulties is that it is easy to be sympathetic and the midwife may identify with her own feelings which the client's message evokes. This transfers the focus from the client to the professional and consequently the listening becomes conversational rather than therapeutic.

Here are some unhelpful classic examples:

- You think that's bad!
- I'll do that for you
- Don't worry
- I remember when I had just the same

All of these impose the midwife's experience on the client. Being sympathetic brings out the meaning for the midwife rather than for the woman.

The difficulty can be putting empathy into practice. Tschudin (1985) suggests a formula for an empathetic approach. First, identify the emotion in the statement made by the client. Then respond to the words spoken and acknowledge them by reflecting back that feeling with a rationale for the feeling if possible. For example, in 'I don't know what to do' the feeling or emotion is confusion or possibly anxiety. The rationale for this is uncertainty about the future. An empathetic reply might be 'You feel confused, because you are not sure what to do'. In summary, Tschudin's (1985) 'formula' for empathy is: you feel . . . because . . .

As you formulated your answers did you notice that these statements are often voiced by clients to midwives? The first client may, of course, simply be enquiring about her blood pressure. However, if there is an underlying emotion you will probably hear it in the tone of their voice. The client may be anxious about their blood pressure or the growth of their baby. 'I'm dying', sometimes heard in childbirth, is probably an expression of primitive fear. 'I can't cope' is a direct request for help, but there may be an underlying sense of desperation. Appropriate empathetic responses might be:

- You feel anxious about your blood pressure
- You feel terrified because the pain is so bad
- You feel desperate because of the responsibility

You now have a tool for practising empathy when you interact with clients, colleagues and families. The key is to practise, even if you begin by listening to conversations on the bus, in the canteen or on television, and rephrasing the responses in an empathic way. For those of us that do not find it natural to be empathic there is a steep learning curve. Learning to be more empathic can also be unsettling for the midwife, because their experiences of expressing emotions were not received sensitively, so the fear of hurting another's feelings can be overwhelming. Sadly, when they do not know what to say, they either say nothing or deny the client's emotions in their response. There is nothing wrong with saying, 'I don't know what to say'. The fear of getting it wrong, voicing the wrong emotion or opening a can of worms is why this needs to be practised. Additionally, the midwife needs to move the conversation to a close sensitively and refer on if needed.

The following activities and comments invite you to exercise the skills described thus far, and illustrate how responses carry on a conversation through sensitive listening and an empathic stance.

They also demonstrate how the responses might draw the conversation to a close.

Activity

Analyse this conversation using the skills discussed so far – listening, questioning and empathy. Then look at what each student might be feeling at the end of the conversation and how you might continue the communication.

Two students have just received their exam results.

Student A: What did you get?
Student B: (sadly) It's a pass.
Student A: What did you get?
Student B: 'C'.
Student A: A 'C'?
Student B: (sounding devastated) Yeah.
Student A: Yeah.

Note the style of the questions; they are not open. Student A uses an echo statement and repeats student B's statement, which can be quite useful when you are not sure what to say. I expect student A also wants to burst out with the news that she has an 'A' grade, but is sensitive enough not too. However, student A has not listened to the sadness and has not been empathic.

Student A may also be feeling bad that she cannot make it better for student B, but also fears she has opened a can of worms for student B. She could try to make it better by saying it's not such a bad grade. But this denies student B's emotion and is unhelpful and is not listening. It is like putting a bandage over a 'wound' to mask the problem.

Examine the next part of conversation in the following activity.

Activity

Analyse this conversation using the skills discussed so far: listening, questioning and empathy.

Student A: You sound disappointed.
Student B: Yeah, well I worked really hard on that assignment.
Student A: It's disappointing only to get a 'C' grade when you've worked so hard.
Student B: (angry) It's just so unfair!
Student A: Do you feel angry because others do not seem to work as hard as you and yet they get a better grade?

Here we observe active listening, open questions and empathic responses. Student B has had her emotion heard and is beginning to feel understood. Notice how the empathic response helps clarify how student B is feeling. She can now think more clearly as she releases some of the emotion.

Now analyse the next part of the conversation.

Activity

Analyse this conversation using the skills discussed so far: listening, questioning and empathy. How do you imagine you might feel if you were student A?

Student B: Oh, maybe they do work hard, it's just that I am a single parent, so I have to find time, whereas others don't have this responsibility.

(Student A wants to bring this to a close, so moves on the interaction)

Student A: You do sound stressed. I wonder if you could get more help from someone.

Student B: Umm, well I cannot afford any more childcare.

Student A: That is difficult; I guess you must have to be very organised. Could you ask for more academic help?

Student B: Well, I always seem to just scrape through. I am concerned I will never finish this course.

Student A: Have you talked to the tutor?

Student A may be feeling anxious that she has opened up herself to being the answer to the problem. Remember, it is not your problem to solve; the other person holds the key. Student A follows with a sensitive answer that demonstrates all the conversation has been heard, and offers some praise for the difficult place student B holds. We can imagine that student B, having been heard, is likely to ask student A about her result.

Moving towards more effective communication would improve midwifery care (Kirkham 1993). Observing mothers and babies communicating and facilitating sensitive care is likely to have an impact not only on midwifery, but also on society, as responding and communicating effectively with 'small babies make a big difference' (Sinclair 2007), which impacts on their sociability and thus society as a whole. It is interesting to note that common errors in communication are also those found in midwifery. As highlighted in official inquiries such as Daksha Emerson (Joyce et al. 2003) and Victoria

Climbié (Laming 2003), the consequences of poor communication can have devastating outcomes. The Nursing and Midwifery Council (2004) standards of proficiency state that communication is a key skill that enables the effective delivery of care and support for women in the pre-conception, antenatal, intrapartum and postnatal periods. Indeed the standard implies adopting the 'bass line' of listening and empathic skills as suggested by Jacobs (2000). It seems clear that much of the issues for midwifery care discussed here would be minimised or prevented if this standard were fully embraced. It follows that midwives would also facilitate parents effectively communicating with their infants as they would be able to demonstrate these skill in their care. Effective communication is the cornerstone of good practice and essential to the provision of good maternity care. This is achieved with intimate and sensitive communication between midwives and their clients.

Acknowledgement

Thanks to Dr Mel Parr, whose ideas contributed substantially to this chapter.

References

Balzer-Riley, J. (1996) *Communications in Nursing*, 3rd edition. Missouri: Mosby-Year Book.

Bolton, R. (1979) *People Skills: How to Assert Yourself; Listen to Others; and Resolve Conflicts*. New York: Touchstone, Simon & Schuster.

Bowlby, J. (1973) *Attachment and Loss. Vol. II: Separation*. London: Hogarth Press.

Department for Education and Skills (2006) *Every Child Matters, Change for Children, Parenting Support, Guidance for Local Authorities in England*. London: DfES.

Department of Health (2004) *The National Service Framework for Children, Young People and Maternity Services*. London: DH.

Eibl-Eibesfeldt, I. (1996) *Love and Hate: The Natural History of Behaviour Patterns*. Trans. Geoffrey Strachan. New York: Aldine De Gruyter.

Gerhardt, S. (2004) *Why Love Matters*. London: Routledge.

Griffin, J. and Tyrrell, I. (2004) *Human Givens*. East Sussex: Human Givens Publishing.

Jacobs, M. (2000) *Swift to Hear: Facilitation Skills in Listening and Responding*. London: SPCK.

John, V. and Parsons, E. (2006) Shadow work in midwifery: unseen and unrecognised emotional labour. *British Journal of Midwifery* 14(5): 266–71.

Joyce, L., Hale, R., Jones, A. and Moodley, P. (2003) *Report of an Independent Inquiry into the Care and Treatment of Daksha Emerson MBBS, MRCPsych, MSc and her Daughter Freya.* London: North East London Strategic Health Authority.

Kagan, C., Evans, J. and Kay, B. (1989) *A Manual of Interpersonal Skills for Nurses: An Experiential Approach.* London: Harper & Row.

Kirkham, M. (1993) Communication in midwifery. In S. Roche and J. Alexander (eds), *Midwifery Practice: A Research-based Approach.* London: Macmillan.

Kirkham, M., Stapleton, H., Thomas, G. and Curtis, P. (2002a) Checking not listening: how midwives cope. *British Journal of Midwifery* 10(7): 447–50.

Kirkham, M., Stapleton, H., Thomas, G. and Curtis, P. (2002b) Stereotyping as a professional defence mechanism. *British Journal of Midwifery* 10(9): 549–52.

Laming, W. H. (2003) *The Victoria Climbié Inquiry Report of an Inquiry by Lord Laming.* London: The Stationery Office.

MacFarlane, A. (1977) Mother–infant interaction. *Dev Med Child Neurol* 19(1) (February): 1–2.

Mapp, T. and Hudson, K. (2005) Feelings and fears during obstetric emergencies – 1. *British Journal of Midwifery* 13(1): 30–5.

Murray, I. and Andrews, L. (2000) *The Social Baby.* Surrey: CP Publishing.

Nichols, P. (1995) *The Lost Art of Listening.* New York: Guilford Press.

Nursing and Midwifery Council (2004) *The Standards of Proficiency for Pre-registration Midwifery Education.* London. NMC.

Paavola, L. (2006) *Maternal Sensitive Responsiveness Characteristics and Relations to Child Early Communicative and Linguistic Development.* Oulu: Oulu University Press.

Pease, A. (1987) *Body Language.* London: Sheldon Press.

Pert, C. (1998) *Molecules of Emotion.* New York: Simon & Schuster.

Ponsford, C. (2006) The emotional needs of the under 3s and good practice in their care. Contributions from professionals interested in child care issues, attending a discussion group *What About The Children?* Annual conference. Kent: WATch.

Ralston, R. (1998) Communication: create barriers or develop therapeutic relationships. *British Journal of Midwifery* 6(1) (8 January): 8–11.

Rowan, J. (1993) *The Reality Game: A Guide to Humanistic Counselling and Therapy.* London: Routledge.

Royal College of Midwives (1999) *Transition to Parenthood.* London: RCM.

Sidgewick, C. (2006) Everybody's business: managing midwifery complaints. *British Journal of Midwifery* 14(2): 70–1.

Sinclair, A. (2007) *0–5: How Small Children Make a Big Difference.* Provocation series 3(1). London: The Work Foundation.

Stapleton, H., Kirkham, M., Thomas, G. and Curtis, P. (2002) Language use in antenatal consultations. *British Journal of Midwifery* 10(5): 273–7.

Steele, H. (2002) Attachment. *The Psychologist* 15(10) (October): 518–23.

Stern, D. (1985) *The Interpersonal World of the Infant.* New York: Basic Books.

Tschudin, V. (1985) *Beginning with Empathy.* London: ENB.

Wave Trust (2005) *WAVE Report, Violence and What to Do about It.* Surrey: Wave Trust Ltd.

Yearwood-Grazette, H. (1978) An anatomy of communication. *Nursing Times* (12 October): 1672–9.

The Aims of Antenatal Care

Laura Abbott

Introduction

This chapter addresses issues involved in the monitoring and assessment of a woman's health during pregnancy. Different assessment methods are used and central to these are history taking and the significance of the booking appointment, as well as important issues concerning screening and the type of screen tests available. Palpation and its importance are included, as well as various pregnancy milestones.

The chapter discusses antenatal care from four key perspectives:

1. *Physiological:* To recognise any deviations from normal, providing management options, treatment and referral as appropriate. To assess mother and fetal well-being
2. *Psychological:* Supporting the transition into pregnancy, providing emotional support and empowerment for women to make their own choices. Giving the women opportunities for fears and anxieties to be expressed. Supporting and assisting with the formulation of a birth plan
3. *Sociological:* Preparation for parenthood to include partners and other children
4. *Economic:* To inform and educate regarding maternity rights, employer's duties and time off work for antenatal visits. To advise and inform women with regards to benefits and entitlements

The midwife's role as antenatal caregiver

To support and act as an advocate in partnership with the woman, providing assessment of maternal and fetal well-being; information in order to make informed decisions and emotional support.

Antenatal assessment and monitoring

The booking visit

Traditionally, the booking visit took place around 12 weeks. From a dietary and minor disorder of pregnancy point of view, contact with the midwife could be much earlier in the first trimester in order to offer support, care and advice. The National Service Framework (NSF) (DH 2004) standard 11 for maternity services suggests that the midwife should be the first port of call for the woman when she finds out she is pregnant. In future, women may well see their midwife earlier than the traditional 12 weeks as government proposals stipulate that the midwife, rather than the GP, should be the first contact a woman has when pregnant.

Case Notes

I was really looking forward to my booking appointment with my midwife. I was 12 weeks pregnant and had finally started to tell all my friends and family. I hate hospitals as my mum died last year and view them as places for ill people and death. My partner and I had read about and researched the area of homebirth and had decided that if all remained well in my pregnancy, I would have liked to give birth at home. I was excited about discussing this with the midwife and had practical questions I wanted to ask her. When I brought this up at my booking appointment, the midwife told me that having a homebirth was out of the question for my first baby. I said that I had done my research and that this was my choice but the midwife was adamant that nobody would support me. I walked out of that appointment feeling disappointed, angry and let down.

Taking a comprehensive history from a woman relies on the midwife having excellent communication skills in order to elicit important information as well as gain the woman's trust. For many, especially first-time mothers, this will be the only time that a woman/

Table 2.1   Booking visit: checklist prompt for midwives

- Be attentive
- Personal details (next of kin, phone numbers)
- Menstrual history, including last menstrual period or date of egg insertion if in vitro fertilisation pregnancy
- Medical history, including any psychiatric illnesses
- Family history
- Known allergies
- Lifestyle, including body mass index, smoking, alcohol and social drug use
- Previous birth history
- Her own mother's birth history
- Physical examination
- Emotional issues, such as relationship difficulties or previous pregnancy losses
- Diet and nutrition, including any eating disorders

couple have met a midwife so this visit is an opportunity to explain the role. The booking visit will paint an overall picture of the woman's physical, psychological and social needs. The woman can refer directly to the midwife and does not need to book in with her GP. National Institute for Health and Clinical Excellence (NICE) antenatal guidelines have endorsed the view that women should have access to antenatal services between 8 and 10 weeks of pregnancy in order to plan care in partnership with the midwife as well as for early consideration of screening options (NICE 2003).

McCourt (2006) undertook a qualitative study examining the antenatal booking interview and interactions between midwives and women using two models of care. It was found that case loading midwives who look after a group of women, giving continuity of care and being on call for their births, were less hierarchical, offered more choice and information than midwives who were delivering a more conventional model of care, such as having different midwives for different stages of pregnancy and birth. Table 2.1 provides a checklist for the booking visit.

Midwifery wisdom

Carry a notebook for prompts to help when you start booking women, ensuring that nothing is written that may breach confidentiality

Opening questions

The opening questions in the booking visit may be related to this pregnancy. Asking the open question 'How are you feeling?' can elicit a variety of responses and information such as whether the woman is experiencing nausea and vomiting, and if appropriate, information about her employment history and if this pregnancy has been planned. It is important to gain information and document it carefully, but not in such a way that a woman/couple feel that this is a box-ticking exercise. The important things to ask are:

- Has she has had any vaginal bleeding?
- Has she suffered from nausea and vomiting?
- Has she had any recent contact with rubella or any other infectious diseases?
- Does she suffer from varicose veins?
- Does she use any 'social' drugs?
- Is she a smoker or a recent smoker – if yes, what type of tobacco and how much?
- What is her weekly alcohol intake?
- How is her home life with regards to relationships and support?
- How is her work life and does her job impact on her pregnancy?
- Does she have any religious and spiritual beliefs?
- Does she have any specific cultural issues and needs?
- Does she have any pets or live on a farm? If yes, advise on hygiene and avoidance of certain animals such as sheep in lambing season due to the risk of disease.

You may find that as the conversation progresses you gain more information that you can use to plan the woman's care and use in your documentation. Try to build on what she is telling you and listen carefully as this will help in your questioning as the consultation continues. McCourt (2006) found that midwives had different styles of questioning during the booking visit. Some were authoritative; others were professional (information-giving) and yet other had a partnership style (offering choice). Midwives who had the partnership style demonstrated most empathy as well as employing a technique of open questioning.

Frye (1998) suggests that midwives observe the woman carefully throughout history-taking as well as using senses such as the sense of smell (for example, does she smell of alcohol or tobacco?), which may give clues as to her lifestyle. The woman should be observed to see if there any scars or bruises and if she displays antagonistic behaviour, in order to try to gain some insight as to why this may be. It is useful to explore diet when discussing body mass index. James (2002) notes that eating disorders are within the spectrum of psychiatric disorders. If there is evidence of this, the woman may or may not need a team approach to care, perhaps including a dietician

Table 2.2   Strategies for effective communication

- Ask open questions
- Make eye contact
- Stay at the same level (with chairs the same height)
- Have a non-judgemental approach
- Observational skills – note any antagonism, bruising, smell of alcohol, for example
- Listen
- Empathise
- Respect choices

or psychologist experienced in eating disorders. By providing education on nutrition in pregnancy the midwife may be a useful resource as well as reinforcing positive eating behaviours.

If the woman works, employment issues can be discussed and the woman may want to know her rights with regard to employment or self-employment. It is important that midwives give up to date and accurate information. Table 2.2 provides some hints and tips concerning effective communication.

Midwifery wisdom

Remember, choice is personal. We all have different preferences, and empathy starts with being non-judgemental.

Emotional well-being

The booking visit can be overwhelming for some women, perhaps because they are receiving a wealth of information. However, it is important to pay attention to their emotional as well as their physical health.

It is useful to explore the labour and birth experiences of the woman's own mother and the mother of her partner as this may have an impact on her hopes and fears and what her influences are with regards to pregnancy and birth. It may encourage further discussion and will also help explore the woman's attitudes to labour and birth. Asking about her family background may also help with exploring feeding issues and attitudes towards breastfeeding as she may come from a family who are very comfortable about breastfeeding or from a family with no close female relatives and who are uncomfortable about it.

A woman may have had a previous difficult or traumatic birth; or she may have suffered a pregnancy loss. The booking visit is an opportunity for the woman to talk about a previous experience; she

Table 2.3   Issues that may be hard for the midwife to raise during a consultation

- Domestic violence
- Previous abuse
- Physical and emotional abuse ('*Has anyone ever sexually, physically or emotionally abused you?*')
- Previous stillbirth/neonatal loss

may be coming to the visit with previous birth issues. Holding the booking visit in the woman's home puts the woman in control and is central to her care with you as her guest. It helps the midwife to assess her social circumstances and affords greater privacy, especially when asking intimate questions. If there are language barriers, it maybe useful to have an interpreter, although this may give rise to confidentiality issues.

Women are entitled to time off work for antenatal visits, but this may be difficult if she has a job with inflexible hours. She could be self-employed so that time off will impact on her business and hence her income. It is important not to pigeonhole women and have an awareness of the great diversity that people have, taking care not to stereotype a woman due to the job that she may do.

Note any hostility. If this is the first time you have met the woman she may not wish to divulge information straight away. Remember that we are all part of a large multidisciplinary team and liaison with other team members such as health visitors and GPs may be needed if you require further information. It is important not to stigmatise or be judgemental by gaining self-awareness and being sure that the care given is not influenced by personal prejudices. Table 2.3 outlines some of the issues that the midwife may find difficult to raise during the consultation.

Midwifery wisdom

Before asking a difficult question make sure you know how to respond to a difficult answer.

Medical and family history

The midwife should assess each woman fully, regarding her medical and family history. It may be that there is nothing significant in her history, but on the other hand the woman may remember something previously forgotten, such as a grandmother with a history of pre-eclampsia. It is essential to gain a medical history from a woman in order to plan her care appropriately. For example, if she has a history of thrombosis, she may be at risk of clotting disorders such as deep vein thrombosis or pulmonary embolism during pregnancy and may need to be offered the services of an obstetrician. If she has a history of serious mental illness such as psychotic disorders or a past history of postpartum illness, a team approach may be needed to offer her appropriate care during her pregnancy and support after her baby has been born.

Examples of questions about her medical history include:

- Any headaches, epilepsy or migraines?
- Any high blood pressure, blood clotting disorders, heart disease or thrombosis?
- Any respiratory problems such as asthma, tuberculosis or chest infections?
- Any digestive disorders, jaundice or anaemia?
- Any diabetes mellitus, thyroid disease or hormonal disorders?
- Any renal problems, kidney disease or recurrent cystitis?
- Any gynaecological disorders, such as pelvic inflammatory disease, sexually transmitted infections, including herpes or thrush, or conception difficulties?
- Is this a planned pregnancy? If it is the result of in vitro fertilisation, does the woman know the conception date?
- Any known allergies, including hay fever, eczema, foods and drugs?
- Any injuries, especially to the back and pelvis?
- Any operations or problems with anaesthetics?
- Any previous blood transfusions?
- Any mental health problems, such as depression, postnatal illness or post-traumatic stress disorder?

Family history

It is important to ask the woman about her family history. You will need to find out whether there is a history of:

- Cardiovascular disorders, such as hypertension, heart disease, stroke and blood clots
- Epilepsy
- Diabetes mellitus or thyroid disease
- Congenital abnormalities such as Down syndrome and spina bifida, or renal and cardiac anomalies, such as tetralogy of Fallot
- Multiple pregnancies
- Partner's health and family history

Blood tests, urine tests and scans offered at the booking visit will include:

- Blood specimens for:
  - Blood group
  - Rhesus status
  - Haemoglobin
  - Hepatitis B, HIV, rubella susceptibility, syphilis
  - Asymptomatic bacteriuria (urine test)
- Ultrasound scan
- Urinalysis

Midwifery wisdom

These tests are not compulsory! Never assume consent . . .

Subsequent visits

NICE's antenatal guidelines (2003) recommend ten visits for nulliparous (no children) women and seven visits for multiparous (one or more births/children) women in the antenatal period. Thorley, Rouse and Campbell (1997) appreciate the need for change in antenatal care, making the woman and her partner the focus of care. However, they criticise the focus on measurement, saying that there is a lack of flexibility and accessibility, and suggest that antenatal care should be available when the woman needs it most rather than attending at fixed intervals. However, NICE (2003) recommends that antenatal visits should be structured and purposeful. Although women may receive fewer midwifery visits, more quality time should be spent at each one (NICE 2003). It is vital that visits are individualised, appropriate and tailored to the individual's needs. The midwife needs to exercise her autonomy and schedule extra visits should the woman's needs dictate this.

In discussing the frequency of antenatal visits, Frye (1998) suggests that reducing the number of visits a woman receives because she is healthy is illogical as midwifery should be about promoting normality. Therefore, if a woman is well and healthy, she still requires her midwife to visit.

Record-keeping

NMC (2002) standards on record-keeping and information-sharing (including confidentiality) point out that the midwife will be judged (amongst other things) on the standards of her record-keeping. The midwife should keep contemporaneous records at all times. The *Confidential Enquiry into Stillbirths and Deaths in Infancy* (DH 1998a), *Confidential Enquiry into Maternal Deaths* (DH 1998c), the NMC (2002) and the Health Service Ombudsman (DH 1999) all cite poor standards of record-keeping in many cases that have been investigated. The NMC's 2003 annual report note that the second highest category for removal from the professional register was failure to keep accurate records and the Health Service Ombudsman (DH 1999) equates poor record-keeping with poor standards of care. (Chapter 10 discusses the important issue of effective documentation further and Chapter 14 explores confidentiality.)

Tests offered at subsequent visits

An anomaly scan is offered between 18 and 20 weeks. No further scanning is recommended. However, if the placenta is low lying at 20 weeks, another scan can be offered at 36 weeks.

- Haemoglobin is assessed at 16 weeks if there is a low Hb (< 11 g/dl) at booking (NICE 2003)
- At 28 weeks, Hb is checked again and anti-D is offered to rhesus-negative women
- At 34 weeks, a second dose of anti-D is offered to rhesus-negative women

At each visit the midwife should undertake a variety of physical checks of the health of the woman and her growing baby, including physical examinations, for example, abdominal palpation, observation of vital signs and the general physical condition of the woman. This care should be tailored for each woman. Cronk (2005) recommends that a woman who has had a previous caesarean section should have her pulse rate checked regularly in order for the midwife to have insight into the woman's healthy heart rate. If a woman has a high BMI, a larger blood pressure cuff should be used because this gives greater accuracy. Urinalysis at each visit should be provided by the production of a mid-stream urine sample in order to avoid contamination and thus an incorrect result.

At each visit the midwife should be alert to conditions such as pre-eclampsia when assessing blood pressure and testing urine for the presence of protein, diabetes mellitus when testing urine for the presence of glucose as well as domestic violence using observational skills and questioning. BP and urinalysis should be taken and documented at each visit. Information should be gained about nutrition, attendance at antenatal classes, place of birth and breastfeeding. Opportunities should be given to the woman to ask questions. NICE (2003) states that there should be continuity of care throughout the antenatal period. This will help the midwife and woman form a trusting partnership.

Assessments at each visit

Palpation

Palpation determines the size, position and growth of the baby by feeling the abdomen with both hands. This should begin at the booking appointment and continue through the woman's pregnancy. The uterus begins to grow and show during the first 20 weeks of pregnancy. As the fetus grows and the pregnancy develops, palpation is essential in assessing the position and movement of the baby, how it is growing and its approximate size.

The midwife must use all of her senses in order to gain skills in palpation, for example:

- Are there are stretch marks (striae gravidarum)?
- Is there a linea nigra (dark line of pigmentation extending from the bikini line to above the naval)?
- Are there any rashes?
- Is there evidence of scarring from previous surgery, or bruising?
- Contour – what is the shape of the uterus – for example, oval or slightly displaced to one side? What is the size and shape of the abdomen? This may give clues as to whether the baby is in a posterior position or presenting in the breech position.

It is vital to gain permission prior to touching the woman. Before palpating the abdomen the midwife's hands must be clean with short fingernails, she should ensure privacy and dignity, make sure the woman has an empty bladder and that she is not flat on her back in order to avoid aortal caval occlusion. NICE (2003) recommends that symphysis-fundal height is plotted on a graph by measuring the uterus from the pubic bone to the height of the fundus.

Abdominal palpation and assessment of the fetal heart

NICE guidance (2003) suggests that it is not necessary to auscultate the fetal heart at antenatal visits because it offers no predictive value. However, some women find it reassuring (NICE 2003). Knowledge of movements, the lie of the baby and if the baby is in an optimal position empowers the woman by explaining ways in which she can

Table 2.4   Using your Pinard's

Why use a Pinard's?

- Some women decline electronic monitoring and it is vital that you have this skill.
- Your batteries may run out.
- Auscultation with the Pinard's gives you more clues as to the position of the baby. This is especially useful if you suspect the baby is in the breech position.
- You can hear the fetal heart (FH) from approximately 28 weeks through the fetal shoulder.

How to use a Pinard's

Five Steps to Pinard Success

1. Palpate to ascertain the baby's position. Ask the woman where she thinks the baby is. Generally, you are aiming to hear the FH through the fetal back (remember that the baby's lungs are not inflated).
2. Use your knowledge and experience to see where the fetal heart might be for the different positions the baby might be in, and choose your target point.
3. Place the Pinard on your chosen spot, put your ear to the 'O', take your hand away from the Pinard, listen – and keep listening.
4. Feel the maternal pulse at the same time. If it coincides, you have the uterine vessels.
5. If after careful listening you really can't hear anything, repeat the palpation and try the Pinard in another spot.

Source: Wickham 2002a

help to encourage the baby into the ideal position for birth. Get used to using your Pinard's, Wickham (2002a) suggests that midwives can learn to hear variability with a Pinard's by adding up the number of heartbeats auscultated in 5-minute intervals (see Table 2.4).

If the number of beats added up in 5-minute intervals differs, variability can be confirmed. Wickham (2002a) explains that if the number of beats is the same, the baby may be asleep. If so, the midwife should try again in 10 minutes.

Midwifery wisdom

The tall woman may feel small for dates.
The short woman may feel large for dates.
Use your senses – your eyes to see, your hands to feel, but sometimes the most useful sense of all is your common sense!

Screening

Midwives need to have skills to impart information about screening options with clarity, sensitivity and in a way that parents can understand. How information is given and the language used can ease anxiety for parents. Parents are faced with having to make decisions about screening for abnormalities as developments in antenatal care mean that there are ever-increasing ways to screen and detect abnormalities in the fetus. The majority of pregnancies will be normal, but for a minority some test results may come back positive, which means that parents face further decision-making about proceeding with more tests.

Referral to other health care professionals is needed if the tests detect an abnormality. Ultimately, the question of whether to continue with the pregnancy may have to be faced. Many Trusts employ a midwife who specialises in screening and abnormalities, supporting parents through their decision-making. If the woman is being cared for by an independent midwife she is still entitled to all the screening options provided by the NHS should she choose to have them. If abnormalities are found, the same options will be discussed and offered.

Screening tests

The following tests are offered to all women:

- Nuchal transclucency at 11–14 weeks to measure the thickness of the back of the fetus's head in order to calculate a risk factor (many Trusts only offer this privately)
- Serum screening at 14–20 weeks for Down syndrome, giving a risk factor or probability of Down syndrome. For example, a 1 : 2800 risk would mean that if the woman was pregnant with the same baby 2800 times, there would be a risk of Down syndrome occurring once
- Anomaly scan at 18–20 weeks (checking for abnormalities) for example, looking at the four chambers of the heart, kidneys, brain, face and limbs.

For women who may be at increased risk only:

- Chorionic villus sampling at 10–14 weeks. A fine bore needle is inserted into the uterus via the cervix and a small piece of developing placenta is taken for analysis. The chromosomes in the cells are looked at to test for abnormalities and inherited disorders
- Amniocentesis at 16–20 weeks. A small sample of amniotic fluid is obtained by inserting a fine bore needle through the abdomen into the amniotic sac via ultrasound guidance, looking for chromosomal abnormalities

Antenatal Results and Choices, a national charity, provides non-directive support and information to parents throughout the antenatal testing process. Visit their website: http://www.arc-uk.org.

Table 2.5 outlines key points that should be taken into account when assessing the women at each visit.

Case Notes

Deborah, aged 32, was pregnant with her second child. Her daughter was a healthy seven year old and this was a much-wanted pregnancy with a new partner, Amir. Deborah decided to have the triple test at 16 weeks and thought of it as just another blood test. The results came back as positive.

Deborah was told this by phone on the Friday of a bank holiday weekend. Deborah and Amir had no idea what this meant for her or her baby and they spent three days desperately worried and frantically searching the Internet for clues. Deborah made an appointment on the Tuesday to see her community midwife who informed her that although the test was positive, it did not mean that her baby had an abnormality. The test result of 1 : 100 meant that there was a higher probability that the baby had an abnormality, but this could only be confirmed by amniocentesis.

Deborah and Amir were faced with a difficult decision as they knew there was a small chance that she could miscarry a healthy baby following an amniocentesis. Deborah felt philosophical and had a 'what will be will be' approach. She would want the baby regardless. Amir, on the other hand, believed that there was no way he could be a father to a child with an abnormality. This resulted in great conflict and arguments. Eventually they decided to go for the amniocentesis. It was stressful for Deborah as she was still uneasy about this choice, but felt she should do it for her partner. The results came back clear – there were no chromosomal abnormalities. Deborah was relieved but also felt angry that she had been through this trauma. She was upset with Amir for persuading her to have such an invasive test that had put their baby at risk. Deborah decided that if she ever became pregnant again she would refuse any screening tests.

Midwifery wisdom

Ask about the baby's movements whilst you are palpating, it will help you in defining the position.

Table 2.5   Key points to be taken into account when assessing at each visit

---

At each appointment you should:

- Observe the woman's appearance: Is she tired? pale? flushed?
- Assess the BP (a large woman may need a larger cuff)
- Undertake a urinalysis
- Observe for signs of oedema in the ankles, legs and hands
- Ask about (assess) gestation

Perform palpation, noting:

- Abdominal appearance: Striae gravidarum? Linea nigra? Bruising?
- Fundal height – is this equal to dates? Give gestation
- Lie: is the baby lying oblique, longitudinal or transverse?
- Presentation: is the baby cephalic? breech?
- Deep palpation: is the presenting part free? How many fifths palpable?

Assess:

- Fetal heart: what is the range? for example, 135–148 beats/min
- Fetal movements? Where? What do they feel like?

Do not forget:

- Date
- Time
- Signature
- Print your name by your signature.

Case Notes

I saw my midwife when I booked at the clinic when I was 12 weeks pregnant and saw another midwife when I was 16 weeks. I had my 20-week scan yesterday and the sonographer said I had a low-lying placenta. My next visit with the midwife is not for eight weeks! Eight weeks! I was told by the receptionist that because this is my second pregnancy, I am entitled to fewer visits than the first time around. How am I supposed to wait until I am 28 weeks pregnant? I have been on the Internet to look at low-lying placentas and am now pretty scared. My friend had a placental abruption last year and her baby died. I just wish I could have a midwife to talk to.

Conclusion

The midwife providing antenatal care needs to understand the physical, psychological, sociological and economic factors that may impact on the woman's care. The needs of the woman from booking throughout pregnancy should be carefully assessed and planned for holistically, using a team approach where appropriate. An in-depth understanding of the physical symptoms of pregnancy at different stages is required in order to be able to educate, inform and reassure the pregnant woman.

Excellent and effective communication skills are vital and the midwife must develop self-awareness in order to be able to provide non-judgemental and unbiased care. Having respect for the choices that women make and valuing the woman as an individual helps in the provision of personalised care. The balance between keeping up to date with the latest guidance and recommendations and developing the midwife's personal art of midwifery leads to providing excellence for the pregnant woman and her family.

References

Cronk, M. (2005) *Mary Cronk's MBE Thoughts on Early Detection of Scar Problems during VBAC.* http://www.caesarean.org.uk/articles/VBACScar-Monitoring.html

Department of Health (1998a) *Confidential Enquiry into Stillbirths and Deaths in Infancy.* 5th Annual Report. Maternal and Child Health Consortium. London: HMSO.

Department of Health (1998b) *Information for Health: An Information Strategy for the Modern NHS, 1998–2005: A National Strategy for Local Implementation.* London: DH.

Department of Health (1998c) *Report on the Confidential Enquiry into Maternal Deaths in the United Kingdom, 1997–1999.* London: HSMO.

Department of Health (1999) *For the Record: Managing Records in NHS Trusts and Health Authorities* (Health Service Circular: HSC 1999/053). London: DH.

Department of Health (2004) *National Service Framework for Children and Young People.* London: DH.

Frye, A. (1998) *Holistic Midwifery: A Comprehensive Textbook for Midwives in Homebirth Practice. Vol. 1: Care during Pregnancy.* Portland, OR: Labrys Press.

James, D. C. (2002) Eating disorders, fertility, and pregnancy: Relationships and complications. *Midirs Midwifery Digest* 12(1) (March): 44–50.

McCourt, C. (2006) Supporting choice and control? Communication and interaction between midwives and women at the antenatal booking visit. *Midirs Midwifery Digest* 16(3): 318–26.

National Institute for Health and Clinical Excellence (2003) *Antenatal Care: Routine Care for the Healthy Pregnant Woman, Clinical Guidelines.* London: NICE.

Nursing and Midwifery Council (2002) *Guidelines for Records and Record Keeping*. London: NMC.

Thorley, K., Rouse, T. and Campbell, I. (1997) Aspects of antenatal care. Results of seeing mothers as partners in antenatal care. *British Journal of Midwifery* 5(9): 546–50.

Wickham, S. (2002a) Pinard wisdom – part 1. *The Practising Midwife* 5(6) (July).

Wickham, S. (2002b) Pinard wisdom – part 2. *The Practising Midwife* 5(9) (August).

Programmes of Care During Childbirth

Laura Abbott

Introduction

This chapter covers a variety of topics exploring programmes of care during childbirth, with choice as its central theme. Place of birth is discussed – hospital, homebirth and birth centre. Choices for women are explored and include reiterating the importance of information-giving to ensure that choices of care are fully informed. Models of care are discussed, including the different types of midwifery care provision available to women. Childbirth preparation classes are explored looking at programmes of education that parents are offered and planning for childbirth.

Midwifery wisdom

How we arrive at our choices may be deep-rooted. Sometimes we don't even know how we get there. It is not our role to judge a woman who makes decisions very different from the ones we would choose for ourselves or our families.

A woman can choose from a variety of models when planning her care during pregnancy and childbirth. A midwife is skilled and qualified to care for the woman from conception through to birth and the postnatal period. However, in the UK most women see their GP as the first point of contact. GPs may not be expert in the different options for maternity care. The House of Commons Health

Committee (2003) describes how some women were frequently referred by their GPs to consultant-led care, thereby limiting choice for women who may be experiencing a normal pregnancy. It was also discovered that women often found it difficult to access maternity care without a referral from their GP. The National Service Framework (NSF; DH 2004) standard for maternity services states that the midwife should be the first port of call for women when they discover they are pregnant. The House of Commons Health Committee (2003) cites several interesting comments regarding consumer organisations and their opinions concerning choice in maternity services – according to Beech, *'Choice is an illusion. The majority of women are conned into thinking they have a choice'*; while Phipps talks of *'informed compliance rather than informed choice'*. It is essential that the midwife is aware of the choices that the woman can make and provides her with up-to-date information so that she can make informed decisions in partnership with the midwife.

The different places where a woman can choose to give birth will now be explored.

Place of birth

A woman has a number of options when thinking about the place in which she wishes to give birth. For most women, pregnancy and birth is a healthy, exciting and special episode in her life. It is important that the woman makes the choice that is right for her and her family. Options need to be woman-centred and focused on meeting the needs of the individual rather than the service as a whole. An Audit Commission report (1997) on women's opinions of maternity care found that although most were happy with the care they received, many wanted more information about their options for care and place of birth.

Hospital with a central delivery suite

A woman may choose to give birth in a hospital and indeed this is where the majority of babies in the UK are born (Birth Choice UK 2007). Women who have complicated or high-risk pregnancies are offered consultant-led care and the consultant obstetrician will be the lead carer. Examples of pregnancies deemed to be high risk are: in women who develop high blood pressure and pre-eclampsia; women with pre-existing medical conditions and women who are carrying more than one baby. However, for women who do develop complications, there needs to be a team approach, bringing together the skills of midwives, obstetricians, paediatricians and anaesthetists to ensure seamless care for the woman. The Department of Health's (2001) report *Why Mothers Die, 1997–1999. Report of the Confidential Enquiry into Maternal Deaths* makes reference to the importance of teamwork in many areas where substandard care has been uncovered.

Healthy women who choose to give birth in hospital do so for a variety of reasons. The woman may feel safer there or wants the reassurance of knowing that an anaesthetist is on hand if she chooses to have an epidural. However, some women may be unaware that they have other options than to go to hospital. In a study about women's choices undertaken by Lavender (2003), it was highlighted that women were reassured by the medical facilities a large consultant unit offered, especially in the event of an emergency. Lavender (2003) attributed this to women's lack of knowledge of the choices available to them and the fact that a medically-oriented approach was perceived to be safer than midwifery-led care. Women should be given the opportunity to familiarise themselves with the delivery suite by having a guided tour with the midwives and midwifery assistants who work there. A woman whose baby is known to be likely to spend time in a Special Care Baby Unit should be offered the chance to visit it and meet members of the team.

Case Notes

My local hospital has a birth centre attached to it. Most of my friends have had their babies there. I must admit that I am petrified of the pain and want to have an epidural as soon as I go into labour! The midwife has said that I should try the birth centre as it is very homely and has two birthing pools. I don't care about the wallpaper, I just care that there is an anaesthetist on standby as soon as I have the first contraction! I want every drug going!

Birth centres

Birth centres are also known as stand-alone birth centres, freestanding birth centres or midwifery led units. They are facilitated and managed by midwives and often have consumer involvement from women who may have used the birth centre previously and members of Maternity Services Liaison Committees (MSLCs) and the National Childbirth Trust (NCT). Staffing usually includes midwives, midwifery assistants and housekeepers. Birth centres often provide antenatal care and postnatal support, as well as facilitating parenthood education. Being midwifery-led, birth centres take the focus away from the medical model and concentrate on the social model of care. With regard to medical facilities should intervention be required, birth centres are the same as what is expected from a homebirth – the woman would be transferred to a hospital just as if she was transferring from home. Birth centres have a wealth of benefits and these have been outlined by Walsh and Downe (2004):

- Increased normal birth rates
- Fewer assisted births using instruments such as forceps and ventouse
- Reduced caesarean section rate
- Fewer women using strong pain-relieving drugs, such as pethidine and diamorphine
- Fewer women using epidurals
- Reduced rates of induction of labour
- Fewer women needing episiotomies
- Fewer vaginal examinations
- Shorter labours
- Reduced incidence of shoulder dystocia (when the baby's shoulder becomes impacted behind the woman's pubic bone)
- More intermittent fetal monitoring and less use of continuous electronic monitoring
- Higher maternal satisfaction
- Increased midwifery job satisfaction
- Increased breastfeeding success
- Cost-effective

Walsh (2005) defines a birth centre as a place that provides midwifery care in childbirth, with importance placed on relationships and the environment rather than on machinery and drama. Many birth centres offer birthing pools or large baths as pain relief and may have options for low lighting, birth balls, birth stools and music. The environment in a birth centre usually facilitates normality. The birth environment is important to women and has been highlighted in the NSF (DH 2004). The NCT issues awards for midwifery-led units that facilitate the best birthing environments for women with the aim of celebrating innovations in practice that enhance women's experience of labour and birth. Lavender (2003) found that many women believed that a midwifery-led unit on the same site as a consultant unit offered safety but with a more homely environment, and 51 per cent said that it was important to them to have a midwife help them to give birth naturally without medical intervention.

Case Notes

I was the 100th mum to give birth in the Hemmingway birth centre. It is such a great environment to give birth. The midwives and staff are so calm and professional and just let you get on with the business of labour. I spent my early labour in the 'sensory room' where it was dark and relaxing with gentle music and aromatherapy oil burning. I had bean bags to lean on and a birth ball to sit on. When I got to 8 cm dilated (with no drugs!) I transferred into the dolphin room (aptly named because of the deep pool). The warm water was just what I needed as I was really howling the place down by then! It wasn't long before my baby boy was born into the water and into my and Lynda's (the midwife) hands. He looked into my eyes and I fell in love instantly and all the pain of labour just melted away. I was on cloud nine. I did it!

Midwifery case loading

Case loading teams of midwives provide total care for women and their babies throughout pregnancy until six weeks post-delivery. They offer hospital, community maternity unit and homebirths. Although this is predominantly primary maternity care, midwives will usually continue caring for women whose pregnancies become complicated but in conjunction with the hospital obstetrician. Case loading midwives will often work in small teams and spend time getting to know a group of women, focusing on their individual needs and working in partnership with the women. Within NHS Trusts this can often be as many as 30 women a year depending on whether the midwife works full- or part-time. In one area of the UK, case loading exists in contract between a group of self-employed midwives and an acute Trust. Walsh (1999) explored case loading midwifery using an ethnographic approach and described the case-load midwife as a 'professional friend' to the woman. One practice in South London (the Albany Practice) was evaluated by Sandall et al. (2001). They describe how the normal birth rate, the home-birth rate and breastfeeding rates all increased for women being case loaded by the midwives at that practice.

Homebirth

Midwifery wisdom

At a homebirth, you are the guest. This puts the woman in control. Homebirth truly empowers the woman and enables the midwife to be 'with woman' without interruption.

There is a large body of evidence that suggests that homebirth is at least as safe as hospital birth for healthy pregnant women (Chamberlain et al. 1997; Ackermann-Liebrich et al. 1996; Olsen and Jewell 2005). Tew (1985), a research statistician, describes how morbidity is higher among women who have babies in an institutionalised setting such as large consultant-led units and a large majority of women who experienced both hospital and home delivery preferred the homebirth. Chamberlain et al. (1994) revealed that there was no evidence to suggest that the safest place for healthy low-risk women to give birth is the hospital, and a Cochrane review by Olsen and Jewell (2005) found no compelling evidence to suggest that hospital birth was safer than homebirth for low-risk women.

Case Notes

I was pregnant with my first baby and really keen to plan a homebirth. However, when I went to see the midwife, she told me that I couldn't have a homebirth with my first child as I had an 'untried pelvis'. She was quite adamant about this. I had really wanted my midwife's support. My partner was nervous about the idea of homebirth and I was hoping that the midwife would put his mind at rest. After the midwife implied it was dangerous, my partner said there was no way he would let me have the baby at home. I ended up in hospital with a ventouse and a third degree tear. I wish I had stayed at home. I wish my midwife had supported my choice. Instead, I felt cajoled into doing something I didn't want to do. I must admit, I felt a bit powerless I am sure my postnatal depression has something to do with feeling as though I had no control over my decisions.

Having a homebirth usually results in fewer unnecessary interventions such as episiotomy or assisted birth, and being in familiar surroundings the woman is more likely to feel relaxed, enabling labour to progress effectively. The National Service Framework (DH 2004) standard 11 states that women should be able to choose their place of birth and that normal childbirth should be facilitated wherever possible. This includes being offered the choice of homebirth. NICE states: 'During their discussions about options for birth, healthy pregnant women should be informed that delivering at home reduces the likelihood for caesarean section' (NICE 2003).

The NMC (2003) says that midwives have a duty to respect women's choices when choosing homebirth. If there is a perceived conflict between risk and a woman's choice, midwives should seek guidance from a Supervisor of Midwives. (The role and function of Supervisor of Midwives is discussed in more detail in Chapter 18.)

Case Notes

Giving birth to my third child at home was an amazing experience for all of us. My older children were there to witness their little sister being born and my midwife was fantastic and so supportive. However, the best part was having a relaxing bath afterwards in my own bath and then snuggling down into my own bed with my gorgeous new daughter!

Women having their babies in a birth centre or at home may choose to labour and/or give birth in water. The Royal College of Midwives (2000) states that 'women experiencing normal pregnancy, who choose to labour or deliver in water should be given every opportunity and assistance to do so'. Birth in water is considered a normal birth and just like homebirth it gives midwives a chance to practise autonomously, using their 'with woman' skills. Women have said that water birth has given a greater sense of control and movement as well as providing good pain relief (Garland and Jones 2000). Researchers such as Burns and Kitzinger (2001) have found water birth to be a safe option. Midwives have a responsibility to ensure they are competent and accountable for their actions and omissions, and all units should be developing guidelines for water birth. Midwives have a responsibility to reflect on rules and ensure accountability for their own practice. One of the roles of the Supervisor of Midwives should be to help other midwives acquire and sustain their skills in water birth.

Table 3.1 provides a list for parents from Independent Midwifery records in order to be prepared for a homebirth.

Table 3.2 describes the contents of a hospital bag.

Midwifery wisdom

Remember to pack some food or drink. The midwife needs to be cared for too!

Midwifery wisdom

Remember, it is the woman's choice to make. Count to ten before you ever hear yourself saying to her 'you can't' or 'you're not allowed'.

Independent midwives

Independent midwives (IMs) are self-employed and work outside the NHS in order to be able to offer continuity of care for a caseload

Table 3.1 Homebirths and equipment

Equipment for parents to provide

- Something waterproof (e.g. waterproof tablecloth, shower curtain) to protect carpet/sofa/bed or wherever you end up (NB. Not all shower curtains are waterproof. Plastic sheets available from garden centres are.)
- Old sheets or linen
- Bin bags
- Torch with spare batteries
- Nourishing, easily digestible food and drink, e.g. bananas, honey, sugary sweets, chocolate, yoghurts, glucose tablets, Lucozade, Ribena and fruit juices.
- Bendy straws to drink from
- Comfortable clothes, e.g. large, baggy T-shirt
- A large soft towel to cover mum and baby together after the birth
- Towels for the baby
- Sanitary pads (large maternity type)
- Two or three new face cloths
- Hot water bottle (to put on back for labour or tummy for after-pains)
- Snacks for your midwife to eat whilst you are in labour!

Optional

- Mirror so that you can see the birth
- Camera/video to record the birth and to take the first pictures of your baby
- Lavender oil, homeopathy, alternative therapies

Equipment provided by the midwife

- Large absorbent pads
- Sphygmomanometer (for reading blood pressure) and a stethoscope
- Thermometer
- Mobile phone in case of emergency
- Pinard's and underwater sonicaid to listen to the baby's heartbeat
- Baby resuscitation equipment, including oxygen, a bag and mask
- An adult bag and mask should oxygen be required
- Entonox (three cylinders) and mouthpieces
- IV fluids, cannulae and giving set
- Syntometrine, syntocinon and ergometrine (drugs used to prevent heavy bleeding)
- Baby weighing scales
- Sterile cord scissors and clamps, episiotomy scissors
- Suturing materials, including local anaesthetics
- Warm electric pad

The majority of equipment provided by the midwife is there as a precaution and is rarely used.

of women throughout pregnancy, birth and for six weeks postnatally, providing women with the care that they choose. This usually involves homebirth. Women choose independent midwives for a variety of reasons. One is to ensure continuity of care and knowing who will be supporting them at the birth. IMs usually support

Table 3.2   Suggested contents of a hospital bag

It is essential to have a hospital bag ready. If you do need to transfer to hospital there will be no time to wait for someone to pack!

- Two or three nightdresses or large T-shirts, dressing gown and slippers
- One pack of night-time or maternity sanitary pads
- Toilet bag with soap, toothbrush, toothpaste, etc., tissues
- Change for the public pay phone (minimum call charge 20 p), list of telephone numbers
- Clothes and shoes to come home in
- Lavender oil, homeopathy
- Large paper pants or old knickers
- Two face cloths
- Camera and several films

For the baby

- Towel
- Nappies
- Cotton wool
- Baby clothes, vest, babygrow and blanket (include warmer clothing for coming home in).

women wanting a homebirth, but may also support her in the hospital if needed.

Any midwife can choose to work in this way whether she has just qualified or has 20 years' experience. IMs work using the *Midwives Rules and Standards* (NMC 2004) as their guide and the latest midwifery evidence to support their practice. IMs, like NHS, agency and bank midwives, have a named Supervisor of Midwives chosen from the local supervisory area that they work in.

Case Notes

I had complications in my first birth, which left me feeling quite distressed. I ended up suffering from post-traumatic stress disorder and it took me some years to decide to get pregnant again. I wanted to know my midwife in my next pregnancy and so we took out a small loan in order to employ an independent midwife to look after us. The visits all took place at our house and lasted at least an hour. I really felt that my midwife spent a lot of time listening to me and respecting my choices. She did all the physical checks, such as assessing the growth of the baby, taking my blood pressure and testing my urine. She also took my blood to test my iron levels and screening tests.

I had not decided where I wanted to give birth but by the time I was 40 weeks chose to have a homebirth. My midwife respected my choice and had always said that it was up to us and she would support me wherever we chose to have our baby.

My labour with my daughter was quite long and tough, but my midwife was by my side the whole time supporting me. The birth of my daughter was so much better than with my first child. I felt that having a trusting and continual relationship with my midwife made all the difference. My midwife visited us for six weeks following birth and was really helpful with assisting me to establish breastfeeding (something I had not managed to do before). She was also able to reassure any concerns I had and check that we were coping psychologically as well as physically.

By the time I was discharged from my midwife's care I felt I had laid to rest the ghost of my first birth and could get on with family life. It was the best money I had ever spent.

The Independent Midwives Association (IMA) has set up an audit of independent midwifery practice in the form of a database project registering clients at the time of initial contact to give the study credibility. The ongoing study has consistently shown that IMs have a high rate of normal births even amongst women who have risk factors (Milan 2005). The IMs also have a 14 per cent caesarean rate compared with a national average of 22 per cent (Birth Choice UK 2007). This is with over 70 per cent of the clients that they book with one or more risk factors (Milan 2005). IMs give informed choice and often support women who have made difficult decisions.

The IMA are respected politically and have members who provide advice and guidance to the Department of Health with issues pertaining to maternity care. Currently, the IMA is proposing that the NHS Community Midwifery Model (NHSCMM) is implemented (Van der Kooy 2005). The NHSCMM proposes that when a woman becomes pregnant, she is given direct access to a list of midwives in her area. The woman then contacts them and chooses the one she feels most comfortable with. That midwife then enters into a standard contract with the NHS who pays on a set fee per case basis. The NHSCMM would be available to those women who want it, no matter where they live or what socio-economic class they come from.

There is much behind-the-scenes work that IMs do. Tables 3.3 and 3.4 are examples of the kind of letters that IMs send to various people/organisations.

Table 3.3 Examples of letters to child health records requesting a NHS number and a request for Guthrie results

Dear Child Health Records,
I am enclosing the birth notification for the baby of Mrs B. Please could you send me the baby's NHS number ASAP in the stamped addressed envelope enclosed in case of admission to hospital /and for neonatal screening.
   Please do contact me if you have any queries.
Yours faithfully,
Independent Midwife

Dear Sir/Madam,
Please could you provide me with a photocopy of the Guthrie results for my records. I have provided a stamped addressed envelope for your convenience.
With many thanks,

Sure Start programmes of care

The NSF (DH 2004) recognises that midwives have an essential role to play in caring for vulnerable women, including those with mental health problems, suffering domestic violence, non-prescription drug users, disadvantaged minority groups and pregnant teenagers. The aim of Sure Start is to help provide a better start in life for children under 4 years who live in disadvantaged areas so that they may have greater opportunities when they start school and better health. Sure Start programmes have developed and children's centres are now opening in many disadvantaged areas where more midwives will be situated.

In an article about Sure Start midwifery, Rosser (2003) outlines an essential area for consideration – the fact that young, vulnerable women living in poverty have urgent needs than can be provided for by the clinical midwife. The problems faced by women offered Sure Start midwifery may be multifaceted. The women and families requiring Sure Start programmes are often disadvantaged. The government has plans to tackle inequalities in health care to ensure a reduction in the mortality rate of babies under 1 year. Policies such as the NSF (DH 2004) and *Tackling Health Inequalities* (DH 2003) have set targets to improve the health of those most disadvantaged. Rosser (2003) poignantly writes of a young woman whom she has helped with some aspects of her life, such as stopping smoking, accessing and using counselling, and help with form-filling in order to write

Table 3.4 Examples of letters to the Supervisor of Midwives and the general practitioner

---

Dear Supervisor of Midwives,
I am writing to inform you that I have been requested to provide midwifery care for:

NAME: Mrs M
ADDRESS:
EDB: 01.01.2008

I have been asked to attend the homebirth of the above named client as well as provide all antenatal and postnatal care.
    In the event of emergency transfer to your hospital I would be grateful if you could provide the direct line numbers for:
Delivery Suite
SCBU
Ambulance Control
I would appreciate it if you could send us some Guthrie cards and an address to which the completed card needs to be sent. Could I also have the address for the Child Health Department in order to send the birth notification after the baby has been born.
    I have completed Intention to Practice notifications which include working in your area.
    Please do not hesitate to contact me if you have any queries.
Thank you.
Yours sincerely,

Regarding: *Mrs B*
ADDRESS: EDB: 01.01.08

Dear Dr.
I have been requested by Mrs B to provide midwifery care and to attend her homebirth. Should a problem arise as a direct result of Mrs B's pregnancy, I will be referring directly to an obstetrician, however if a non-pregnancy health-related issue should occur, I hope to refer directly to you. If there are any health issues that you feel would be useful for me to be aware of please do get in touch. Please do not hesitate to contact me if you have any queries.
Thank you.
Yours sincerely,

---

off debts and apply for benefits to buy food and a cooker. Sure Start is an area where the public health role of the midwife and clinical midwifery really combine.

See Tables 3.5 and 3.6 for the seven Sure Start principles of care and the Sure Start targets.

Midwifery wisdom

We cannot fix everyone, but the small gestures that go beyond the call of duty may make a difference to the woman who is vulnerable.

Table 3.5 The seven Sure Start principles of care

1. Working with parents and children
2. Services for everyone
3. Flexible at the point of delivery
4. Starting very early
5. Respectful and transparent
6. Community driven and professionally co-ordinated
7. Outcome driven

Source: DfES 2002

Table 3.6 Sure Start targets

• 10 per cent reduction in children admitted to hospital with gastroenteritis, severe injury or respiratory infection
• Support and guidance on breastfeeding
• Identifying and supporting women with postnatal depression
• 100 per cent contact of all families within two months of birth
• Smoking reduction of at least 6 per cent
• Antenatal information and support for parents.
• Increased incidences of children having normal levels of language, communication, speech and literacy.
• A 12 per cent reduction in children who live in households in which neither parent works.

Source: Sure Start 2003

Parenthood education programmes

There is a variety of ways that parents can have childbirth education. This section outlines the options available to parents. Parenthood education classes are also discussed. Parenthood education is a helpful way for prospective parents to meet others and build up a support network for the latter stages of pregnancy and after the baby is born. Parents can access parenthood education and attend child-birth classes in a number of ways and it is important that the midwife offers different choices to the woman and her partner.

NHS classes

These classes are facilitated by midwives and occasionally have input from other health care providers, such as health visitors and physiotherapists. The classes are often held at the local hospital, birth centre or GP surgery; they are free and available in the evenings when both parents can attend. Midwives may also run parenthood education for different groups of women, such as teenage mums, lone mothers, couples or parents wanting to achieve a vaginal birth after a caesarean section.

Active birth classes

Active birth classes are fee-based and are run by antenatal teachers who have been trained by the Active Birth Centre. Yoga is usually included, with an emphasis on relaxation, breathing and self-help methods for coping with labour. Many of the exercise and yoga classes are for women, incorporating the couple in the childbirth preparation and education classes.

National Childbirth Trust classes

Classes run by the NCT are provided by antenatal teachers trained by the NCT. They are are kept to a minimum of around six couples and are held in community centres or at the teacher's home. The fee may be negotiated if a woman is on a low income. The focus is on informed choice and decision-making and issues such as pain relief, positions for labour and life with a new baby are addressed. There is also discussion around the medicalisation of birth and how to avoid a cascade of intervention and plan for a natural birth.

Parenthood education classes provide an opportunity to ask questions and explore areas of concern. As the classes usually involve couples, it is a way of including the partner in the pregnancy and birth, as well as providing information associated with support for the woman.

Birth plans

A birth plan is a means by which a woman can communicate her wishes to her midwives and hospital doctors. It may include choices such as wanting to use water for birth, avoiding the use of pethidine and wanting skin-to-skin contact with the baby immediately after birth (NCT 2004). The midwife can help the woman write her birth plan. Midwives need to ensure that they are the woman's advocate and that the woman is given balanced, non-judgemental and appropriate information at every stage so that she is able to make informed choices. Midwifery records should reflect discussions and plans of how choices can be implemented. The latest NMC guidance determines that it is the midwife's duty to support and respect the woman's choice. The Supervisor of Midwives should support the midwife in facilitating the woman's choice (NMC 2006). The NMC (2006a; http://www.nmc-uk.org/aFrameDisplay.aspx?DocumentID =1680) notes that to withdraw a woman's choice of a homebirth is similar to an NHS Trust withdrawing hospital services. Midwives need to have the courage to be advocates for the women they are supporting.

When to call the midwife

When discussing choices and birth plans, it is useful for the woman to have information about when to call her midwife. They should be given information on how to make contact with her midwife and when to call, particularly when symptoms such as severe headache or reduced fetal movements may indicate that there could be a problem (see Table 3.7). It is useful for women and couples to know what is normal and when to call the midwife if they think labour has started.

Midwifery wisdom

Birth wishes may not always go to schedule for a couple, but always respect the woman's birth plan. She has thought long and hard about what she wants and has taken the time to write it down. That in itself deserves your attention and respect.

Table 3.7 Advice for women on when to call the midwife

- Baby's movements reduced
- Severe headache
- Severe itching
- Visual disturbances
- Epigastric (upper abdominal) pain
- Bleeding
- Abnormal discharge
- Spontaneous rupture of the membranes
- Contractions have started
- Needing reassurance

Conclusion

Choice for pregnant women is a key issue which the current government is keen to promote (DH 2004). The midwife has a responsibility to inform women of their choices. This is particularly important when it comes to place of birth. Women may not know that they have the option of a birth centre or a homebirth, and these options should be given from the first booking appointment. Once the place of birth had been decided, the woman needs to know she can change her mind should she wish. A woman should be encouraged to write down or communicate her plans for birth. This can help her in exploring the options available and outline her wishes in respect of labour and the birth of her baby.

Parenting education is an important way of giving information to couples to help them arrive at their choices. There are many ways that women can access classes and the midwife can inform her of what is available in her area. Models of care vary in each area. There are different ways that midwives can practise midwifery, from working within a hospital or birth centre to working outside of the NHS as an independent midwife or case loading for a group of women. Models of care may vary, but all women require information, respect and to be given the opportunity to make choices that meet their individual needs.

References

Ackermann-Liebrich, U., Voegeli, T., Gunter-Witt, K. et al. (1996) Outcomes of planned home versus hospital deliveries: Follow-up study of matched pairs for procedures and outcomes. *British Medical Journal* 313(7088): 1313–18.

Audit Commission (1997) *First Class Delivery: Improving Maternity Services in England and Wales.* Abingdon: Audit Commission Publications. http://www.birthchoiceuk.com/Frame.htm (accessed 3 March 2007)

Birth Choice UK (2007) http://www.birthchoiceuk.com/.

Chamberlain, G., Wraight, A. and Crowley, P. (1997) *Report of the 1994 Confidential Enquiry by the National Birthday Trust Fund.* London: Parthenon Publishing.

Department for Education and Skills (2002) *About Sure Start. Sure Start Unit.* www.surestart.gov.uk (accessed 1 March 2007).

Department of Health (2001) *Why Mothers Die. 1997–1999. Report of the Confidential Enquiry into Maternal Deaths.* London: RCOG Press.

Department of Health (2003) *Tackling Health Inequalities: A Programme for Action.* London: DH.

Department of Health (2004) *National Service Framework for Children and Young People.* London: DH.

Garland, D. and Jones, K. (2000) Waterbirth: Supporting practice with clinical audit. *MIDIRS Midwifery Digest* 10(3): 333–6.

House of Commons (1992) *Maternity Services: Government Response to the Second Report from The Health Committee, Session 1991–1992.* London: HSMO.

House of Commons Health Committee (2003) *Choice in Maternity Services.* Ninth Report of Session 2002–2003, Vol. 1. London: The Stationery Office.

Lavender, T. (2003) *Report to the Department of Health Children's Taskforce from the Maternity and Neonatal Workforce Group.* London: DH.

Milan, M. (2005) Independent midwifery compared with other caseload practice. *MIDIRS Midwifery Digest* 15(4): 548–54.

National Childbirth Trust NCT (2004) *Your Birth Year: Understanding the Choices you have in Pregnancy, Birth and Motherhood.* London: NCT.

National Institute for Health Clinical Excellence (2003) *Antenatal Care: Routine Care for the Healthy Pregnant Woman. Clinical Guidelines.* London: NICE.

Nursing and Midwifery Council (2004) *Midwives Rules and Standards.* London: NMC.

Nursing and Midwifery Council (2006) *Midwives and Homebirths Circular.* http://www.nmc-uk.org/aFrameDisplay.aspx?DocumentID=1680 (accessed 11 March 2007).

Olsen, O. and Jewell, M. D. (2005) *Home versus Hospital Birth: In the Cochrane Database of Systematic Reviews* (Issue 2).

Rosser J. (2003) How do the Albany midwives do it? Evaluation of the Albany Midwifery Practice. *MIDIRS Midwifery Digest* 13(2): 251–7.

Royal College of Midwives (2000) *The Use of Water in Labour and Birth.* Position Paper 1a. London: RCM.

Sandall, J., Davies, J. and Warwick, C. (2001) *Evaluation of the Albany Midwifery Practice.* Final Report, March. London: King's College.

Shearer, J. M. (1985) Five-year prospective survey of risk of booking for a home birth in Essex. *Br Med J (Clin Res Ed)* 291(6507) (23 November): 1478–80.

Sure Start (2003) *Sure Start Guidance 2004–2006.* Section 1. www.surestart.gov.uk/aboutsurestart (accessed 10 March 2007).

Tew, M. (1985) Place of birth and perinatal mortality. *Journal of the Royal College of General Practitioners* 35 (August): 390–4.

Van der Kooy, B. (2005) The NHS Community Midwifery Model (NHS CMM) London: The Independent Midwive Association. www.independentmidwives.org.uk.

Walsh, D. (1999) An ethnographic study of women's experience of partnership caseload midwifery practice: the professional as a friend. *Midwifery* 15: 165–76.

Walsh, D. (2005) Birth Centre Care: a review of the literature. *Birth Issues* 13(4): 129–34.

Walsh, D. and Downe, S. (2004) Outcomes of Free-Standing, Midwifery-Led Birth Centres: A Structured Review of the Evidence. *Birth* 31(3): 222–9.

Interdisciplinary Working: Seamless Working within Maternity Care

Eileen Huish and Lisa Nash

Introduction

In response to service users' demands and the need to improve safety, there is a drive for services to join up to provide integrated care (DH 2005). Services that women need for their maternity care may be provided by the NHS, social care, the voluntary sector or organisations such as Sure Start. For some women care will be provided in the community or in the hospital setting by midwives and obstetricians, but for those with complex social needs maternity care should be provided in partnership with other agencies such as children's services, domestic abuse teams, drug and alcohol teams, learning disability and mental health services (DH 2007). The aim of this chapter is to prepare readers to provide seamless care by exploring various aspects of collaborative working, including the possible consequences when collaborative working is absent.

Seamless care

Seamless care is delivered by building robust lines of communication and professional working relationships. But first, what is meant by 'seamless care'?

As a client moves through the health and social care system for whatever reason the client and their family/carers will experience the services provided by different agencies/professions. This journey is often referred to as a care pathway. Instead of clients being passed from one agency to another all working completely independently, clients should have access to an integrated system.

Figure 4.1 shows one possible care pathway for a woman with a confirmed eight-week pregnancy who is admitted to hospital. Read the boxes and follow the arrows.

Each of the arrows in Figure 4.1 represents a point when a breakdown in providing seamless care between departments may occur. The arrows represent a delay in the provision of care or a breakdown in communication and information-sharing. It used to be the case that a pregnant woman needing an ultrasound scan at the weekend would have to wait until the following Monday because there were not enough ultrasonographers to provide an out-of-hours service. However, this care pathway has been improved in many Trusts by training midwives in early pregnancy ultrasound. Now, if a woman needs an ultrasound scan at the weekend she does not need to wait.

Activity

Draw a care pathway that you are familiar with. Each time you use an arrow consider how information is shared, how well the agencies work together, whether clients usually experience delays and what the possible causes for the delays are. Then, most importantly, consider how improvements can be made.

This may seem difficult if you are at the start of your education. Consider it again when you are about to qualify.

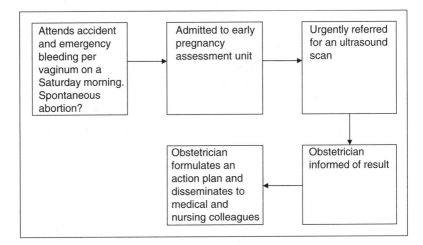

Figure 4.1   An example of a woman's possible care pathway

Here are some examples of health care professionals midwives work with:

- The general practitioner (GP) in the community. The midwife may refer the pregnant woman to the GP from the antenatal clinic – for example, when a woman is symptomatic of a urinary tract infection
- Health visitors in the community, when the midwife hands over the care of the women to the health visitor and when discussing newly booked clients. The health visitor will have a wealth of information about the family, such as a history of domestic violence, child protection issues, and so on. This information should be shared on a need-to-know basis so that confidentiality is maintained whilst ensuring the safety of the woman and her family
- Social workers. Where there are child protection issues, housing concerns and benefit queries the midwife may seek advice from the social worker. All pregnant women under 16 years of age will be referred to a social worker
- The obstetric physiotherapist, for advice on postnatal exercises, symphisis pubis dysfunction, back pain
- The obstetrician to refer women whose pregnancy is deviating from the norm
- The paediatrician for neonatal examination and resuscitation in emergency situations. In some units the midwife will perform the neonatal examination on neonates who have had a normal delivery, but they will always refer if an abnormality is detected
- The ultrasonographer, who performs routine and urgent scans. It is important to remember that antenatal scans are always performed when required, irrespective of the ultrasonographer's workload
- The dietician, particularly for a woman who has diabetes, is obese or has an eating disorder
- The paramedic who brings a woman in labour into the maternity unit, or whom you meet as a community midwife attending an unexpected home delivery or a life-threatening situation, for example cord prolapse

- The psychiatric nurse if you are caring for a woman with a mental health illness
- The medical team if you are caring for a woman with a medical condition
- The surgical team if you are caring for a woman who needs surgery during her pregnancy or postnatally
- The infection control nurse to maintain infection control standards

The Northwick Park Report

To illustrate the importance of effective interdisciplinary and team working, the Northwick Park Report (Healthcare Commission 2006) will be discussed so that the reader may benefit from the lessons learnt from the Healthcare Commission's findings and recommendations.

The Healthcare Commission conducts investigations into health care provision in England and Wales, usually following allegations of serious failings. If there are concerns about patient safety, the Healthcare Commission will undertake an investigation to discover whether this is the case and to identify possible causes for the deficiencies. Recommendations will also be made in order to help the organisation improve the quality of care it provides and to restore public confidence in its services. Lessons learnt from these investigations are shared throughout the NHS in order to promote best practice and ensure that patient safety is maintained nationwide.

The Northwick Park investigation was commissioned following ten maternal deaths between April 2004 and April 2005 at Northwick Park Hospital and a higher than expected number of neonatal deaths. The aim of the investigation was to uncover the factors surrounding this disproportionately high number of deaths. Following the investigation the Trust was put onto special measures. These are imposed to ensure that any deficiencies in the services are remedied by appropriate means through an action plan.

Issues concerning staffing were raised and included:

- A high attrition rate of midwives, with 72 vacancies in December 2004
- The consultants had been allowed to specialise in gynaecology

- Additional obstetricians were not appointed
- The consultants were not always available
- Lack of clarity regarding the consultants' duties
- Temporary medical staff were not allowed to work on the labour ward
- If medical staff went sick they had to cover each other's workload
- Medical staff experienced difficulties attending training because of their heavy workload
- Consultants criticised each other in front of staff
- Not all consultants supported changes introduced by the clinical director
- Poor communication and working relationships were found across all staff groups, which exacerbated the high attrition rate

(Healthcare Commission 2006)

The following recommendations were made:

- Improvement to communication with women and their families
- The Trust to take on board the views of the women
- All staff to attend cultural awareness training
- All complaints to be responded to appropriately
- Address shortage of staff urgently
- Training and skills for staff caring for women post-surgery or who require invasive monitoring
- Improve communication and working relationships of all staff groups
- Attendance and records for mandatory training to be improved
- The new clinical maternity information system to be introduced immediately, along with appropriate training of staff
- Clinical audit should be developed and findings communicated to staff
- Trust should work with local health care partners to commission additional capacity on a temporary basis while recommendations acted upon
- Trust should ensure effective communication with Primary Care Trusts and the Strategic Health Authority about quality, including the routine reporting of any serious untoward incident

(Healthcare Commission 2006)

Activity

Consider whether the Northwick Park Report recommendations will improve team working.

You may find it useful to read the full report to gain greater understanding and find out more about the work of the Healthcare Commission. From consideration of the Northwick Park Report (Healthcare Commission 2006) it is apparent that effective collaboration and good team working across disciplines is required to maintain standards and ensure continued patient safety.

Collaborative working

The aim of all health and social care professionals is to provide collaborative, patient-centred care. Collaborative working and the concept of teams will now be considered. Collaborative working has many benefits, including improved client satisfaction, improved clinical outcomes, reduction of mortality rates and improved staff morale (Jeffrey and Dichter 2003; Sloper 2004). Key elements for collaborative working are mutual trust and respect across disciplines and an understanding of the roles and responsibilities of other professions. Understanding other departments' operational needs and issues that they face on day-to-day basis assists cooperation and cross-disciplinary support. However, there are barriers to collaborative working which will now be considered.

Barriers to collaboration

To engage in collaborative working an awareness of barriers needs to be developed so that individual practitioners can work to overcome them.

Language
During uni-professional working a unique language is developed. Some of this may be clinical terms used solely in midwifery, but it may include abbreviations or jargon. Try to imagine how difficult it is for someone from another discipline to understand this sort of language. For example, a midwife may use the abbreviation IUD to mean intra-uterine death, but another discipline may understand it to mean intra-uterine device. However, a midwife might use IUCD as an abbreviation for intra-uterine contraceptive device. This

demonstrates how a breakdown in communication can occur through the use of language.

We are taught not to use jargon with patients and this good practice should be extended to other professionals to prevent misunderstandings (see Chapter 1). Language is therefore a potential barrier to collaborative working. It is interesting to note that Allan et al. (2006) suggest that interprofessional working develops a shared language and conversely that a shared language is a basic step towards collaborative working.

Attitudes/preconceptions to other professions

Sloper (2004) identified negative professional stereotyping as a barrier to inter-agency working. Many people have attitudes towards and preconceptions about other professions, which may be positive or negative. Barr et al. (2005) discusses research which shows that inter-professional education (IPE) may not improve negative stereotyping, but professionals can examine and acknowledge their own attitudes so that they do not inhibit their ability to work with others.

Activity

Which words would you use to describe each of the following professions?

- Obstetrician
- General practitioner
- Social worker
- Physiotherapist
- Nurse
- Ultrasonographer

Did you include caring, practical, team player, good communicator, leader, intelligent, hardworking, unapproachable, inefficient, arrogant, unsupportive, offhand, rude, aggressive, bully (Tunstall-Pedoe et al. 2003)? Try to think of more.

Activity

Thinking about the words you use to describe a profession will help you to begin to explore your own attitudes and preconceptions.

- How were they formed?
- Are they positive or negative?

Professionalism dictates that the same standard of care should be delivered to a service user regardless of the practitioner's attitude to that individual. Equally, practitioners should be able to work cooperatively with any other profession. Try to foster a positive attitude by respecting and valuing the contribution that other professions make to care pathways.

Throughout your education and future career, endeavour to identify barriers to collaborative working and seek to overcome them. During your education Interprofessional Education (IPE) will help you to prepare for collaborative working and will be discussed in more detail later in this chapter.

Conceptualising teams

Activity

Consider the following:

- Who makes up the team you work in?
- Are women and their families/carers part of that team?
- How are women involved in their care?
- What is your role in the team?
- What are the roles of others in the team?

Do you consider the people that you work with every day to be part of your team? Is this team uni-professional? Does it include administration and clerical staff, or does it include people from another professional discipline? For example, in the community a midwife works closely with health visitors and GPs on a daily basis. However, in a complex pregnancy (for clinical and/or social reasons) the team that needs to work together may be very transient. That is to say, it is formed for a limited period to care for one woman and her family. The example given here concerns a single diabetic woman of 32 weeks' gestation who has an 18-month-old daughter. The woman develops pre-eclampsia and needs to be admitted to hospital, but she has no one who can look after her daughter for a long period of time.

The team involved in this woman's care may be made up of a midwife, a social worker, an obstetrician, a dietician and staff involved with fostering. In cases such as this clear lines of communication need to be formed and a case manager may be assigned who is responsible for ensuring that multi-agency service delivery is coordinated (Sloper 2004).

Service user involvement

Women were surveyed as part of the Northwick Park Report (Health-care Commission 2006) on how and where improvements should be made. Service user involvement is now a Department of Health requirement in the provision of maternity care, service improvement and research. Involving a woman in a decision about her care demonstrates respect for her values. The benefits to her are increased confidence, reduced anxiety and better relationships with professionals (DH 2004). Any feedback from women, whether in the form of complaints or recommendations, should be regarded as a positive contribution to service improvement (HM Government 2007). Service users and carers are an integral part of service delivery and design, and as such should be considered as part of the team.

Functioning teams

Activity

What does a team need to function?

Teams are important as they allow seamless care; a breakdown in the team will disrupt this process.

Activity

Think of a situation where you have had to work as part of a team. Reflect on the following:

- Who led the team?
- How did the team leader manage the team/delegate duties to other members?
- How did the team interact?
- What went well?
- What did not go quite so well?
- What could have been done differently?

Every team has to develop and goes through certain behavioural stages. Tuckman (1965) developed a model based on these stages – forming, storming, norming and performing. He added adjourning in the 1970s.

Forming

In the 'forming' stage the team depends on its leader. It may help if you think back to your first day at university when you did not know anyone and would have (we hope) been impressed with your lecturer. At this stage in the team's development individual roles and responsibilities are unclear, and the leader will have many questions to answer regarding the direction and purpose of the team. The leader will tell the team what to do, whilst the team will test the leader.

Storming

During the storming stage the individuals are competing with each other for their position in the team. As the term suggests, the team does not function smoothly – various sub-groups form and it is easy for them to be distracted from achieving their common goal. Again, think about the early days of your course and how cliques were formed in your group. Some groups can get stuck at this stage and it is important for them to stay focused on their goal or they will be easily distracted.

Norming

During the norming stage everything becomes clear. The roles and responsibilities within the group are formed and the leader becomes the facilitator, gaining more respect. The group becomes cohesive and make decisions unanimously, further developing their style. This could be akin to when you have settled into university life and you know what is expected of you.

Performing

In the performing stage the team has a clear path to follow. Any disagreements are resolved within the team and the leader to set tasks for individuals. The team will now look after each other and require little active participation from the leader. They will socialise together and are concerned with the development of their team. Think about when you started socialising as a large group with your university colleagues.

Adjourning

The adjourning stage, as the term suggests, is when the group disbands. This is usually when the project has finished (as at the end of your programme). At this stage the team members should have achieved their goal (for example, successfully completed your programme) and are ready to move on to new projects. Some people have a sense of grief in this stage and the sensitivity of the situation should be recognised as members may feel insecure. This may occur towards the end of your midwifery education when it is usual for students to feel a sense of loss and find themselves in a working environment on their own. Many people find the changes difficult and it is well known that it increases stress.

Activity

Consider the consequences if the team never get beyond the storming stage and refer back to the Northwick Park report.
    Do you think that these multidisciplinary teams never progressed beyond this stage?

Individual practitioners have a responsibility to the multidisciplinary team; they should be working towards the same goal, ensuring that their individual tasks have been completed on time and should understand the purpose of a multidisciplinary team (Atwal and Cauldwell 2006). Your midwifery educational programme may include working in teams with other students either uni-professionally or multi-professionally. Try to transfer what you have learnt about team working in the classroom to the practice setting.

Team roles

Farmer et al. (2003) discussed the findings of a study conducted in Scotland, which explored the role of midwives and GPs in the rural community. Their study found that the implementation of midwives taking the lead in low-risk pregnancies was variable. The reasons were numerous, but included GPs' intransigence to the role of midwives, and where midwives were taking the lead GPs were left uncertain of their own role. The study highlighted the need for clear boundaries for all staff involved with care because roles which are open to interpretation may lead to poor inter-professional working, which will ultimately compromise the quality of care. The findings of this study can be transferred to other situations. For example, new ways of working are continuously being developed and new roles emerging. Where the new role of the midwifery care assistant is being introduced, all staff should clearly understand the role and the impact that this has on themselves. There is also a requirement for role flexibility and team members may need to adopt different roles in different situations. For example, in the community setting where some Trusts have begun to integrate the role of the health care assistant, the midwife no longer needs to lead on certain responsibilities, such as facilitation of breastfeeding and demonstration baby bathing.

Referral and handover

One aspect of providing a seamless service is to know when to refer, to whom and the agreed mechanism for doing so. It is accepted that when a referral has been discussed and agreed between a client and a practitioner a certain amount of information will be shared. This includes name, date of birth and contact details as a minimum; but what further information does the agency/professional need to act on the referral? If all the appropriate information is included in the referral, the woman will experience a seamless service. However, if essential information is omitted, the woman will experience unnecessary delays. For example, when referring to a geneticist about a possible inherited condition the geneticist will need to know the family history, whether the woman is already pregnant and the gestation of her pregnancy in order to prioritise the appointment. On the other hand, it is not necessary to share every piece of information in a referral and this may be considered to be a breach of confidentiality (see Chapter 14). A midwife, for example, may be aware that the woman's partner is a transsexual, but not every health care professional involved in the woman's care needs to know this. Information such as this can become gossip.

Activity

Think back to a referral that you were involved in and the information that you passed on. Did you include all the relevant information and was it all pertinent?

The art of referring has its own set of knowledge and skills. However, receiving a referral also needs to be considered. When you receive a written referral do you read *all* the information? Or do you look at it then dismiss it, perhaps thinking that you know better? The same questions need to be asked for written and verbal handovers. For example, during a handover from a paramedic, do you value the contribution that the paramedic is making? Remember, a paramedic has observed the woman in a completely different situation and may have vital information that should not be ignored. For example, the paramedic may have witnessed the woman's partner behaving aggressively, so that domestic violence is suspected.

Interprofessional education

Interprofessional education (IPE) is defined as 'occasions when two or more professions learn with, from and about each other to improve collaboration and the quality of care' (Freeth et al. 2005). For IPE to be achieved there must be interaction between the participants. This is what differentiates IPE from common/shared learning. Because care pathways can break down between clinical and non-clinical staff and between non-clinical staff from different departments, the definition applies to all staff in health and social care and the word 'profession' in the definition should be thought of in broad terms. A porter, cleaner or a member of clerical staff may work in a professional manner. IPE in the workplace should include opportunities for all types of staff to interact. Another term often used is interprofessional learning (IPL). This is the learning that comes from the interaction between professions (Freeth et al. 2005). The aim of IPE during educational programmes is to prepare practitioners for collaborative working and it lays the foundation for continuing IPE throughout your career. It should take place in both the classroom and the workplace, although some educational institutions may find it difficult to introduce IPE into the classroom, if for example they only deliver nursing programmes. The benefits of IPE for all types of staff can go beyond improving care; it can improve working relationships, build mutual respect and consequently improve job satisfaction and reduce stress.

Freeth et al. (2005) describe four types of interprofessional learning:

1. Exchange-based
2. Action-based
3. Simulation-based
4. Observation-based

Some of these activities require organisation and facilitation; however, students and practitioners can take responsibility/ownership of interprofessional learning in the practice setting. This can be achieved by shadowing other professionals, joint patient consultations and making the most of opportunities during everyday, work-based activities. It may, for example, be useful to spend an hour or two shadowing an ultrasonographer, a social worker or a mental health nurse. A final-year student midwife could spend time working with a medical student during their obstetric placement – a patient consultation, ongoing assessment of a lady during labour or a first assessment of a newborn baby could be conducted together. This enables both students to learn about each other's roles and responsibilities along the care pathway.

Discuss your IPL opportunities with your mentor/link lecturer at the start of each of your practice placements. Find out what is available and when you may be invited to take part in an activity that has been organised for you; alternatively, you may need to initiate an activity for yourself. Before undertaking any IPE activities, agree with your mentor the aims and learning outcomes, and after the activity discuss any uncertainties or queries.

Interprofessional learning takes place during multidisciplinary working, but only if you are conscious of it and make the most of it.

Activity

During your practice placements you will work with or come into contact with other disciplines.

- Reflect on a recent experience of working with another discipline.
- What did you learn about the other discipline?
- How can you use this knowledge to improve the client experience?
- Will this new knowledge/understanding alter your own practice – clinical or non-clinical?

Practice is made up of clinical and non-clinical tasks – for example, administration or passing on a message – and care pathways may break down due to poor execution of such tasks.

Reflection

Reflection is used to maintain and improve our own practice; however, reflection also needs to be used to improve women's experiences of moving through the health and social care system. Consider keeping reflective accounts of your interprofessional learning in your practice portfolio as this will provide evidence of your learning to work collaboratively. Working in collaboration to provide seamless care is an employment skill and therefore any improvement in knowledge or skills as a result of IPE should be included in your personal development plan to help you to write a CV and prepare for interviews.

The Health Sciences and Practice Subject Centre of the Higher Education Academy has published a *Midwifery Student Employability Profile* (2005). This includes a list of reflective questions that students may use as a prompt to reflect on their developing skills. One of the sets of questions is about teamwork and working with others, but there are several sets of questions each exploring a different topic. Consider using this document to assist you with work applications and interviews.

Practice, both clinical and non-clinical, impacts on other departments and professionals. The way we work, the actions we take or do not take or the information that is not passed on may cause delays in the woman's care pathway or the service may appear unprofessional. For example, if the ultrasound department is expecting a woman for an anomaly scan and has not been told that she has had a miscarriage, she may be caused unnecessary distress and valuable ultrasound appointment time may be lost as the department will have allocated an appointment to a woman who no longer needs it. There must be robust lines of communication between departments along care pathways.

The NMC's *Standards of Proficiency* state that a midwife must *'contribute to the development and evaluation of guidelines and policies and make recommendations for change'* (NMC 2004). Guidelines and policies often affect another department or profession and therefore this type of improvement activity should be done in consultation, involving other members of staff. IPL can take place during this type of service improvement activity and this is one way in which practitioners can continue to learn about other professions throughout their career. IPL, multidisciplinary working and service improvement are closely linked, support each other and are described by Barr et al. (2005) as being three cogs in a machine which drive each other.

Conclusion

IPE and uni-professional education support one another. Both are necessary so that practitioners recognise when collaboration is required and when responsibility for an aspect of care is theirs alone (Freeth et al. 2005). It has been demonstrated that good interdisciplinary team working is essential for client care and safety, and key elements required for successful collaboration have been discussed. Continue to reflect on your IPE experiences and interprofessional working throughout your career as this should be part of your continuing professional development. Your goal should now be to develop beyond professionalism to interprofessionalism.

References

Allan, C., Campbell, W., Guptill, C. et al. (2006) A conceptual model for interprofessioanl education: The international classification, disability and health. *Journal of Interprofessional Care* 20(3): 235–45.

Atwal, A. and Cauldwell, K. (2006) Nurses' perception of multidisciplinary team work in acute health care. *International Journal of Nursing Practice* 12: 359–65.

Barr, H., Koppel, I., Reeves, S. et al. (2005) *Effective Interprofessional Education: Argument, Assumption and Evidence.* Oxford: Blackwell.

Department of Health (2004) *Patient and Public Involvement in Health: The Evidence for Policy Implementation.* http://www.dh.gov.uk (accessed March 2007).

Department of Health (2005) *Creating a Patient-Led NHS: Delivering the NHS Improvement Plan.* http://www.dh.gov.uk (accessed April 2007).

Department of Health (2007) *Maternity Matters: Choice, Access and Continuity of Care in a Safe Service.* http://www.dh.gov.uk (accessed April 2007).

Farmer, J., Stimpson, P. and Tucker, J. (2003) Relative professional roles in antenatal care: Results of a survey in Scottish rural general practice. *Journal of Interprofessional Care* 17(4): 351–62.

Freeth, D., Hammick, M., Reeves, S. et al. (2005) *Effective Interprofessional Education: Development, Delivery and Evaluation.* Oxford: Blackwell.

Health Sciences and Practice Subject Centre (2005) *Midwifery Student Employability Profile. The Higher Education Academy.* http://www.health.heacademy.ac.uk (accessed March 2007).

Healthcare Commission (2006) *Investigation into 10 Maternal Deaths at, or Following Delivery at, Northwick Park Hospital, North West London Hospitals NHS Trust, between April 2002 and April 2005.* London: Commission for Healthcare Audit and Inspection.

HM Government (2007) *Learning from Tragedy: Keeping Patients Safe.* London: The Stationery Office.

Jeffrey, R. and Dichter, M. (2003) Teamwork and hospital medicine. *Critical Care Nurse* 23(3): 8–11.

Nursing and Midwifery Council (2004) *Standards of Proficiency for Pre-registration Midwifery Education.* London: NMC.

Sloper, P. (2004) Facilitators and barriers to coordinated multi-agency services. *Child: Care, Health and Development* 30(6): 571–80.

Tuckman, B. (1965) Developmental sequence in small groups. *Psychological Bulletin* 63(6): 384–99.

Tunstall-Pedoe, S., Rink, E. and Hilton, S. (2003) Student attitudes to interprofessional education. *Journal of Interprofessional Care* 17(2): 161–72.

Intrapartum Care

5

Annabel Jay and Cathy Hamilton

Introduction

The midwife is the expert in normal childbirth. It is her role to promote and support the normal physiology of labour, whilst noting any signs of variations from the norm that might harm the woman or her baby. The *Midwives Rules and Standards* (NMC 2004) require the midwife to report any deviations from the norm to another suitably qualified health professional (who may be a doctor) with the necessary skills required to manage the situation. In order to do this, the midwife should have a clear understanding of what is meant by a 'normal' labour and birth. The focus of this chapter will be on the midwife's role in the promotion of a normal labour resulting in a safe and memorable childbirth experience for the woman and her family.

Management strategies which a midwife can employ in order to provide choice for women in her care will also be discussed. This will include a discussion of the different forms of pain relief available to women giving birth in the UK today.

It is assumed that the reader has a basic knowledge of the anatomy and physiology underpinning the reproductive system.

Definitions of 'normal'

There is currently no standard or universally acceptable definition of a 'normal' birth. The term has different meanings for

Table 5.1   Definition of normal birth

Definition of normal birth
Birth without caesarean section Birth without assisted delivery (ventouse or forceps) No induction of labour No regional anaesthesia (epidural or spinal block)

Source: BirthChoice UK 2003

Table 5.2   What normality excludes

Normality excludes
Induced and augmented labour Timing of labour Medical methods of pain relief Withholding food and fluid in labour Artificial rupture of membranes Restricted mobility Clinical environment Continuous fetal monitoring Routine vaginal examination Routine episiotomy

Source: Bates 1997

obstetricians, midwives and members of the public. Even within the midwifery profession, individuals may hold different definitions, ranging from anything short of a caesarean section at one end of the scale to a totally physiological birth without any intervention at the other. Most people, however, would probably consider normal birth to be somewhere between these two extremes (Mead 2004).

There is a gulf between the understanding of 'normality' and what is perceived as 'the norm'. The latter refers to statistical norms for commonly used procedures such as an epidural or cardiotocography (the electronic monitoring of the fetal heart) (Mead 2004), which fall outside many people's concept of what constitutes 'normal' labour.

For the purpose of statistics, the government has adopted the definition of normal birth proposed by BirthChoice UK (see Table 5.1).

The World Health Organisation (1996; cited in Mead 2004) advises that interventions to the physiological process of birth should not occur without good cause. To this may be added the RCM's description of what normality excludes (see Table 5.2).

Stages of labour

Labour has been traditionally divided into three stages:

1. The onset of labour to the time when the cervix (neck of the womb) is fully opened to allow the fetus to move down into the birth canal
2. From when the cervix is fully open to the birth of the baby
3. From when the baby is delivered to the expulsion of the placenta (afterbirth) and membranes from the woman's body

The organisation of labour into these three stages has been challenged by some writers, who suggest that labour should be considered as a continuum, with physiological, physical and emotional factors playing an integral part in the process (Walsh 2004).

This chapter will now consider how the midwife can promote a normal, physiological labour, with reference to the criteria in Table 5.2.

Promoting spontaneous labour – avoiding induction of labour

Around 20 per cent of pregnant women have their labour induced (NICE 2001). In most cases this is because the pregnancy is prolonged, but is otherwise normal. It is current practice in most maternity units to offer routine induction of labour to women whose pregnancy goes beyond 41 weeks (NICE 2001). Whilst there is little argument against induction for serious obstetric complications, it should be remembered that the process is an invasive procedure requiring many interventions. When the only reason for induction is post-term pregnancy, it may be preferable to encourage the onset of spontaneous labour with natural methods. These include:

- *Sexual intercourse without use of a condom or diaphragm* if this is aesthetically acceptable to both the woman and her partner. It is thought that the prostaglandins in semen help to speed the process of cervical effacement. However, this is not recommended if the membranes have ruptured, as there is a risk of ascending infection.
- *Spicy foods.* The maxim 'hot sex and a hot curry' is sometimes used! It is thought that the spices in curry or similar dishes provoke bowel activity, which in turn promotes the onset of contractions. Similar properties are linked to fresh pineapple. It is not known whether there is any empirical evidence to support

this, but it is unlikely to cause harm as long as the woman enjoys the food and is not allergic to any of the ingredients.

- *'Sweeping the membranes'*. This process involves the midwife inserting a gloved forefinger through the cervical os and rotating it in a circular fashion to separate the membranes from the lower uterine area. This causes prostaglandins to be released which promote cervical effacement (thinning and stretching) and dilatation. Research shows that a sweep increases the chances of labour starting spontaneously within the next 48 hours and can reduce the need for other methods of induction (NICE 2001). It is only possible if the cervix is already open sufficiently to admit a finger. This should never be forced. This process may be carried out in the antenatal clinic or the woman's home and may result in a 'show' (a lightly blood-stained mucous discharge) and some mild cramps afterwards. The current NICE guidelines recommend that a sweep should be offered prior to any induction process (NICE 2001).

Onset of spontaneous labour

The timing of the start of labour in humans is less precise than it is in other species. It is suggested that the average day of onset is 39.6 weeks (Ndala 2005a). The underlying theory of labour is still not fully understood although the timing of its onset is thought to be related to fetal brain activity. It is suggested that adrenocortioctrophic hormone (ACTH) is released from the fetal pituitary gland which causes the woman's hormone progesterone to be converted to oestrogen. This in turn increases the sensitivity of the uterus to prostaglandins and oxytocin, which are produced by both the mother and the fetus (Ndala 2005a). These hormones cause the uterine muscle fibres to contract and shorten, so stimulating the beginning of the labour process. Studies have shown that where there is an abnormality in the fetal hypothalamus and pituitary gland, prolonged pregnancy may follow (Johnson and Everitt 2000).

It is usually the woman who will notice that labour has begun. Traditionally, there are certain cardinal signs of impending labour which women are told to expect. However, research has shown that regardless of whether a woman has given birth before, individual women will experience the onset of labour in a variety of ways. As well as this, many women report a process which bears little resemblance to the classical diagnosis of labour onset (Gross et al. 2006). It is important to bear in mind that labour is unique to each woman and that the pain and discomfort of early labour may be perceived differently by different individuals.

Case Notes

Fiona was three days overdue. That morning she was very excited when she noticed a small amount of blood in her underwear. She felt sure that she was going into labour and would probably give birth that night. Indeed, as the day went on she began to experience regular contractions, which became more and more painful and that night she was unable to sleep. However, in the morning the contractions subsided and for the rest of the day she felt no further pain. She felt disheartened and wondered if she would ever go into labour.

She spent the day in bed and slept deeply. At midnight, contractions resumed and became longer stronger and more frequent. She went into hospital at 0200 h and eventually gave birth at 1100 h. This was almost three days after she had first noticed the show and to Fiona seemed like a very long time.

Signs that labour has started

Onset of uterine contractions

As labour begins, the formerly painless uterine tightening (Braxton Hicks contractions) increases in frequency and the woman starts to perceive the contractions as uncomfortable. This discomfort may be felt in the lower abdomen or in the lower back or both. Some women also experience pain at the top of their legs. The woman will eventually notice that this discomfort coincides with a tightening of her uterus. If the midwife were to put her hand on the fundus (top) of the uterus then these contractions would be readily felt as a hardening. At first, the uterine contractions occur every 15–20 minutes and may only last 20–30 seconds. However, as labour progresses they begin to increase in length, strength and frequency, leading to effacement and dilatation of the cervix.

Passage of a mucus 'show'

During pregnancy, the cervical canal contains a plug of mucus (the operculum), which is believed to protect the fetus from infection. As the cervix begins to dilate in early labour, this mucus plug will often be dislodged and the woman will notice a bloodstained discharge in her underwear or after she has passed urine. This is often the first sign that labour is imminent, although it may still be some hours before it begins in earnest. Some women are never aware of the passage of this show.

Spontaneous rupture of the membranes ('the waters breaking')

This may occur before the onset of labour or any time during labour. It is not a true sign that labour has begun unless it is accompanied by dilatation of the cervix.

Approximately 6–19 per cent of women will experience spontaneous rupture of the membranes before labour begins (Tan and Hannah 2002). Spontaneous rupture of the membranes can be recognised by the sudden loss of a significant amount of clear fluid from the vagina. However, for some women this may not be instantly recognisable if only very small amounts of fluid are lost. If the fetal presenting part is engaged deeply in the pelvis then this could well be the case. Small amounts of fluid loss could be mistaken for urinary incontinence, which is common in the latter stages of pregnancy due to excessive pressure of the fetus on the bladder. The midwife will need to take a careful history from the woman and usually continued observation of fluid lost from the vagina will lead to a definite confirmation that spontaneous rupture of the membranes has indeed occurred.

Other signs

Some women feel slightly nauseous as labour approaches and others experience diarrhoea. There may also be a tendency for some women to become preoccupied with cleaning and tidying their homes. This is referred to as the 'nesting' instinct and is representative of the woman preparing her immediate environment for the impending birth and her newborn baby (Odent 2003; Johnston 2004).

Activity

Discuss with as many women as possible how their labour started.

- What signs and symptoms did they experience?
- When were they certain that they were in true labour?

Midwifery care in early labour

Women should receive information from the midwife caring for them during pregnancy about how to recognise the onset of labour and when to contact the midwife well in advance of the event. The onset of labour is a time of excitement but also uncertainty and fear for women, particularly if they are expecting their first baby. In today's society, many women live some distance from their immediate family and they may feel isolated and unsure of what do to or who to contact when labour starts. They may be new to the area or new to the country, and language difficulties may lead to further anxiety and lack of understanding of what they should do.

For these reasons it is important that women are given appropriate written instructions and contact telephone numbers by the midwife who is providing their care during the pregnancy. Many women will also attend preparation for parenting sessions when these issues will be discussed. Usually if they are planning a hospital birth, women will be asked to contact the maternity unit by telephone and discuss their progress with the midwife. A woman opting for a homebirth will contact the appropriate midwife so that they can decide together whether a home visit is required.

When the midwife receives a call from a woman in early labour, she needs to take a history to ascertain whether the woman should come directly into hospital for assessment or whether she can stay at home and await further events. If the woman has no complications and is in early labour with contractions occurring irregularly and infrequently (maybe every 15–20 minutes) then it is better if she remains at home. This is known as the latent phase of labour. Research studies have demonstrated a significant link between later admission to the labour ward and a positive birth outcome (for example, a reduced caesarean section rate) (Hemminki and Simukka 1986; Ghacero and Enabudosco 2006).

Increased levels of stress which a woman may experience on admission to the unfamiliar and often frightening environment of the modern labour ward may lead to the increased production of catecholamines. These are the 'fight or flight' hormones (adrenaline and noradrenaline) and research has demonstrated that they tend to inhibit the production of oxytocin (Wuitchik et al. 1989; Peled 1992). As oxytocin causes contraction of the uterine muscle it follows that a reduction in oxytocin leads to diminished (i.e. weaker and fewer) contractions and a slowing down of the progress of labour. It is suggested that paying attention to the physical environment in hospital labour wards and ensuring that it is as calm, peaceful and as private as possible will lead to better birth experiences and outcomes (Page 2003).

The midwife could suggest to the woman that she has a warm bath to help her relax, that she tries to get as much rest as possible and that she has a light meal and drinks plenty of fluid in order to prepare herself for the onset of the active phase of labour. The woman should be advised to contact the delivery suite again when the contractions become stronger and harder to cope with, or if she has any concerns. Sometimes despite being in early labour a woman may feel that she wants to go into hospital for reassurance from a midwife that all is progressing normally.

If the woman reports any complications such as vaginal bleeding which appears to be more than a 'show', or if she has any medical disorders such as diabetes, cardiac problems, pregnancy-induced hypertension or a known malpresentation such as breech, she should be asked to come directly to the labour ward. This is in accordance with the *Midwives Rules and Standards* (NMC 2004), which state that where a deviation from the norm becomes apparent a practising midwife should inform an appropriately qualified health care professional.

Women are also usually asked to come into hospital if they think that their membranes have broken. This is so that the midwife can exclude any signs of infection, such as a raised temperature and pulse rate, which are a potential risk when the membranes rupture before the onset of labour. Women with ruptured membranes are often discharged home to await the onset of labour, once they have been assessed by the midwife. In 86 per cent of these women, labour begins spontaneously (Savitz et al. 1997). If it does not occur spontaneously, then induction of labour will be considered (NICE 2001).

Activity

Find out what your unit's policy is regarding women whose waters break (prelabour rupture of membranes) before labour starts.

Initial examination

On arrival at the labour ward, the woman and her partner (if she has one) should be welcomed by the midwife who will be caring for them. In most labour wards today the woman will not know her midwife and this initial meeting is of great importance. The midwife needs to make an assessment of the woman's physical and emotional condition, but the woman also needs to feel reassured that she is in a caring and supportive environment.

Pregnancy history

Before examining the woman, the midwife should review her medical records. Most women will bring them to the labour ward on their admission. The progress of the current pregnancy should be ascertained as well as the outcome of any previous pregnancies, as this may have a bearing on the current one. The woman's general health and any medical history of note should also be considered. The woman's birth plan, if she has one, should be looked at in conjunction with the woman and her partner so that any special requests or needs can be highlighted and discussed. If a woman has not made a birth plan, then the midwife will need to discuss with her any significant issues, such as what methods of pain relief are available, if she has any preference for a particular birth position and how she would like the third stage of labour managed. This is because it is easier to discuss these kinds of issues with a woman before she is in very strong labour, when she may be unable to make an informed decision about options which are available to her.

Physical examination

The midwife should observe the general condition of the woman. This includes an assessment of how she is coping with the contractions and whether she appears anxious or fearful. The midwife should also look for any indication that the delivery of the baby is imminent so that appropriate preparations for the birth can be made. This includes getting equipment ready to receive the newborn baby and ensuring that the room is warm.

The general colour of the woman should be noted. Extreme pallor, flushed skin or cyanosis could be an indication that there are underlying medical problems, such as anaemia, heart disease or infection, which might impact on the management of care. Signs of oedema should be also noted. It is very common for women in the latter stages of pregnancy to have slightly swollen fingers and feet. However, if the oedema is marked, and particularly if it involves the face (the woman's birthing partner could be asked for his or her opinion in relation to this), this may be a sign of pregnancy-induced hypertension (PIH) which could have serious implications for the woman and her baby.

Physical examination includes taking the woman's pulse, blood pressure and temperature. These recordings should be noted in the woman's records as they will act as baseline readings as the labour progresses. Traditionally, these readings are taken every four hours throughout labour although this timing is not evidence-based, but should be based on the woman's condition.

A sample of the woman's urine should be tested on admission and then regularly throughout the labour. If protein is detected, then this may also indicate the presence of PIH, although it may also be due to contamination with amniotic fluid if the membranes have broken.

Glucose in the urine (glycosuria) could indicate gestational diabetes, which may also be suggested by the medical history if there has been persistent glycosuria throughout the pregnancy. The presence of ketones (ketonuria) suggests that the woman has not eaten for some time or has suffered from excessive vomiting. Ketonuria is an indication that the body is using fat as a major source of energy rather than carbohydrate.

A small amount of ketonuria is to be expected during labour as a physiological response to the increased energy demands within the body at this time. However, if large amounts of ketones are present, this may indicate a severe depletion of the body's energy source which could lead to a reduction in uterine activity and a slowing down of the progress of labour. This can be corrected by giving the woman fluids directly into her veins (intravenously) via a plastic cannula.

An abnormality in any of these readings should be reported to the obstetrician as they may indicate an underlying problem with the general health of the woman or with the progress of her labour.

Assessment the progress of labour

There are many ways of assessing a woman's progress in labour, requiring midwives to draw on their knowledge, skills and experience. A holistic practitioner will assess progress not only through physical examination, but also by observing subtler outward signs, including the woman's behaviour and psychological state (Mander 2002). The main difference between active and expectant management of labour is the level of confidence that the midwife has in the woman's physiology (Sookhoo and Biott 2002). In active management, progress of labour is prescribed and charted against an expected trajectory. If labour fails to follow the expected pattern, intervention occurs. In expectant management, the condition of mother and fetus is the main point of reference and different rates of progress are accepted as variations in normal physiology (Sookhoo and Biott 2002).

Midwives often refer to the three 'P's as the main factors involved in the progress in labour: the 'powers' (contractions), 'passage' (the bony pelvis) and 'passenger' (the fetus). This approach may be helpful to some as a methodical way of assessing the progress of labour, but has been criticised for reducing the woman to a set of body parts rather than a whole person (Kitzinger 2005).

Observation of the woman's behaviour

A woman in the latent first stage of labour may not display any outward signs. As cervical dilatation advances and the woman enters the active phase of labour, she may become restless, uncomfortable and suffer pain. Unless a woman has had epidural anaesthesia (this will be discussed later in this chapter), she will probably want to change position frequently, often finding a mobile, upright or forward-leaning posture more comfortable. It is thought that this instinctive behaviour assists the descent and rotation of the fetus.

Vocal changes are often noted as labour progresses. In early labour, conversation and interaction are usually unhindered, but as the frequency and intensity of contractions increases, women find it increasingly difficult to hold a conversation and will often close their eyes in concentration until the pain passes. The level of breathing changes as contractions intensify: as the second stage approaches, women are often heard to make a deep, slow 'mooing' sound which is associated with the urge to bear down. This may increase in intensity as the fetus is expelled. Women should not be discouraged from vocalising in labour and indeed it may be unhelpful to attempt to do so (McKay and Roberts 1990).

The urge to bear down, or push, is usually automatic and beyond the woman's conscious control. As the second stage intensifies, the urge will become overwhelming and women may briefly hold their breath and bear down, often several times, during the peak of each contraction. However, when the baby is in an occipito-posterior position, this may cause an urge to push well before full cervical dilatation, therefore the presence of an urge to push in the absence of other signs of progress is not a reliable indicator of the onset of second stage. If in doubt, a vaginal examination should be undertaken to confirm full dilatation (Enkin et al. 2000).

Some women will be distressed and give the impression of being in advanced labour when they are not. There may be psychological reasons for this, such as fear, or physical reasons, such as an occipito-posterior position of the fetus, causing intense pressure on the lower sacral region. It is important that the midwife makes use of a range of observations to get an accurate picture of progress in labour, rather than relying on a single factor.

Outward signs

Natal line

One non-invasive means of estimating progress is to observe the 'purple line' that slowly ascends from the anal margin to the top of the natal cleft (skin between the buttocks). It is generally supposed that this line moves at the roughly same rate as the cervix dilates, reaching the top of the natal cleft at full dilatation (Hobbs 1998). Although many midwives use this technique, it may not be regarded as a clinically acceptable means of assessing progress in some maternity units. The purple line can only be viewed if the woman is not sitting or lying on her back and may be harder to see in very dark-skinned women.

The rhombus of Michaelis

The rhombus of Michaelis is a kite-shaped area over the lower back that includes the lower lumbar vertebrae and sacrum (see Figure 5.1). It is believed that this area of bone moves backwards during the second stage of labour, pushing out the wings of the ilea and increasing the pelvic diameter (Wickham and Sutton 2005). This allows more space for the fetus to descend through the pelvis. Sutton notes that when in a forward-leaning posture, a lump appears on the woman's back, at and below waist level. This happens at the

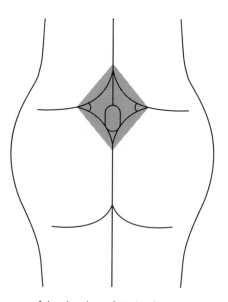

Figure 5.1 Diagram of the rhombus of Michaelis

start of the second stage. This is thought to be the reason why, if a woman is labouring in a semi-supine position, she may automatically reach up to find something to hold on to and arch her back. This phenomenon is absent in women who have had epidurals, as the anaesthesia blocks the nerve impulses that cause the rhombus to move (Wickham and Sutton 2005).

Anal dilatation

As the presenting part reaches the pelvic floor and begins to displace the muscle and tissue, anal dilatation may be noted. This is usually a sign that the second stage of labour is reaching its culmination. The woman may pass an involuntary bowel motion at this time if her rectum is full, as the pressure of the presenting part flattens the rectum against the sacral bone, expelling any contents. Women may be unaware of this happening due to the intensity of the contractions and the concentration of pushing. The midwife should remove any faecal matter swiftly and discretely.

Anal dilatation may alternatively be caused by deep engagement of the presenting part or premature pushing (Ndala 2005c), so should not be taken as a definitive indicator of progress if other signs are not present.

Vulval gaping/appearance of the presenting part

At the same time as anal dilatation occurs, vulval gaping may be noted. The vaginal opening stretches and the perineal body flattens and distends. The presenting part may be visible on parting the labia. This is usually a sure sign of progress when noted for the first time. However, if there is a lot of caput and moulding (swelling and distortion of the fetal skull) this may be misleading, as the bony part of the fetal skull may be much higher in the birth canal than it appears and may even protrude through the cervix prior to full dilatation, as may a breech (Ndala 2005c).

Spontaneous rupture of membranes

The most common time for the woman's membranes to breaks *naturally* is at the end of the first stage of labour when the cervix is fully dilated and thus unable to support the forewaters against the force of uterine contractions (Ndala 2005b). Therefore, spontaneous rupture of membranes in an uncomplicated labour which has hitherto progressed normally may well indicate the end of the first stage of labour. Some midwives will confirm this by vaginal examination, which can also be used to rule out cord prolapse. Others will choose to watch and wait.

Observation of woman's psychological state

The transitional phase

The definition of the transitional phase varies, but it is commonly used to describe the period from the end of the first stage of labour to full dilatation of the cervix. It is not commonly described in midwifery or obstetric textbooks (Mander 2002), nor is it routinely documented in written labour records. It is essentially a midwifery observation and relies on the midwife's knowing the woman and recognising changes in her behaviour that indicate the baby's imminent arrival. Kitzinger (1987) identifies transition as the most difficult part of labour for many women and it undoubtedly represents one of the most challenging aspects of the midwife's role.

During the transitional phase, a woman's behaviour and mental state may change suddenly. Mander (2002) believes that the transitional phase often represents a psychological low point when the woman despairs of being able to give birth unaided and becomes overwhelmed by both physical and emotional pain. She may become very agitated and restless, display aggression, irritability and irrational behaviour, such as wanting to go home or demanding a caesarean section. It is important to remember that this phase is temporary and not a reflection of her true personality. Many women are extremely apologetic after the birth and should be reassured that their behaviour was natural and no cause for embarrassment.

Another manifestation of the transitional phase is an apparent withdrawal of the woman into herself. She may close her eyes, cease talking and appear unaware of what is happening around her. Leap (2000) explains that the woman is focusing her energy and concentration in preparation for the supreme effort of giving birth.

Although not every woman displays obvious signs of the transitional phase, it is important that the midwife is able to recognise them and supports and encourages the woman through to the second stage of labour. Continuous care in labour allows the midwife to note behavioural changes, to act appropriately and to avoid unnecessary intervention (Mander 2002).

Pain/sensation

As labour progresses and contractions become stronger and longer, pain and discomfort increase. Anecdotal evidence suggests that a small minority of women experience very little pain and may not even be aware that they are in labour until the urge to push is felt. However, a woman's psychological state will often influence her perception of pain; therefore, pain is not a reliable indicator of progress without other signs.

Abdominal palpation and auscultation

The purpose of abdominal palpation during labour is to assess the lie, presentation, position, flexion and descent of the presenting part (usually the head). These findings are significant when done repeatedly over a period of time, as an indicator of how far labour has progressed and give some indication of how it is likely to continue. Again, continuity of carer is important and findings may be subjective.

The most common findings of abdominal palpation in early labour are a fetus that is in a longitudinal lie, a cephalic (head down) presentation and a left occipito anterior (LOA) position. The head is normally flexed and descent is measured in fifths palpable above the symphysis pubis. When 2/5th or less is palpable, the head is said to be engaged. Engagement is defined as the widest part having passed through the pelvic brim (Ndala 2005b). In primiparous women, the head is normally engaged well before labour commences, whereas in multiparous women, the head may still be free at the start of labour. As labour progresses, the fetus will gradually move into a direct occipito anterior (OA) position and the head will descend further until no fifths are palpable through the abdomen.

When the same midwife uses her skill of palpation at intervals throughout labour, it is possible to track the progress of the fetus through the pelvic canal. The midwife will always palpate prior to any vaginal examination so that the findings of both can be related to each other, thus giving a more accurate overall picture of progress.

In women of African ancestry, descent of the presenting part may not occur until later in labour, when descent may happen rapidly (Vincent 2003). This is due to their pelvic structure, which often differs from that of Caucasian women.

Listening to the fetal heart not only allows the midwife to assess fetal well-being, but also allows descent of the fetus to be tracked. The point at which the heart sounds are loudest will gradually change as the fetus rotates and descends. Once deeply engaged, it may be difficult to auscultate the heart sounds with a Pinard stethoscope, due to the positioning of the fetal chest behind the symphysis pubis.

Monitoring of contractions

Contractions generally begin as mild, period-type cramps that are often irregular and intermittent and may continue thus for hours or even days (Vincent 2003). This happens as the cervix is effacing and beginning to dilate. This very early period is often referred to as the latent phase and varies in length, as many women will not be aware of exactly when it began. Some women may believe that they are in established labour. The midwife will need to use tact and careful explanation to help her understand what is actually happening to her body.

Eventually, the latent phase of labour merges into the active phase, and contractions generally start to become regular and closer together. The active (or established) phase of labour is defined by the National Institute of Clinic Excellence (NICE 2007) as progressive cervical dilatation with regular, painful contractions. In the earlier part of the active phase, contractions may be as little as 2 : 10 (i.e. twice in 10 minutes), lasting 30 seconds. They gradually increase in length, strength and frequency as labour progresses, up to a maximum of around 5 : 10 (five times in 10 minutes), lasting over a minute with barely a break in between.

The midwife may need to place her hand on the woman's abdomen at fundal level in order to assess the length and frequency of contractions, especially if the woman has an epidural in situ. It is difficult to assess the strength of a contraction through palpation – the woman herself is a better judge of that. By assessing the length, strength and frequency of contractions intermittently over a period of time, the midwife can make an estimate of how the woman's labour is progressing.

Some women experience a temporary lull in contractions at the end of the first stage of labour, but prior to the onset of expulsive contractions. This coincides with the presenting part descending and rotating as it reaches the pelvic floor (Ndala 2005c). This period is sometimes referred to as the latent phase of second stage, before contractions begin to feel expulsive and it should not be assumed that labour has slowed down or ceased. Once the woman starts to display expulsive contractions, often described as an overwhelming urge to push or open her bowels, it is likely that she has reached the second stage of labour.

Vaginal examination

Many hospitals will have a policy of performing regular vaginal examinations (VE) throughout labour, regardless of the risk status of the woman. Midwives are increasingly working in an environment in which the evidence from VE supersedes all other indications of progress. There is thus a risk that midwives and students will lose confidence in other means of assessing progress (Sookhoo and Biott 2002).

The first VE is often carried out soon after admission to the delivery suite. However, depending on local policy, the midwife may wait until she is sure that the woman is in active labour. It is common practice to carry out a VE to confirm onset of the second stage of labour, though this may not be necessary if the presenting part is already visible. However, if the woman displays an urge to push when there is doubt about progress in labour, a vaginal examination should be carried out (Enkin et al. 2000). All VE are invasive procedures and risk introducing bacteria to the genital tract. They also compromise the woman's dignity and sense of autonomy, so should not be undertaken without good reason. Many midwives working in the community or birth centres will operate a policy of conducting a VE only if there is a clear indication to do so.

VE allows the progress of labour to be assessed through a number of indicators. These are:

The state of the cervix

The midwife will assess the position, effacement, consistency and dilatation. In early labour, these findings may be expressed using the Bishop's Score system, a tabular representation which allocates points to each factor (see Table 5.3). The higher the number of points, the more advanced the state of cervix towards established labour.

The station of the presenting part

Even if the cervix is closed, the midwife will be able to ascertain the descent of the presenting part (PP) through the pelvis. This should have been estimated by abdominal palpation prior to commencing the VE. The PP is measured in relation to the ischial spines (see Figure 5.2) and is estimated in centimetres. The ischial spines may

Table 5.3 Bishop's score

Parameter	0	1	2	3
Dilatation	<1 cm	1–2 cm	2–4 cm	>4 cm
Length	>4 cm	2–4 cm	1–2 cm	<1 cm
Consistency	Firm	Average	Soft	–
Position	Posterior	Mid	Anterior	
Station	–3	–2	–1, 0	+1, +2

http://www.perinatal.nhs.uk/main.htm
accessed 22.10.07

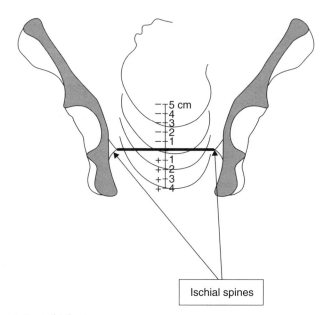

Figure 5.2 Ischial spines

be felt as blunt, bony prominences on stretching the examining fingers to the sides of the vaginal wall. Thus a position of 0 means that the PP is level with the ischial spines: −1 means one cm above the ischial spines; +1 means 1 cm below (Allotey 1996) (see Figure 5.2). The midwife would expect the PP to descend steadily throughout labour as the cervix dilates. However, midwives may have difficulty locating the ischial spines and the use of this landmark is highly subjective and therefore may not be a very accurate tool for measuring descent (Allotey 1996).

Position of the cervix

Prior to the onset of labour, the cervix points towards the posterior vaginal wall. On VE it may be very difficult to locate. From the end of pregnancy until the onset of established labour, it gradually becomes central and eventually anterior facing. Thus the ease with which the cervix can be reached is an indicator of progress in the latent or early phase of labour.

The size and shape of the bony pelvis

The midwife conducting the VE will note any unusual findings such as a narrow pubic arch or a prominent sacrum, either of which might impede the progress of labour. A higher than expected PP coupled with an unusual pelvic structure is a likely indicator that labour will not progress to delivery, regardless of the strength of contractions. This must be reported urgently to the senior obstetrician as a caesarean section is likely to be needed.

The position of the presenting part

If the cervix is sufficiently dilated, it will be possible for the midwife to assess the attitude (flexed or deflexed) of the fetal head by feeling for the fontanelles. A deflexed head at the start of labour would be expected to gradually flex, so that the posterior fontanelle becomes readily palpable. Lack of flexion may be an indicator of poor progress due to an unfavourable fetal position or to inefficient contractions.

The position of the fetus can be determined through palpation of the sutures on the fetal skull. By noting the position and direction of the sutures, the midwife can assess whether the fetus has rotated into a good position for birth. If VEs are repeated over a period of time, the midwife should be able to track the progress of the fetus as it rotates and descends through the birth canal. These are important signs of progress in labour and a lack of rotation, flexion and descent may indicate an obstruction to normal labour.

The partogram

The standard tool in hospitals for assessing the progress of labour is the partogram (sometimes known as the partograph). This maps cervical dilatation and descent of the PP along a time-scale, with space to include basic observations such as temperature, pulse, urine output and blood pressure (Duff 2002). It is commonly used once a woman is in 'established' labour – local policies may differ in their definition of this term, but it usually refers to a state of regular contractions becoming longer, stronger and closer together with progressive dilatation of the cervix and descent of the PP. The partogram requires the midwife to undertake physical observations and document the findings at regular intervals throughout labour. The woman's progress is thus represented in the form of a graph, allowing her carers to see at a glance how she has progressed, which may give an indication of the normality of her labour. However, the value of the partogram depends on an accurate diagnosis of the onset of labour and this is often unknown. The purpose of a partogram is to detect dysfunctional physical patterns in labour, thereby allowing early intervention before the mother or fetus becomes compromised. Despite its widespread use, the partogram is controversial as it depends on clock-watching and demands regular physical

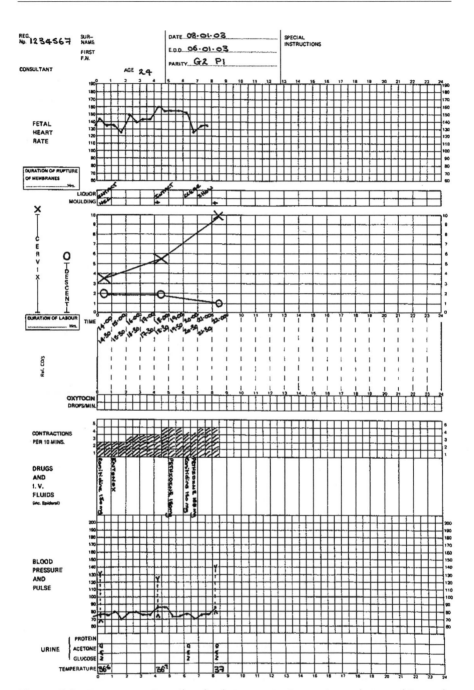

Figure 5.3   A partogram. Reproduced with permission. Source: Symonds, M. and Symonds, I.M. (2003) *Essential Obstetrics and Gynaecology* 4th Edition. Churchill Livingstone, London.

interventions (Duff 2002) (see Figure 5.3). It takes no account of the subtler signs of progress.

The assessment of progress in labour is rarely achieved through a single observation. The midwife must take into account several factors and build an overall picture of the woman's progress, comparing this to previous observations and to current expectations. A judgement based on a single observation is unlikely to give a true picture of progress and may result in either unnecessary intervention or failure to intervene when indicated.

Medical forms of pain relief

Although labour is a physiological process many woman feel the need to resort to different methods of pain relief to help them cope with what can be the overwhelming pain of labour.

The exact definition of what constitutes a medical form of pain relief is open to debate. Most practitioners would take it to include all drugs, whether taken orally, by injection, by inhalation or by regional block. Other methods of pain relief are less easy to categorise. These include transcutaneous electronic nerve stimulation (TENS), acupuncture, aromatherapy and other alternative or complementary therapies. It may be argued that any form of pain relief, whether drug-related or not, that involves an invasive procedure is 'medical'. However, a woman who is enabled to use her own choice of alternative therapy during labour will probably feel that she has laboured 'naturally' and without medical pain relief.

An analgesic can be defined as a drug which reduces the pain sensation but without causing a loss of consciousness or touch (Ndala 2005d). The most desirable characteristic of an analgesic given during labour is that it should provide maximum pain relief with minimal adverse effects on the woman and her baby. Unfortunately, as will be seen, the perfect labour analgesic is not currently available!

It is important, however, that the midwife remains up to date with the current methods of analgesia and is able to inform women of their potential benefits and side-effects. This information should be given in a clear, unbiased way during the antenatal period so that women and their families have time to consider their options.

Nitrous oxide/Entonox

Entonox is a colourless, odourless gas which consists of nitrous oxide and oxygen in equal parts. It is colloquially referred to as 'gas and air' or sometimes 'laughing gas'. It is approved for use by midwives and can be used throughout labour, although a woman inhaling it continually throughout a long labour may start to tire and be unable to use it effectively.

Entonox is provided by piped supply directly into the delivery room or stored in portable cylinders which may be carried by midwives and used in the home setting. The gases start to separate if stored at a temperature below –7 °C. For this reason it is important that cylinders are stored at a temperature of at least 10 °C and inverted several times before use in order to ensure that the gases are adequately mixed (Ndala 2005d).

Women inhale the gas by breathing it in via a mouthpiece or a face mask. As the analgesic effect of the gas does not take effect until after about 20 seconds, the woman should be encouraged to start inhaling as soon as she feels the contraction beginning. In this way, the maximum effect of the analgesic will coincide with the peak of the contraction.

The midwife can assist the woman by helping her to breathe the gas in effectively. It is suggested that taking short panting breaths is not efficient and the woman should be encouraged to take deep breaths at the normal breathing rate (Bryant and Yerby 2004). Rapid breathing should be discouraged as it can lead to hyperventilation and less oxygen getting to the baby via the placenta (Gamsu 1993).

A notable advantage of Entonox during labour is that it is excreted rapidly via the maternal lungs so that toxic levels do not accumulate and affect the fetus adversely. If a woman does not like the sensations evoked by using the gas, she simply stops inhaling it and the effect is soon lost. Some women report feeling dizzy and nauseous while inhaling entonox, although the majority find that the sense of euphoria evoked, coupled with the lessened pain sensation, make it a popular pain-relieving choice.

Entonox is not, however, the perfect analgesia for labour in that while it helps many women cope with the pain of the contractions it does not take away the pain sensations completely and in this sense is not a true analgesic (Bryant and Yerby 2004).

Epidural analgesia

Epidural analgesia involves the introduction of a local anaesthetic into the epidural space around the spinal cord. Drugs which have been used include opiates such as diamorphine, morphine and fentanyl. It has been found that mixing an opiate with a local anaes-

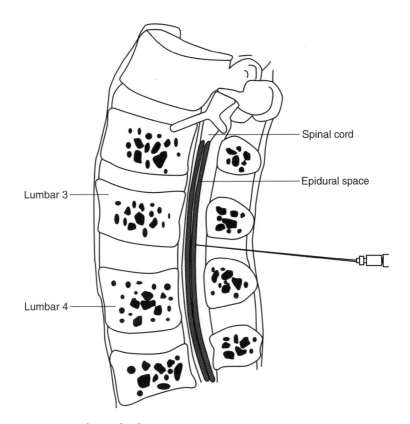

Figure 5.4 The epidural space

thetic gives longer, more effective pain relief with less loss of movement in the lower limbs (Collis et al. 1993). This is known as the 'mobile epidural' and it means that potentially women are able to walk about as their labour progresses. The initial study used an injection of the combined drugs straight into the cerebrospina fluid via the subarachnoid space followed by an insertion of an epidural catheter. It was also known as a 'combined spinal epidural' (Collis et al. 1993). However, this method has largely been discontinued and anaesthetists tend to use the combined drugs directly into the epidural space (Eisenach 1999). The drugs commonly used are bupivacaine (the local anaesthetic) and fentanyl (the opiate).

The epidural space (see Figure 5.4) is approximately 4 mm wide and located around the dura mater (the outermost layer of the meninges surrounding the spinal cord). It contains a number of blood vessels, fatty matter and spinal nerves. During pregnancy and more specifically labour, the size of the space is reduced considerably by the engorgement of the veins which occur during pregnancy. The local anaesthetic is inserted into the space with the aim of surrounding the fibres of the spinal nerves in order to block the pain sensations. It is usual practice for the lumbar route to be used and usually the anaesthetic is introduced between the lumbar vertebrae 2 and 4 or 2 and 3.

An epidural may be indicated in the following situations:

- It is the woman's choice as an effective method of pain relief
- During prolonged labour as this method is usually very effective and will allow an exhausted woman a chance to rest and recuperate
- A malposition such as occipital-posterior which often leads to severe back pain and an early need to push before the cervix is completely open
- A malpresentation such as a breech where certain manipulations are likely to be required during the second stage of labour and there is a higher risk that a caesarean section might be indicated
- Multiple pregnancy for reasons as above
- A woman who has very high blood pressure. The use of epidural analgesia may lead to a reduction in blood pressure as the local anaesthetic blocks the transmission of both motor and sensory nerves as well as having an effect on the sympathetic nervous system. This will cause dilation of the veins and a subsequent fall in blood pressure
- Pre-term labour in order to avoid the use of narcotic drugs which will pass through the placenta and may have an adverse effect on the fetus
- For instrumental (forceps and ventouse (suction) deliveries and operative deliveries (caesarean section)

(Ndala 2005d).

On the other hand, an epidural is not recommended if a woman has chronic backache or a spinal deformity, as this could lead to difficulties during the procedure. If she has a blood clotting disorder this might lead to excessive bleeding around the site where the needle is introduced into the spinal cord. Due to the effect which this type of anaesthesia has on blood pressure, it is not recommended if a woman has low blood pressure or a low blood volume (Ndala 2005d). In this situation, the woman would be advised to use another method of pain relief such as pethidine or diamorphine.

Administration of epidural anaesthesia: the procedure

The introduction of anaesthesia into the epidural space is a skilled procedure which should only be carried out by a suitably qualified anaesthetist. The role of the midwife in this case is to support the woman in her choice, and to ensure that she has all the information she needs about the risks and disadvantages associated with this method of pain relief. The midwife will also be required to assist the anaesthetist in the preparation of the necessary equipment and drugs, as well as ensuring that the woman is lying in the most appropriate position. The midwife will also need to monitor the condition of the woman and fetus during and following the procedure and report any deviations from the norm to the anaesthetist.

Disadvantages of epidural use

Effect on the progress of labour

The epidural usually gives a high degree of pain relief, but it is believed to prolong labour and lead to more intervention, including operative and instrumental deliveries (Hawkins et al. 1995; Lieberman et al. 1996). The problem in identifying the disadvantages of epidural use lies in the fact that women usually request an epidural when their labour is becoming particularly difficult or prolonged, possibly due to the fetus lying in a difficult position (such as the occipito-posterior position) As a result it is difficult to say whether it is the epidural which is complicating labour or whether the labour is complicated anyway (Fogel et al. 1998).

Lowering of blood pressure (hypotension)

As epidural anesthesia lowers blood pressure, this effect can cause a problem at the start of the procedure. The woman is likely to feel faint, dizzy and sick (nauseous) as her blood pressure falls. Hypotension can be rectified by ensuring that sufficient intravenous fluids are given.

Inability to pass urine

Women may be unable to pass urine with an epidural in place due to the loss of sensation in the bladder area. A full bladder can lead to a delay in the labour and the possibility that the bladder will be damaged if an instrumental delivery is later required (Bryant and

Yerby 2004). This could lead to problems such as urinary infection or incontinence in the postnatal period.

The midwife should remind the woman of the need to pass urine regularly and her abdomen should be palpated at regular intervals to assess for signs of a full bladder. If the woman is unable to pass urine, then a urinary catheter may be necessary.

Dural tap

This complication occurs when the dura is pierced by the needle and anaesthetic is injected inadvertently into the cerebrospinal fluid (CSF). As the CSF leaks out, it causes a fall in pressure in the brain which results in the woman experiencing a severe headache, which is worse when she sits up. Eventually the dura will heal, but this can take several days and may mean that the woman has to lie flat, unable to take care of her baby. An alternative method of treatment is for the anaesthetist to inject 10–20 ml of the woman's own blood back into the epidural space. This will seal over the puncture in the dura and will alleviate the problem (Ndala 2005d).

Total spinal block

This is a rare but serious complication which is caused by the inadvertent injection of anaesthetic into a vein. This causes a loss of sensation and movement in the upper part of the woman's body and will affect the muscles required for breathing. The midwife needs to be alert to the fact that that this has occurred, the first sign being that the woman complains of a slight tingling sensation in her tongue followed by a very rapid deterioration in her general condition. Immediate resuscitative steps will be needed urgently in this case.

Long-term backache

Research has shown a higher incidence of backache in women who have received epidural anesthesia during labour (MacArthur et al. 1990). It is suggested that the loss of sensation during labour results in an unusual strain on the ligaments of the back which can lead to long-term backache. The woman might have been sitting in an awkward position for some time but felt no discomfort and as such did not alter her position. Other studies do not show an increased incidence of backache in women who had received epidurals when compared with women who had received other methods of pain relief (Howell et al. 2002). Research is ongoing, but women need to be aware that there is a suggestion that they may have a greater chance of experiencing backache in the future if they have an epidural.

Opioid analgesia

Opioids are drugs derived from the opium poppy (papaver somniferum). They bring about a sense of well-being and drowsiness. They are also known as narcotic drugs. Women in labour have used opioid drugs for pain relief since the 1950s and they have been widely used in midwifery because they are readily available and can be administered intramuscularly. Three opioids are commonly used in labour in the United Kingdom:

1. Pethidine
2. Meptazinol
3. Diamorphine

Pethidine

Pethidine is a controlled drug which a midwife can administer without the need for a prescription from a doctor (see Chapter 9).

It is a synthetic substance which has strong pain-relieving and sedative properties. It works by attaching itself to receptor proteins and then diffusing through cell membranes where it affects the central nervous system. It does this by changing the sensitivity of the nerves to pain perception and actually reducing the pain sensation (Yerby 2000).

Once in the muscle, pethidine has a rapid onset with the effect lasting up to four hours. It can also be injected straight into a vein. The dose is usually 50–200 mg depending on the weight of the woman, the progress of her labour, the degree of pain she is experiencing and the route of administration (Bewley 1997).

Side-effects include nausea, vomiting, a fall in blood pressure, excessive sweating and sometimes may lead the woman to feel that she is 'out of control'. Some women may be unable to pass urine because the smooth muscle in the bladder sphincter contracts as a result of the drug. Pethidine also causes delayed stomach emptying which may put the woman at risk of inhaling some of the contents of her stomach (gastric aspiration) should a general anaesthetic be required during labour (Jordan 2002). Indeed, some women report that these side-effects outweigh any pain relief which pethidine may give them (Beech 1998). Further research (Oloffson et al. 1996) suggests that pethidine is only effective as a sedative and not as an analgesic. A more recent randomised controlled trial demonstrated that pethidine was more effective than a placebo in relieving labour pain but that this effect was only slight (Tsui et al. 2004).

Another disadvantage of the use of pethidine during labour is that it readily crosses the placenta. Studies have shown that two hours after intramuscular administration of pethidine, the drug begins to transfer back to the mother via the placenta (Cawthra 1986). Pethidine is broken down in the liver and as the fetal liver is immature, it takes longer to be broken down and this makes the fetus even more susceptible to side-effects of the drug (Hunt 2002).

In the fetus these side-effects include a change in the heat rate pattern and a loss of the variability of the heart rate. It also affects the respiratory centre in the fetal brain and can lead to a decrease in the respiratory rate at birth. For this reason, it is preferable not to give pethidine if delivery is expected within 2–3 hours. If, however, it is given within one hour of the birth or more than six hours prior to the birth, the effect on the neonatal respiratory rate is minimal (Belfrage et al. 1981).

Rosenblatt et al. (1981) observed that babies whose mothers had received pethidine during labour were less alert, quicker to cry and unsettled up to seven days after birth. Barrett (1983) suggests that such babies were less efficient at attaching to the nipple and sucking at the breast.

If a baby does have difficulty breathing at birth, then the antidote to pethidine – naloxone – can be given by intramuscular injection. This has the effect of blocking the protein receptors which pethidine binds to so stopping the action of the drug and the subsequent effect on respiration. Naloxone can be given in doses of 1 mg per kg of body weight (Bryant and Yerby 2004). The effects of naloxone wear off quickly – usually after an hour. For this reason it is important that the newborn baby is observed carefully as the respiratory depression effect of the pethidine may remain problematic once the naloxone has ceased working (Bryant and Yerby 2004).

Although the side-effects of pethidine to both the woman and fetus are noted, for some women it is an effective form of pain relief and means that they may not need to resort to the more invasive epidural method. However, it is important that they are aware of the potential difficulties, particularly in relation to breastfeeding, so that they can make an informed choice about what method is most appropriate for them (Wood and Soltani 2005). The role of the midwife includes ensuring that women and their families have the up-to-date information they need in order to make the appropriate choice for them.

If pethidine has been used during labour, this should be high-lighted by the midwife during the postnatal period so that appropriate support can be given to the mother and baby (Hunt 2002). This may include teaching the woman to hand express her milk and to recognise when a drowsy baby is ready to feed (Hunt 2002).

Meptazinol (Meptid)

Meptazinol is a synthetic substance which is similar to pethidine (although it is not classified as a controlled drug) but has less effect on the woman's cardiovascular and respiratory functions (Ndala 2005d). It is given intramuscularly and the usual dose is 100–150 mg (Heywood and Ho 1990). The effect begins approximately 15 minutes after administration and lasts for up to four hours (Park and Fulton 1991). It has been demonstrated that there are no significant differences in the analgesic and side-effects of the two drugs, but that meptazinol caused more vomiting (Sheikh and Tunstall 1986). However, the use of meptazinol resulted in the baby being born more alert and with an improved respiratory function compared with pethidine (Park and Fulton 1991; Reynolds 1998).

Diamorphine

Diamorphine, another controlled drug, may be given intramuscu-larly during labour and it has been shown to have certain advantages over pethidine in terms of better pain relief, less nausea and vomiting, and less effect on the baby's respiratory rate at birth (Fairlie et al. 1999).

The suggested dosage of diamorphine is 2.5–7.5 mg (Park and Fulton 1991), with the drug taking effect in 5–10 minutes and lasting around three hours. Since 2004, midwives have been able to use it on their own initiative in their professional practice without the need for a prescription from a doctor (see Chapter 9).

Midwifery care in the first and second stages of labour

Avoiding unnecessary time restrictions in labour

The current practice of timing each stage of labour – especially the active second stage – reflects the predisposing medical models of care in operation since the early twentieth century. The aim is to reduce adverse outcomes to mother and baby by detecting early signs of deviation from the norm, which may be indicated by an unusually prolonged labour. However, there is no evidence to impose arbitrary time limits on labour or to justify intervention unless there are clear signs of fetal or maternal compromise or a lack of progress (Janni et al. 2002; cited in RCM 2005). There may, however, be an increased risk in maternal morbidity when the second stage of labour exceeds two hours (Janni et al. 2002; Myles and Santolaya 2003). The midwife must decide whether the possible risk to the mother of a prolonged second stage outweighs the possible risks to the mother and baby of a curtailed second stage through the intervention of medical procedures. Recent guidelines by the National Institute for Clinical Excellence (NICE 2007) advise that normal progress in first stage labour is identified by cervical dilatation of 2 cm or more every 4 hours. Once active second stage has been identified, birth should be expected within 3 hours for primiparous women and 2 hours for multiparous women.

Some maternity units impose strict time limits, particularly on the active second stage of labour, whilst others allow the midwife to use her discretion. An example of this might be a woman who is making steady progress, although at a slower than average rate. In this case, interventions may be withheld, providing that both mother and fetus remain well. To reduce the likelihood of intervention in the second stage of labour, the midwife can use her skills to encourage the passive descent of the presenting part, thus shortening the active pushing phase (Roberts 2002). This might include encouraging the woman to adopt different postures to reduce the urge to push or employing distraction techniques such as back massage.

Movement and posture

Case Notes

Julie arrives in the delivery suite in established labour with her first baby. She is well and there is no evidence of fetal compromise. Julie has seen babies being born on television where the woman is lying in bed. On entering the labour room, Julie automatically gets undressed and into the bed. Her partner helps her lie down and arranges pillows around her, as he has seen people do on television.

Julie's contractions are becoming increasingly painful and she is unable to get comfortable. She is thinking about asking for an epidural.

Women, like most female mammals, are not physiologically designed to give birth in a supine position. Adopting an upright, forward-leaning posture is more natural for birthing. This allows gravity to assist with the descent and rotation of the PP and pressure on the internal cervical os to promote dilatation. There are other physiological advantages to adopting an upright posture for labour. These include a reduction in aorto-caval compression, better alignment of the fetus and an increased pelvic outlet (MIDIRS and the NHS Centre for Reviews and Dissemination 2003).

When the woman adopts an upright or forward-leaning posture with her legs slightly apart, the ligaments between the sacro-iliac joints and the pubic symphysis, already softened by the effects of the hormones progesterone and relaxin, allow the bones of the pelvis to separate slightly. This can create up to 28 per cent more space in the pelvic outlet (Robertson 2001), allowing for an easier birth. When a woman is upright, the natural tilt of the pelvis guides the fetus in a downward direction, whereas a woman in a semi-supine position must push her baby uphill. Postures which interfere with the physiological progress of the fetus through the pelvis are likely to lengthen labour, which in turn may lead to fetal compromise and maternal exhaustion.

An upright position in the first stage of labour is associated with less need for narcotic pain relief and epidurals (Williams et al. 1980) and a shorter first stage (Roberts, Mendez-Bauer and Wodell 1983). A systematic review by Gupta and Hofmeyr (2004) showed that women who adopted upright postures for the second stage of labour tended to have shorter second stages, fewer assisted births and episiotomies, less severe pain and fewer fetal heart rate anomalies. There is little evidence comparing different upright positions for giving birth. However, a study by Ragnar et al. (2006) considered sitting and kneeling postures in the second stage of labour and found that although there was no difference in the length of the second stage of labour, the kneeling position was associated with less pain and a more favourable experience for the woman.

Until the advent of modern obstetric practices, it was normal for women to give birth standing, squatting, on all fours or in some other supported upright posture (Coppen 2005). Twentieth-century hospital practices changed this in order to facilitate the midwife's and obstetrician's role with regard to examinations in labour. Unless the woman has an epidural block in situ or other medical impediment, she should be encouraged to move freely and adopt whatever posture is comfortable. The RCM evidence-based guidelines (RCM 2005) note that women's choice of position for labour is strongly influenced by what they feel is expected of them. It is therefore incumbent on the midwife to promote the use of different positions. It is not acceptable to impose restrictions based on the midwife's own comfort. Even where continuous fetal monitoring is necessary, the woman need not be restricted to the bed. Unless there is a medical reason to the contrary, women should be encouraged to mobilise freely during labour.

Women giving birth at home may adapt their surroundings to suit their needs. There should be no reason why women undergoing normal labour in hospital should not be encouraged to do likewise: hospital beds can be moved, mats or mattresses can be placed on the floor, a birthing ball or beanbag may be placed on the bed or the floor, a birthing stool may be used if available (MIDIRS and the NHS Centre for Reviews and Dissemination 2003).

Activity

Take a good look around the delivery rooms in your maternity unit. Think about how easy it would be for women to adopt various postures in labour.

- Could the furniture be adapted or moved to facilitate upright, forward-leaning postures?
- Does the unit supply birthing balls or a birthing stool, and if so, what restrictions are there on its use?

Eating and drinking in labour

Case Notes

Julie has been in active labour for several hours. There are no complications. Julie's last full meal was at 1900 h yesterday evening and, after a restless night, she had only a cup of tea and a bowl of cereal before coming into hospital five hours ago. Julie has been drinking water freely, as the Entonox makes her thirsty. She is now starting to feel very weary and a little dizzy. Her contractions have slowed down and she is beginning to feel discouraged.

The case note above is a typical scenario of a labouring woman who needs food.

In the latter half of the twentieth century, many maternity units imposed restrictions on eating and drinking in labour. This was based on the principle that reduced gastric motility during labour increases the risk of vomiting. In the event of a caesarean section, acid stomach contents could be inhaled, a condition known as Mendelsohn's syndrome (Mendelsohn 1946). However, improvements in anaesthesia in the last 50 years have seen this almost eradicated (Parsons and Nagy 2006). There is currently no good evidence to support the restriction of food and drink in labour in preventing Mendelsohn's syndrome. Furthermore, the aspiration of undiluted, acidic gastric fluids is far more dangerous than when diluted by food or drink (Parsons and Nagy 2006). It is common practice on labour wards to give antacids to all labouring women. However, there is no strong evidence to suggest that this has any effect on maternal mortality and morbidity (Pengelley 2002).

Narcotic drugs used in labour have the effect of delaying gastric emptying time (Broach and Newton 1988). If these are used, the woman should be advised to have sips of water only, otherwise, there is no evidence that withholding food and drink is beneficial and indeed this practice is likely to be harmful (Broach and Newton 1988). If a woman is allowed to remain hungry, her blood glucose level will fall, leading to ketosis, which, combined with starvation and fatigue, may lead to reduced uterine action and therefore the likelihood of medical intervention. In addition, hunger may adversely affect the woman's sense of well-being and mood. Current evidence suggests that labouring women who feel hungry should be encouraged to eat as their appetite dictates, providing there is no likelihood of their needing general anaesthesia (Baker 1996).

The above notwithstanding, there are some simple precautions which the woman should be advised of to limit the risk of nausea and vomiting. Although vomiting is common in labour, it is unpleasant for the women who experience it. Examples of suitable foods and drinks include low-residue, low-fat, easily absorbed foods such as bananas, 'smoothies', cereal bars, toast, yogurts or isotonic sports drinks. Foods which are high in fat or energy content tend to slow gastric emptying (Micklewright and Champion 2002) and may increase nausea.

Whilst most women appreciate the option of eating and drinking in labour (Newton and Champion 1997) some will neither wish nor need to do so. If this is the case, she should not be enticed to eat against her will. Odent (1994) notes that once in active labour, most women choose not to eat. In short, the labouring woman's appetite is usually the best judge of whether or not she needs to eat in labour.

Activity

Read the literature on Mendelsohn's syndrome.
Find out what your local maternity unit policy says about eating and
   drinking in labour.

Support in labour

Case Notes

A midwife is giving an antenatal class about labour. Several of the
women present have asked who they can have as their birth partner.
Some want to have their mother present as well as their husband or
partner. One woman wants to bring her doula (a non-medical assistant,
who provides physical and emotional support). Another woman is
anxious about the midwifery support she will receive in labour.

Most women will instinctively seek support and help in labour. In
times past, this support was traditionally the role of female atten-
dants such as lay midwives and family members. Since the 1970s,
male partners have become commonplace in the birthing room. It is
widely recognised that labouring women perceive a need for
empathic companionship and support (DH 1993) and that their reactions to labour may be influenced by the support they receive (Enkin
et al. 1996). Midwives are ideally placed to offer support in terms of
physical care and information-giving and should also be able to offer
emotional support and advocacy (MIDIRS and the NHS Centre for
Reviews and Dissemination 2003). However, not all midwives are
able to fulfil the support needs of women. There are many reasons
for this, not least of which is the increasing pressure that midwives
are under to care for several labouring women at once. Therefore
most maternity units welcome one or more close companions to
offer emotional support to the labouring woman.

There is evidence that women who receive continuous support in
labour require less pharmacological analgesia, have fewer operative
births and are more satisfied with the outcome of their labour
(Hodnett et al. 2004), while women who perceive little professional
or lay support in labour appear more likely to suffer post-traumatic
stress six weeks postnatally (Czarnocka and Slade 2000). Spiby et al.
(2003) note that women expect midwives to offer coping strategies
for pain and that these help to enhance the experience of labour and
reduce distress.

Continuity of care and continuous care

In reviewing current evidence, Sandall (2004) concludes that there is convincing, research-based evidence that women receiving continuity of care from a team of midwives are less likely to need pharmacological pain relief in labour or to have technical intervention. Maternal satisfaction is also increased. However, there is good evidence that *continuous* support during labour has more of a positive impact on childbirth outcome and on women's perception of labour than *continuity* of support alone (Sandall 2004). This may include advice, information, physical assistance or emotional support and may be from either a midwife or a layperson, such as a friend of family member. The Cochrane review of support for women during childbirth (Hodnett et al. 2002; cited in Sandall 2004) demonstrated that women who have continuous support during labour are less likely to have an operative birth, analgesia or report dissatisfaction with their experience. However, the benefits of continuous support were shown to be greater when the supporter was not a member of the hospital staff.

There is ample evidence that physical, emotional and psychological support in labour enhances the experience for the woman and reduces the likelihood of intervention (Enkin et al. 1996). Midwives should therefore allow the labouring woman her choice of birth partner throughout labour.

Activity

- Find out what the policy on your maternity unit says about birth partners.
- Not all women are accompanied by a birth partner. Consider how a midwife can give additional support to an unaccompanied woman.
- Some birth companions are not there through the woman's own free choice. Consider situations when this might arise and how, as the midwife, you would handle it.

Pushing in second stage

Case Notes

The midwife has just examined Julie and found her cervix to be fully dilated. Julie is experiencing frequent, strong contractions and is starting to get an urge to bear down. Julie's partner wants to know what he should do – should he encourage her to push?

A typical childbirth scene as portrayed by the media includes a doctor or midwife urging a labouring woman to take a deep breath, hold it as long as possible and push with all her might. This was once common practice in the UK, but there is no current evidence to support it. Indeed, this Valsalva manoeuvre, as it is known is now associated with fetal compromise due to the reduction in oxygenated maternal blood crossing the placenta during the manoeuvre (Thompson 1993; Roberts 2002). Current evidence suggests that instinctive, physiological pushing behaviour is less harmful to the fetus and the woman (Sleep 1990).

Midwifery care in the third stage of labour

Physiological or expectant management of the third stage

Activity

Sita had a managed third stage following the birth of her first baby three years ago. She has requested a physiological third stage this time as the oxytocic drugs she received made her extremely nauseous.

- What information can the midwife give her in order to help her make an informed decision about the management of the third stage of labour?

As the term implies, physiological management of the third stage of labour relies on the normal physiological processes within the body to facilitate expulsion of the placenta and membranes. The woman takes an active role in this process with the midwife observing her condition and providing support and encouragement as required. The midwife is also required to maintain her records in relation to time of delivery of the placenta and condition of the woman through out.

The main principle of physiological management is that there is no intervention on the part of the midwife unless the woman begins bleeding heavily or the baby needs urgent separation from its mother for resuscitation (Baston 2004). The process can take up to an hour although research suggests that an average time is about 15 minutes (Rogers and Wood 1999). However long the process takes, if the woman's condition remains stable and she does not begin to bleed heavily, there is no cause for concern. There is a suggestion that blood loss in the postnatal period is less for women who have had a physiological third stage (Wickham 1999), although it is clear from the evidence that a physiological third stage is associated with a higher blood loss during the actual delivery (Prendeville et al. 2004).

There is some debate about when is the best time for the umbilical cord to be clamped and cut, and further research is needed. As Inch (1985) points out in keeping with the principles of expectant management, the cord should not be clamped and cut until after the placenta and membranes have been expelled. It has been shown that there are benefits to doing this in relation to the baby continuing to receive oxygenated blood via the cord (Harris 2004). This is of particular importance if the baby is born prematurely (Kinmond et al. 1993). However, if the cord is particularly short, then not cutting it means that the woman is unable to hold her baby. A compromise in this situation is for the midwife to wait until the cord has stopped pulsating (usually after 5–10 minutes) and then clamp and cut it.

The woman should be encouraged to breastfeed her baby as soon as possible while waiting for the placenta to be delivered as the natural oxytocin released as the baby sucks will stimulate contraction of the uterine muscle.

The maternal end of the cord should not be clamped but should be left to drain into a suitable receptacle. This will mean that blood can drain from the placenta and reduce its overall size which will further help to facilitate delivery (Johnson and Taylor 2006). However, any blood which drains from the placenta should not be included in the final estimate of blood lost during the delivery as it is placental rather than maternal blood (Johnson and Taylor 2006).

When the uterus contacts the woman may feel some abdominal pain and will then have an urge to bear down again. She should be encouraged to do this and she may want to move into a more upright position (standing or squatting) so that gravity can assist the process (Rogers et al. 1998). A rush of blood will be seen and the cord may appear to lengthen as the placenta moves into the vagina. The woman will then spontaneously push the placenta and membranes out.

Active management of the third stage of labour

Active management of the third stage of labour includes giving the woman an oxytocic drug, the early clamping and cutting of the umbilical cord and controlled cord traction (Baston 2004).

A systematic review of four studies comparing active management of labour with physiological management suggests that active management should be the recommended option in the hospital setting (Prendeville et al. 2004). The review concluded that there was an overall reduction in maternal blood loss in those women having active management of the third stage compared with those women undergoing physiological third stage with no intervention. The rate of postpartum haemorrhage was also significantly lower in the actively managed women. The situation regarding the homebirth or birth centre setting is less clear (Enkin et al. 2000). The review also showed that side-effects of the oxytocic drugs used in the third stage include severe nausea and vomiting for some women, headache and raised blood pressure. Women who receive oxytocic drugs also sometimes complain of abdominal pain ('after-pains') due to the sustained contraction of the uterus which these oxytocic drugs induce.

The midwife must ensure that the woman knows what options are available to her in relation to the third stage of labour and that this information is presented in a clear, unbiased way so that she can make an informed decision (Anderson 1999; Rogers and Wood 1999). For some women, it is very important that they experience the whole childbirth process with minimal intervention and studies have highlighted the great satisfaction that a totally drug-free labour may give (Rogers and Wood 1999). The choice of whether to have a physiological third stage may be the only one left to a woman who has had to abandon her ideal birth options. For example, a woman may have hoped for a homebirth but due to slow progress in labour may have been transferred to a hospital unit (Baston 2004). Other women may be concerned about the unpleasant side-effects of the oxytocic drugs and for this reason would prefer to avoid them.

For these reasons, it is preferable that care options are discussed with the woman during the antenatal period so that she has time to consider the issues and include her wishes on her own birth plan. It is suggested that it is the midwife's role to discuss the advantages and disadvantages of the available options with their clients and then to ensure that they are suitably skilled to support the women in whatever choice they eventually opt for (Anderson 1999).

Syntometrine (1 ml) is an oxytocic drug often used in active management of the third stage. It contains 500 μg of ergometrine and 5 units of oxytocin. The oxytocic component of the drug induces a strong contraction of the upper uterine segment after approximately 2–3 minutes of administration. This effect lasts 5–15 minutes (Baskett 1999). In contrast the ergometrine component induces a strong sustained contraction of the uterine muscle 6–8 minutes after administration (Sorbe 1978). This effect lasts for approximately 60–90 minutes.

If a woman is known to have raised blood pressure or cardiac problems, then syntocinon is the drug of choice (DH 1994) as it does not cause sustained contraction of muscle fibres in the way that the ergometrine component of syntometrine does. If a women with a raised blood pressure is given an oxytocin-containing ergometrine, then contraction of muscles within her blood vessels will lead to her blood pressure being raised even more. Syntocinon can be given either intravenously (5 iu) or intramuscularly (5–15 iu). Syntocinon also has fewer side-effects such as the nausea and vomiting associated with syntometrine.

If a woman is to have an active management of the third stage, the oxytocic drug is traditionally administered intramuscularly by the midwife as the baby's anterior shoulder delivers. It is usually given in the upper outer part of the woman's leg. However, if the midwife is alone during the birth, then giving the drug at this precise time is not possible. In this case the midwife will administer the drug following the birth of the baby. In either case, the drug should always be given following the delivery of the baby's shoulder to ensure that shoulder dystocia (the shoulders trapped behind the woman's pubic bone) is not a possibility (Baston 2004).

The umbilical cord should be clamped using specially designed umbilical clamps and then cut as soon as possible after the delivery of the baby. This is because the oxytocic drug causes a contraction of the uterus which forces placental blood into the baby's circulation. This overloads the infant's circulatory system (indeed the baby can receive up to half of his whole blood volume again) and may cause hyperbilirubinaemia (high levels of bilirubin in the blood stream), leading to neonatal jaundice (Johnson and Taylor 2006).

The woman's partner may ask to cut the cord and this request can usually be facilitated with the support of the midwife. In cases of an instrumental delivery, the midwife may need to remind the obstetrician who is undertaking the delivery of the couple's request so that it can still be accommodated if the condition of the woman and her baby allows. As Baston (2004) points out, the memory of the birth and the couple's involvement in it will remain with them forever so it is important to respect such requests if possible.

Following clamping and cutting of the cord, the midwife should place her hand on the woman's abdomen and wait for signs that the uterus has contracted. She will feel that this has occurred when the uterus hardens underneath her hand; it will feel like a smooth hard, cricket ball. It is important at this time that the midwife avoids so-called 'fundal fiddling' (that is unnecessary touching of the uterus) which may lead to the placenta only partially separating from the uterine wall (Johnson and Taylor 2006), which may in turn be a cause of excessive bleeding and postpartum haemorrhage. Spencer (1962) suggested controlled cord traction (CCT) should be commenced as soon as the uterus contracts and this was a traditional aspect of an actively managed third stage. However, since then Levy and Moore (1985) have suggested that it is preferable to wait for further signs that placental separation has occurred.

Signs of separation include the rising of the fundus and the hardening of the uterus as described above, coupled with a gush of blood from the vagina and a lengthening of the umbilical cord. Levy and Moore (1985) found no significant difference in the incidence of postpartum haemorrhage (PPH) or the length of the third stage between those who commenced CCT immediately they felt the uterus contract and those who waited for signs of separation. However, the incidence of PPH did increase significantly when the midwife unsuccessfully applied CCT without waiting for signs of placental separation.

CCT involves the midwife either wrapping the cord around her fingers or using a clamp to apply downward, sustained pressure until the placenta becomes visible at the vulva. Once the placenta can be seen, the traction is applied upwards to follow the curve of the vagina. The placenta is then delivered into a bowl. Care should be taken of any trailing membranes and the midwife may need to use forceps to gently tease the membranes out of the vagina. Alternatively, twisting the trailing membranes into a rope may be useful and some midwives ask the woman to cough gently to assist this process.

Some midwives place their hand above the symphysis pubis while undertaking CCT and push the uterus upwards. This is known as 'guarding the uterus' and is thought to prevent the uterus being pulled inside out (uterine inversion). However, there is no evidence to suggest that this is necessary (Harris 2004).

Midwifery care after birth

Following delivery of the placenta, the midwife documents how long it took. Rogers et al. (1998) suggest that the average length of the third stage using active management is 6–8 minutes. The midwife should also palpate the uterus to ensure that it remains contracted and the amount of vaginal blood loss is estimated and recorded.

The woman's vagina and external genitalia should then be examined for signs of trauma and a decision needs to be made as to whether suturing of the area is needed. This is often an uncomfortable examination and the midwife should make sure that the woman has Entonox to use if required and that she understands why she is being examined. All effort should be made to reassure and relax her. It may be helpful if the partner holds her baby close to her as a way of distracting her from the examination.

Conclusion

This chapter has focused on the physiological aspects of labour with an emphasis on the role of the midwife in promoting normality. For issues relating to care of women in high-risk situations the reader is referred to the obstetric literature. Emergency scenarios are discussed in Chapter 6. The role of the midwife in empowering the woman to cope with the tremendous physical and emotional demands of childbirth has also been highlighted. It is acknowledged that labour is a complex, multifaceted process with physical, psychosocial and emotional elements underpinning it. As the *Midwives Rules and Standards* (NMC 2004) emphasise, childbirth is much more than simply the act of giving birth. It is a continuous process from conception, through pregnancy, labour, birth and beyond. Many factors unique to the individual woman will impact on the process and it is essential that midwives are competent to provide effective and appropriate care during this time. The midwife will need to use her skills to support the individual needs of each woman she cares for in whatever setting she is working (for example, the home, the hospital or birth centre) and regardless of the woman's cultural background and individual preferences.

References

Allotey, J. C. (1996) The use of the ischial spines to determine descent of the fetus: a hazardous practice? *The Art and Science of Midwifery gives Birth to a Better Future.* Proceedings of the International Confederation of Midwives 24th Triennial Congress, 26–31 May, Oslo. London: International Confederation of Midwives: 577–9.

Anderson, T. (1999) Active versus expectant management of the third stage of labour. *The Practising Midwife* 2(2): 10–11.

Baker, C. (1996) Nutrition and hydration in labour. *British Journal of Midwifery* 4: 568–72.

Barrett, J. W. H. (1983) Prenatal influences on adaptation in the newborn. In P. Stratton (ed.), *Psychobiology of the Human Newborn.* Chichester: John Wiley.

Baskett, T. E. (1999) *Essential Management of Obstetric Emergencies*, 3rd edition. Bristol: Clinical Press.

Baston, H. (2004) Midwifery basics: care during labour: third stage. *The Practising Midwife* 7(4): 31–6.

Bates, C. (1997) *Debating Midwifery: Normality in Midwifery*. London: Royal College of Midwives.

Beech, B. (1998) A little shot of something (not so) nice. *Association for Improvement in Maternity Services Journal* 10(1): 7–8.

Belfrage, P., Boreus, L. O., Hartvig, P. et al. (1981) Neonatal depression after obstetrical analgesia with pethidine. The role of the injection-delivery time interval and plasma concentrations of pethidine and norpethidine. *Acta Obstetricia et Gynaecologica Scandinavica* 60(1): 43–9.

Bewley, C. (1997) Injectable methods of pain relief in labour. In J. Alexander, V. Levy and S. Roch (eds), *Midwifery Practice: Core Topics 2*. Basingstoke: Macmillan: 38–50.

BirthChoice UK (2003) *Normal Birth Rate 1990–2001*. www.birthchoiceuk. com/Professionals/NormalBirthHistory.htm.

Broach, J. and Newton, N. (1988) Food and beverages in labour. Part II: the effects of cessation of oral intake during labour. *Birth* 15: 88–92.

Bryant, H. and Yerby, M. (2004) Relief of pain during labour. In C. Henderson and S. Macdonald (eds), *Mayes' Midwifery A Textbook for Midwives*, 13th edition. London: Bailliere Tindall: 458–74.

Cawthra, A. M. (1986) The use of pethidine in labour. *Midwives Chronicle and Nursing Notes* 99(1183): 178–81.

Collis, R. E., Baxendall, M. L., Srikantharajah, I. D. et al. (1993) Mobility during labour with combined analgesia. *Lancet* 341(8847): 767–8.

Coppen, R. (2005) *Birthing Position: Do Midwives Know Best?* London: Quay Books Division, MA Healthcare Ltd.

Czarnocka, J. and Slade, P. (2000) Prevalence and predictors of post-traumatic stress symptoms following childbirth. *British Journal of Clinical Psychology* 39: 35–51.

Department of Health (1993) *Changing Childbirth: Report of the Expert Maternity Group*. London: HMSO.

Department of Health (1994) *Confidential Enquiry into Maternal Deaths in the UK 1988–90*. London: HMSO.

Duff, M. (2002) Labour behaviours: a method of assessing labour progress. International Confederation of Midwives. *Midwives and Women Working together for the Family of the World*: ICM proceedings. CD-ROM, Vienna.

Eisenach, J. (1999) Combined spinal epidural analgesia in obstetrics. *Anaesthesiology* 91(1): 299–302.

Enkin, M., Keirse, M. J. N. C., Renfrew, M. and Neilson, J. (1996) *A Guide to Effective Care in Pregnancy and Childbirth*, 2nd edition. Oxford: Oxford University Press.

Enkin, M., Kierse, M. J. N. V., Neilson, J. et al. (2000) *A Guide to Effective Care in Pregnancy and Childbirth*, 3rd edition. Oxford: Oxford University Press.

Fairlie, F. M., Marshall, L., Walkers, J. J. et al. (1999) Intramuscular opioids for maternal pain relief in labour: a randomized controlled trial comparing pethidine with diamorphine. *British Journal of Obstetrics and Gynaecology* 106(11): 1181–7.

Fogel, S. T., Shyken, J. M., Leighton, B. L. et al. (1998) Epidural analgesia and the incidence of cesarean delivery for dystocia. *Anesthesia and Analgesia* 87: 119–23.

Gamsu, H. (1993) The effect of pain relief on the baby. In G. Chamberlain, A. Wraight and P. Steer (eds), *Pain and its Relief in Childbirth*. Edinburgh: Churchill Livingstone.

Ghacero, E. P. and Enabudosco, E. J. (2006) Labor management: an appraisal of the role of false labor and the latent phase on the delivery mode. *Journal of Obstetrics and Gynecology* 26(6): 534–7.

Gross, M. M., Hecker, H., Maltern, A. et al. (2006) Does the way that women experience the onset of labour influence the duration of labour? *British Journal of Obstetrics and Gynaecology* 113(11): 289–94.

Gupta, J. K. and Hofmeyr, G. J. (2004) Positions for women during second stage of labour (Cochrane review). *The Cochrane Library*, Issue 1. Chichester: John Wiley.

Harris, T. (2004) Care in the third stage of labour. In C. Henderson and S. Macdonald (eds), *Mayes Midwifery: A Textbook for Midwives.* London: Bailliere Tindall: 507–23.

Hawkins, J. L., Hess, K. R. and Kubicek, M. A. (1995) A reevaluation of the association between instrumental delivery and epidural analgesia. *Regional Anesthesia* 20: 50–60.

Hemminki, E. and Simukka, R. (1986) The timing of hospital admission and the progress of labour. *European Journal of Obstetrics and Gynaecology and Reproductive Biology* 22: 85–95.

Heywood, A. M. and Ho, E. (1990) Pain relief in labour. In J. Alexander, V. Levy and S. Roch (eds*), Intrapartum Care: A Research-based Approach.* Basingstoke: Macmillan.

Hobbs, L. (1998) Assessing cervical dilatation without VEs: watching the purple line. *Practising Midwife* 1(11): 34–5.

Hodnett, E. D., Gates, S., Hofmeyr, G. J. and Sakala, C. (2002) Continuous support for women during childbirth (Cochrane review) In: *The Cochrane Library*, Issue 1. Chichester: John Wiley.

Howell, C. J., Dean, T., Lucking, L. et al. (2002) Randomised study of long-term outcome after epidural versus non-epidural analgesia during labour. *British Medical Journal* 325(7360): 357–9.

Hunt, S. (2002) Pethidine: love it or hate it? *Midirs Midwifery Digest* 12(3): 363–5.

Inch, S. (1985) Management of the third stage of labour – another cascade of intervention. *Midwifery* 1(2): 114–22.

Janni, W., Schiessl, B., Peschers, U. et al. (2002) The prognostic impact of a prolonged second stage and the effects on perinatal and maternal outcomes. *Acta Obstetrica Gynaecologica Scandinavica* 81: 214–21.

Johnson, M. H. and Everitt, B. J. (2000) *Essential Reproduction*. 2nd edition. Oxford: Blackwell Science.

Johnson, R. and Taylor, W. (2006) *Skills for Midwifery Practice*, 2nd edition. London: Elsevier.

Johnston, J. (2004) The nesting instinct. *Birth Matters* 8(2): 21–2.

Jordan, S. (2002) *Pharmacology for Midwives (Evidence Base for Safe Practice)*. Basingstoke: Palgrave.

Kinmond, S., Aitchison, T. C., Holland, B. M. et al. (1993) Umbilical cord clamping and preterm infants: a randomized trial. *British Medical Journal* 306(6871): 172–5.

Kitzinger, S. (1987) *Giving Birth: How it Really Feels*. London: Gollancz.

Kitzinger, S (2005) *The Politics of Birth in Edinburgh and Elsewhere*. London: Elsevier Butterworth Heinemann.

Leap, N. (2000) Pain in labour: towards a midwifery perspective. *MIDIRS Midwifery Digest* 10(1): 49–53.

Levy, V. and Moore, J. (1985) The midwife's management of the third stage of labour. *Nursing Times* 81(39): 47–50.

Lieberman, E., Lang, J. M., Cohen, A. and D'Agostino, R. (1996) Association of epidural analgesia with cesarean delivery in nullipara. *Obstetrics and Gynaecology* 88(6): 993.

MacArthr, C., Lewis, M., Knox, E. G. et al. (1990) Epidural and long-term backache after childbirth. *British Medical Journal* 301(6742): 9–12.

Mander, R. (2002) The transitional stage. In S. Wickham (ed.), *Midwifery Best Practice*, vol. 3. Edinburgh: Elsevier Butterworth Heinemann: 127–30.

McKay, S. and Roberts, J. (1990) Obstetrics by ear: maternal and caregiver perceptions of the meaning of maternal sounds during second stage of labour. *Journal of Nurse-Midwifery* 35: 266–73.

Mead, M. (2004) Midwives practices in 11 UK maternity units. In S. Downe (ed.), *Normal Childbirth: Evidence and Debate*. Edinburgh: Churchill Livingstone.

Mendelsohn, C.L. (1946) The aspiration of stomach contents. In M. Parsons and S. Nagys (2006) Anaesthetist's perspective on oral intake for women in labour. *British Journal of Midwiery* 14(8): 488–91.

Micklewright, A. and Champion, P. (2002) Labouring over food: the dietician's view. In P. Champion and C. M. Cormick (eds), *Eating and Drinking in Labour*. Oxford: Books for Midwives.

MIDIRS and the NHS Centre for Reviews and Dissemination (2003) *Support in Labour*. Informed choice for professionals leaflet. Bristol: MIDIRS.

Myles, T. and Santolaya, J. (2003) Maternal and neonatal outcomes in patients with a prolonged second stage of labour. *Obstetrics and Gynaecology* 102: 52–8.

National Institute for Health and Clinical Excellence (2001) Induction of labour. *Clinical Guideline D, 1*, London: NICE.

National Institute for Health and Clinical Excellence (2007) Intrapartum Care: Care of healthy women and their babies during childbirth. *NICE clinical guideline 55* London: NICE.

Ndala, R. (2005a) The onset of labour. In D. Stables and J. Rankin (eds), *Physiology in Childbearing with Anatomy and Related Biosciences*, 2nd edition. London: Elsevier. p. 471.

Ndala, R. (2005b) The first stage of labour. In D. Stables and J. Rankin (eds), *Physiology in Childbearing with Anatomy and Related Biosciences*, 2nd edition. London: Elsevier. p. 479.

Ndala, R. (2005c) The second stage of labour. In D. Stables and J. Rankin (eds), *Physiology in Childbearing with Anatomy and Related Biosciences*, 2nd edition. London: Elsevier. p. 509.

Ndala, R. (2005d) Pain relief in labour. In D. Stables and J. Rankin (eds), *Physiology in Childbearing with Anatomy and Related Biosciences*, 2nd edition. London: Elsevier. p. 495.

Newton, C. and Champion, P. (1997) Oral intake in labour: Nottingham's policy formulated and audited. *British Journal of Midwifery* 5: 418–22.

Nursing and Midwifery Council (2004) *Midwives Rules and Standards*. London: NMC.

Odent, M. (1994) Labouring women are not marathon runners. *Midwifery Today* 31: 23–51.

Odent, M. (2003) Preparing the nest. *Midwifery Today* 68: 13–14.

Oloffson, C. H., Ekbolom, A., Ekman-Ordenberg, G. et al. (1996) Lack of analgesic effect of systemically administered morphine or pethidine on labour pain. *British Journal of Obstetrics and Gynaecology* 103: 968–72.

Page, L. (2003) Creating a better birth environment. *British Journal of Midwifery* 11(12): 714.

Park, G. and Fulton, B. (1991) *The Management of Acute Pain*. Oxford: Oxford University Press.

Parsons, M. and Nagy, S. (2006) Anaesthetists' perspective on oral intake for women in labour. *British Journal of Midwifery* 14(8): 488–91.

Peled, G. (1992) Birth and the Gulf War. *MIDIRS Midwifery Digest* 3(1): 54.

Pengelley, L. (2002) Eating and drinking in labour: the consumer's view. In P. Champion and C. McCormick, *Eating and Drinking in Labour*. Oxford: Books for Midwives.

Prendeville, W. J., Elbourne, D. and McDonald, S. (2004) Active versus expectant management in the third stage of labour (Cochrane review). *The Cochrane Library*, Issue 1. Chichester: John Wiley.

Ragnar, I., Altman, D., Tyden, T. and Olsson, S. E. (2006) Comparison of the maternal experience and duration of labour in two upright delivery positions – a randomized controlled trial. *British Journal of Obstetrics and Gynaecology* 113: 165–70.

Reynolds, F. (1998) Effects of analgesia on the baby. *Fetal and Maternal Medicine Review* 10: 45–59.

Roberts, J. (2002) The 'push' for evidence: the management of the second stage. *Journal of Midwifery and Women's Health* 47: 2–15.

Roberts, J. E., Mendez-Bauer, C. and Wodell, D. A. (1983) The effects of maternal position on uterine contractility and efficiency. *Birth* 10(4): 243–49.

Robertson, A. (2001) *Skills for Childbirth Educators. Volume 1: Learning about the Pelvis* (video). Australia: Birth International. Available from www. Birthinternational.co.

Rogers, J. and Wood, J. (1999) The Hitchingbrooke third stage trial. What are the implications for practice? *The Practising Midwife* 2(2): 35–7.

Rogers, J., Wood, J., McCandlish, R. et al. (1998) Active versus expectant management of third stage of labour: the Hinchingbrooke randomised controlled trial. *The Lancet* 351: 693–9.

Rosenblatt, D., Belsey, E. M., Lieberman, L. et al. (1981) The influence of maternal analgesia on neonatal behaviour. *British Journal of Obstetrics and Gynaecology* 88(4): 407–13.

Royal College of Midwives (2005) Positions for labour and birth practice points. *Evidence-based Guidelines for Midwifery-led Care in Labour*. www. rcm.org.uk.

Sandall, J. (2004) Promoting normal birth: weighing the evidence. In S. Downe (ed.), *Normal Childbirth: Evidence and Debate*. Edinburgh: Churchill Livingstone.

Savitz, D. A., Anath, C. V., Luther, E. R. and Thory, J. M. (1997) Influence of gestational age on the time from spontaneous rupture of the chorioamniotic membranes to the onset of labor. *American Journal of Perinatology* 14: 129–33.

Sheikh, A. and Tunstall, M. E. (1986) Comparative study of meptazinol and pethidine for the relief of pain in labour. *British Journal of Obstetrics and Gynaecology* 93(3): 264–9.

Sleep, J. (1990) Spontaneous delivery. In J. Alexander, V. Levy and S. Roch (eds), *Intrapartum Care: A Research-based Approach*. Basingstoke: Macmillan Education.

Sookhoo, M. L. and Biott, C. (2002) Learning at work: midwives judging progress in labour. *Learning in Health and Social Care* 1(2): 75–85.

Sorbe, B. (1978) Active pharmacologic management of the third stage of labour. *Obstetrics and Gynaecology* 52(6): 694–7.

Spencer, P. M. (1962) Controlled cord traction in management of the third stage of labour. *British Medical Journal* 1(5294): 1728–32.

Spiby, H. et al. (2003) Selected coping strategies in labour: an investigation of women's experience. *Birth* 30: 189–94.

Sutton, J. and Scott, P. (1996) Understanding and teaching optimal foetal positioning. Tauranga, New Zealand: Birth Concepts.

Tan, B. P. and Hannah, M. E. (2002) Prostaglandins versus oxytocin for prelabour rupture of membranes at or near term. *Cochrane Database Systematic Review, The Cochrane Library* Issue 3 Chichester: John Wiley.

Thompson, A. M. (1993) Pushing techniques in the second stage of labour. *Journal of Advanced Nursing* 18: 171–7.

Tsui, M. H. Y., Kee, W. D. N., Ng, F. F. et al. (2004) A double-blind randomised placebo-controlled study of intramuscular pethidine for pain relief in the first stage of labour. *BJOG: An International Journal of Obstetrics and Gynaecology* 111(7): 648–55.

Vincent, M. (2003) Progress in a pocket. *Midwives* 6(2): 82–4.

Walsh, D. (2004) Care in the first stage of labour. In C. Henderson and S. Macdonald (eds), *Mayes' Midwifery A Textbook for Midwives*, 13th edition. London: Bailliere Tindall.

Wickham, S. (1999) Further thoughts on the third stage of labour. *The Practising Midwife* 2(10): 14–15.

Wickham, S. and Sutton, J. (2005) The rhombus of Michaelis. In S. Wickham (ed.), *Midwifery Best Practice*, volume 3. Edinburgh: Books for Midwives Press/Elsevier Butterworth Heinemann.

Williams, R. M., Thorn, M. H. and Studd, J. W. W. (1980) A study of the benefits and acceptability of ambulation in spontaneous labour. *British Journal of Obstetrics and Gynaecology* 87: 122–6.

Wood, C. and Soltani, H. (2005) Does pethidine relieve pain? *The Practising Midwife* 8(7): 17–25.

Wuitchik, M., Kakal, D. and Lipshitz, J. (1989) The clinical significance of pain and cognitive activity in latent labour. *Obstetrics and Gynaecology* 73(1): 35–42.

Yerby, M. (2000) *Pain in Childbearing: Key Issues in Management.* Edinburgh: Bailliere Tindall.

Effective Emergency Care

Caroline Duncombe, Meryl Dimmock and Sarah Green

Introduction

This chapter aims to provide readers with evidence-based knowledge to strengthen the skills required in emergency situations. It will facilitate readers' ability to provide safe and effective care to women and babies if faced with an emergency. It is also intended to provide an understanding of how emergency care is supported by the Nursing and Midwifery Council (NMC) through the *Midwives Rules and Standards* (2004a). Having to manage an unexpected emergency is a daunting prospect. However, by being familiar with the scenario and attending regular 'skills and drills' updates, fears and anxieties should be reduced and the ability to achieve a successful outcome increased.

Rule 6 of the *Midwives Rules and Standards* (NMC 2004a) identifies midwives' responsibility and sphere of practice. It states that:

> *'In an emergency, or where a deviation from the norm which is outside her current sphere of practice becomes apparent in a woman or baby during the antenatal, intranatal or postnatal periods, a practising midwife shall call such qualified health professional as may reasonably be expected to have the necessary skills and experience to assist her in the provision of care.'*

The standard that accompanies this rule states that a midwife *'is responsible for maintaining and developing her own competence'*. Guidance to the midwife includes: *'You should be appropriately prepared and clinically up to date to ensure that you can carry out effectively, emergency procedures such as resuscitation, for the woman or baby'*. This rule therefore implies that in an emergency a midwife should have the skills to give the immediate care necessary to benefit the woman and her baby, and that help should be requested from other appropriate health care professionals when available.

A number of organisations provide multidisciplinary courses and guidelines to follow in emergency situations. These include the Resuscitation Council UK, Advanced Life Saving in Obstetrics (ALSO), Advanced Life Support (ALS), Advanced Paediatric Life Support (APLS) and Neonatal Life Support (NLS). These promote multidisciplinary teamwork, which is a requirement of the Clinical Negligence Scheme for Trusts (CNST).

CNST is a scheme set up by the NHS Litigation Authority to handle clinical negligence claims against member NHS bodies. CNST requires annual multidisciplinary practice sessions or 'drills' in maternity units, as they help all members of staff, especially new and junior staff, know and understand their specific roles and responsibilities in an emergency. It specifies that obstetricians and midwives should be involved in these, together with other staff relevant to the situation, whether working in the hospital or the community (CNST 2006). These drills should include the identification of the equipment required and methods for ensuring that appropriate emergency assistance, including cardiac arrest teams, arrive promptly (CEMACH 2004).

The emergency situations to be discussed are those identified in the Standards of Proficiency for Pre-registration Midwifery Education (NMC 2004a), and in the report *Why Mothers Die* (CEMACH 2004). They are:

- Maternal resuscitation
- Neonatal resuscitation
- Shoulder dystocia
- Vaginal breech delivery
- Manual removal of the placenta
- Manual examination of the uterus
- Management of postpartum haemorrhage
- Management of an eclamptic seizure

With each of these emergency situations, factors that increase the risk of occurrence will be identified. This will facilitate anticipation of problems that might affect delivery and enhance the ability to give the correct guidance regarding place of birth as recommended in *Why Mothers Die*. It identifies that women who are known to be at higher risk of developing problems during labour or birth should be advised to deliver in a consultant obstetrician-led unit (see Chapter 3).

Maternal resuscitation

Incidence: Cardiac arrest is rare in pregnancy, but it is estimated that it happens to 1 : 7692 women from pregnancy to one year after birth. Approximately half are due to substandard care (CEMACH 2004).

Risk factors: The most common cause of maternal cardiac arrest, regardless of aetiology, is hypovolaemia and hypotension (Morris and Stacey 2003).

The factors that increase the requirement for maternal resuscitation vary, but include those identified by CEMACH (2004) as being the leading causes of direct maternal death (due to pregnancy), shown in Figure 6.1.

Certain physiological changes that occur in pregnancy may have an impact on maternal resuscitation. These include:

- *Increase in cardiac output by 30–40 per cent.* This starts as early as four weeks' gestation to promote maternal adaptation to pregnancy, as well as the blood supply to the enlarging uterus.

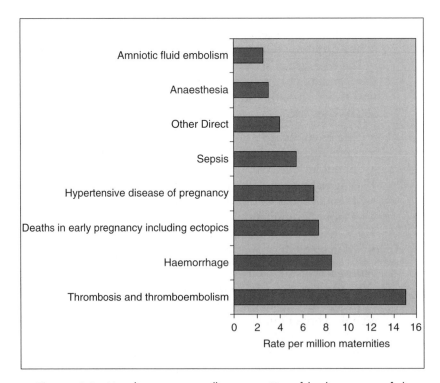

Figure 6.1 Mortality rates per million maternities of leading causes of direct deaths; United Kingdom 2000–2002 (CEMACH, 2004)

- *Increase in blood volume by up to 50 per cent.* The uterine blood flow increases from 100 ml/min at the end of the first trimester to 500 ml/min by term (Stables 1999). It results in a fall of haemoglobin due to the effect of haemodilution.
- *Increased oxygen consumption of 20 per cent.*
- *Decreased peripheral resistance.* This is due to both the development of the uteroplacental circulation, and the relaxation of the peripheral vascular tone.
- *Decreased residual capacity of the lungs of 25 per cent.*
- *Delayed emptying of stomach contents.* This leads to an increase in volume and acidity of the gastric contents.
- *The weight of the pregnant uterus.* This can lead to aortocaval compression when a woman is lying in a supine position, particularly after 20 weeks' gestation. The weight presses on the aorta and vena cava, restricting blood flow to vital organs such as the brain and heart, causing a reduction in cardiac output and hypotension.

The Resuscitation Council (UK) currently sets the standard for maternal resuscitation in the United Kingdom and produces training aids and literature. These are available to health care professionals and lay people through resuscitation trainers. The aim is to establish and maintain standards for resuscitation and to foster good working relations between all disciplines involved. Figure 6.2 shows the algorithm for basic adult resuscitation.

In pregnancy physiological changes can complicate the resuscitation procedure, and particular attention should be made to minimise aortocaval compression. The uterus needs to be tilted to the left by 25–30°. This can be achieved by:

- Using a firm triangular wedge present in many maternity units, or a pillow
- Using a human wedge, i.e. knees
- Using a tipped up chair
- Performing manual uterine displacement. This is when an attendant (who may be the midwife or another helper, e.g. doctor, health care assistant or partner) manually lifts the weight of the uterus to the left, off the woman. Aortocaval compression will be relieved by this method and cardiac output increased by 20–25 per cent, but it may interfere with effective chest compressions. It is important to remember that cardiac output is reduced to approximately 30 per cent of the normal output during effective cardiopulmonary resuscitation and its effectiveness depends on the efficacy of external chest compressions (Ueland et al. 1972; Lee et al. 1986; Resuscitation Council (UK) 2005).

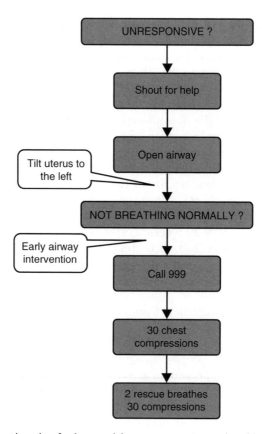

Figure 6.2 Algorithm for basic adult resuscitation (Reproduced by kind permission of the Resuscitation Council (UK) 2005)

- Perimortem (near the time of death) (Webster's New World Medical Dictionary 2003) caesarean section may have to be undertaken early in the resuscitation attempt in order to relieve aortocaval compression, increase venous return and increase cardiac output. If it is done within 4–5 minutes, the likelihood of maternal and neonatal survival is increased. Due to the length of time it may take to get a theatre ready, it may be appropriate to undertake the procedure on the spot. The only vital equipment required for this is a scalpel. In a hospital setting, equipment to enable intravenous access, administration of fluids, endotracheal intubation, a method for closure of the wound and neonatal resuscitation should be immediately available.

In all cases it is imperative that staff with the appropriate experience are present when dealing with a cardiac arrest in a pregnant woman as soon as possible. These are an obstetrician, anaesthetist and neonatologist. Particular attention should be made to effective cardiac compressions. A rate of 30 compressions to 2 breaths is recommended.

Once expert help arrives:

- Incorporate early advanced airway intervention
- Apply pressure to the cricoid cartilage to occlude the upper end of the oesophagus against the vertebrae and prevent the acid gastric contents from being aspirated
- Treat causative factors such as hypovolaemia, toxicity
- Communicate with relatives
- Maintain record keeping and documentation

If the situation occurs in an out-of-hospital setting, then the emergency services need to be mobilised and basic resuscitation must continue with the woman tilted to the left until expert help is available.

Neonatal resuscitation

Incidence: A large study in Sweden indicated that 10 per 1000 babies over 2.5 kg required either mask inflation or intubation. Of these, 8 per 1000 responded to mask inflation and 2 per 1000 required intubation (Palme-Kilander 1992). There is no information available for the UK.

Risk factors: The factors that increase the requirement for neonatal resuscitation vary. Many labour ward policies require a trained resuscitator to attend deliveries for all emergency caesarean sections, breech births, multiple births, instrumental deliveries, preterm births, anticipated fetal distress and in the presence of meconium. However, it is not easy to predict which babies will require resuscitation at birth. Therefore, everyone who attends births should be trained in newborn life support.

Babies who require resuscitation do so for different reasons from an adult. Physiologically, a newborn baby is prepared to withstand a lack of oxygen for periods during labour and birth. Generally, they are born with strong hearts, and the initial help they need is with respiration. Their lungs are filled with fluid at birth, so to resuscitate a newborn baby it is usually sufficient to inflate the lungs with air or oxygen. The heart will normally still be pumping and so will bring oxygenated blood back to the heart from the lungs, leading to

Newborn Life Support

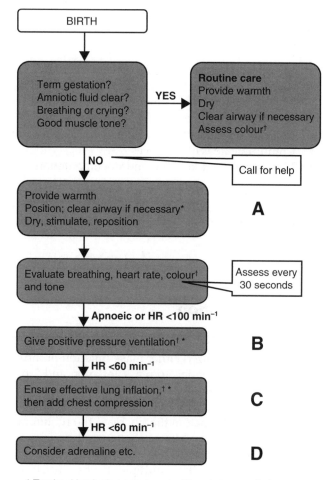

Figure 6.3 Newborn life support (Reproduced by kind permission of the Resuscitation Council (UK) 2005)

recovery. Rarely the heart may need to be 'bump' started. Figure 6.3 shows the algorithm for newborn life support.

Newborn life support consists of the following:

* *Drying and covering the baby to conserve heat.* The priority is to keep a baby dry and warm. Drying the baby will provide stimulation and allow time for assessment of colour, tone, breathing and heart

rate. Putting a hat on the baby's head will help to maintain a warm temperature, as the hair can stay damp. Babies who become cold following birth are less able to maintain oxygen levels and become hypoglycaemic. The use of food-grade plastic wrapping is recommended by the Resuscitation Council (UK) (2005) to maintain body temperature in significantly preterm babies

- *Assessing the need for any intervention.* Most babies when dried and kept warm will spontaneously start to breathe within 60–90 seconds of birth. A normal heart rate is 120–150 beats/min. This is best judged by listening with a stethoscope

If *meconium* is present, do not aspirate it from the nose and mouth while the head is on the perineum as it is of no benefit and does not prevent meconium aspiration syndrome. Do not remove meconium from the airways of crying babies for the same reason. However, if babies are *not* crying at birth and meconium is seen in the oropharynx, this can be cleared with the use of a stiff yankaur sucker, although there is no evidence of the efficacy of this practice

- *Opening the airway.* The baby should be placed on its back with its head in the neutral position, i.e. with the neck neither over- nor under-extended. A folded towel may be placed under the shoulders to aid positioning if the baby has a prominent occiput (back of head). However it is important to ensure the neck is not overextended when doing this. If the baby's tone is very poor, it may also be necessary to apply a chin lift or jaw thrust. This may be enough to enable air to enter the lungs to initiate the process of life
- *Rescue breathing.* If a newborn does not make an effort to breathe, it will be appropriate to assist the process by giving up to five rescue breaths which need to last for 2–3 seconds each to be effective. This is because there may be no or limited chest movement for the first two to three inflations due to the movement of fluid from the lungs, or poor positioning of the mask
  - By aerating the lungs, the neural centres in the brain, which are responsible for normal breathing, will function again and the majority of newborns will recover. Air may be used initially, although oxygen should be available if there is no rapid improvement in the newborn's condition.
  - If the baby's heart rate increases, but spontaneous breathing is not initiated, then regular breaths should be provided at a rate of approximately 30–40/min until the baby starts to breathe on its own.
- If there is no evidence of lung inflation, consider:
  - Is the baby's head in the neutral position?

 – Do you need jaw thrust?
 – Do you need a longer inflation time?
 – Do you need a second person's help with the airway?
 – Do you need to remove an obstruction in the airway using a laryngoscope and wide bore suction?
 – What about an oropharyngeal (Guedel) airway?
 There is no point in progressing until there is evidence that air is entering the lungs.

- *Chest compression.* In a few cases, the cardiac function will have deteriorated so that oxygenated blood is not transferred from the aerated lungs to the heart. If the heart rate remains below 60 beats/min following effective rescue breaths, chest compressions will be required. The recommended method of delivering chest compressions is to grip the chest with both hands so that the two thumbs can press on the lower third of the sternum, with the fingers over the spine at the back. The chest should be compressed quickly and firmly by about one third of the depth at a ratio of 3 : 1 compressions to inflations. A rate of 90–120 compressions/min should be aimed for. The aim is to move oxygenated blood from the lungs back to the heart. It is important to allow enough time during the relaxation phase of each compression cycle for the heart to refill with blood.

- *Administration of drugs* (rare). In the rare event that lung inflation and chest compressions are insufficient, drugs may be required to restore the circulation. The outlook for this group of babies is poor

- The Resuscitation Council (UK) (2005) states that '*If there are no signs of life after ten minutes of continuous and adequate resuscitation efforts, then discontinuation of resuscitation may be justified*'. However, the midwife's responsibility is to continue resuscitation until care is transferred to an appropriate practitioner (NMC 2004a)

As in all emergency situations, it is imperative that staff with the appropriate experience are called as soon as possible, and particular attention should be made to:

- Communication with the parents
- Record keeping and documentation

Shoulder dystocia

While caring for mothers in labour midwives are constantly monitoring progress in order to predict and react to unfolding events.

The rate of progress in labour and particularly the second stage is predictive of the possibility of obstruction during the delivery. Shoulder dystocia is one such delay.

Active childbirth encourages mothers to be upright, mobile and in control. The midwife works with the mother, engaging her trust, and this relationship is essential when faced with an emergency situation.

Definition: Shoulder dystocia is best defined as an impaction of the anterior shoulder of the fetus against the maternal symphysis pubis after the fetal head has been delivered. Any measures aimed at expediting delivery concentrate on changing the relationship between the two bony parts. Gibb (1995) described three types of shoulder dystocia, increasing in severity:

1. A tight fit when delivering a big baby
2. A unilateral dystocia, where the anterior shoulder becomes impacted above the maternal symphysis pubis
3. A bilateral dystocia, where both the shoulders have become arrested above the pelvic brim

Incidence: The incidence of dystocia is generally agreed to be between 0.2 per cent and 0.3 per cent at term (Eden et al. 1987), increasing to 1.3 per cent by 42 weeks. These figures may vary due in part to midwives' reluctance to diagnose true shoulder dystocia.

Risk factors: Although it is known that the following risk factors are predictive of shoulder dystocia, it is also acknowledged that they are of reasonably poor predictive value. Current practice encourages midwives and obstetricians to attempt to anticipate difficulty using these triggers:

- *Prior shoulder dystocia.* This is predictive of a further risk of dystocia with a reoccurrence rate of 10 per cent in subsequent deliveries (Smith et al. 1994)
- *Diabetes.* With its association with larger babies, diabetes is a significant risk factor for both pre-gestational and gestational diabetes
- *Post-dates pregnancy.* As a pregnancy continues past 40 weeks there is a correlation with larger babies
- *Prolonged first stage.* A longer first stage, or one that has been augmented, may be symptomatic of a fetus that is large in proportion to the mother
- *Prolonged second stage.* A second stage that is longer than expected, i.e. in a multiparous mother, is indicative of a larger baby

- *Operative vaginal delivery.* Either forceps or ventouse deliveries are associated with a higher incidence of difficulty with the fetal shoulders

Management

The manoeuvres described here are the currently recommended management for shoulder dystocia. They are described from the simple to the more complex, but this order is not prescriptive. They can be undertaken in any order, but for midwives the simple manoeuvres are the starting point. Organisations such as ALSO recommend the use of a mnemonic HELPERR.

Help
Evaluate for episiotomy
Legs (McRoberts position)
Pressure (suprapubically)
Enter (for manoeuvres)
Remove (the posterior arm)
Roll (the patient either into all fours or through 360 degrees)

The first action of the midwife is to confidently diagnose a shoulder dystocia and call for assistance, i.e. more midwives, obstetricians and paediatric support. Once help is on its way the measures described below should be commenced. In a community setting or a midwife-led unit the measures can be undertaken in any order, commencing with simple measures such as rolling the patient onto all fours. In a birthing pool, the mother should be encouraged to stand up and place one foot on the edge of the pool to allow for delivery.

- *McRoberts manoeuvre.* This involves placing the mother flat on her back and putting her knees on her chest. Once she is in this position attempts should be made to deliver the baby. It should be possible for the midwife to deliver the baby as normal. The manoeuvre is aiming to:
  - Rotate the symphysis pubis anteriorly
  - Push the posterior shoulder over the sacrum
  - Open the pelvic inlet to its full capacity
  - Correct any maternal lordosis
  - Remove the sacral promontory as an obstruction

  If the manoeuvre in unsuccessful it is suggested that it is repeated before moving on to another. The McRoberts position is a relatively safe intervention with a good rate of success of 40–50 per cent

- *All fours position.* When there is the suspicion that a mother is at risk of a shoulder dystocia the midwife may suggest that the delivery is conducted with the mother on all fours. This position optimises the sacral curve and is in effective McRoberts upside down. With the mother on all fours she can be encouraged to rock, thereby mimicking the movement of the legs when put into the McRoberts position. This is therefore a useful tool when delivering in a birth centre or in the mother's home
- *Suprapubic pressure.* This is aimed at displacing the anterior shoulder from the symphysis pubis to allow it to enter the pelvis. It is also referred to as Rubins 1:
  - Pressure is applied by the midwife or an assistant to the mother's abdomen, above the baby's back, in a downward direction towards the side of the mother that the baby is facing
  - Whilst this pressure is applied the delivering midwife will continue to try to deliver the baby. The pressure should be continuous initially. If unsuccessful the assistant can be asked to provide pressure in a rocking movement
  These manoeuvres have been shown to be effective in 67 per cent of cases of shoulder dystocia. (Luria et al. 1994)
- *Episiotomy.* It is widely accepted that in the event of a shoulder dystocia occurring, an episiotomy is desirable to prevent further damage to the mother's pelvic floor and to provide space for the 'enter' manoeuvres. However, as routine episiotomy is not current practice it is difficult to know when the optimum time to perform it is. Once the baby's head has delivered it is technically very difficult to ensure the procedure does not damage the baby
- *Rubins 2 and the wood screw manoeuvre* – the 'enter' manoeuvres. These aim to rotate the shoulders into the oblique diameter and are often combined to expedite delivery. The wood screw involves the midwife inserting as much of her hand as possible into the vagina in order to apply pressure to the posterior aspect of the anterior shoulder to turn it to the oblique. During this manoeuvre the mother should be placed in the lithotomy position, or if at home, the McRoberts position. Suprapubic pressure can also be continued. The midwife can also enter her other hand to apply pressure to the anterior aspect of the posterior shoulder in order to provide better rotation. If at any time during the manoeuvre it is seen that the baby has moved, an attempt to deliver should be made. Rubins 2 concentrates on reducing the diameter of the shoulders. Working from behind the baby a shoulder is located and pushed into the oblique. These two procedures can be used together in order to be of most effect

- *Delivery of the posterior arm.* If the previous endeavours have been unsuccessful the last of the 'enter' manoeuvres is when an attempt to deliver the posterior arm is made. The midwife enters in front of the baby's body and locates the lower arm. Pressure is exerted on the elbow to try to make the lower arm raise, this is then grasped and gently pulled across the baby's face in a 'cat lick' motion thereby delivering the posterior shoulder

If the above manoeuvres are unsuccessful the whole round of procedures should be performed again. It is recommended that this is undertaken by another midwife or obstetrician.

Documentation

Every obstetric emergency must be carefully documented after the event. This can be aided by using the mnemonic and writing the time each manoeuvre is performed and by whom. This will enable good debriefing of the parents when they are ready to talk about the event.

Risk management

With the advent of clinical governance, professionals are more accountable to the mothers and are encouraged to learn from events. Reporting forms for all obstetric risk events are available in all units across the country. They allow for accurate audit of events and aid the planning of training programmes designed to keep professionals up to date with current practices in maternity care.

Vaginal breech delivery

Incidence: Babies present by the breech in 15 per cent of babies at 29–32 weeks, and 3–4 per cent of pregnancies at term (Enkin et al. 2000). The later they stay breech, the less likely they are to turn spontaneously.

Risk factors: In the majority of cases there is no explanation why a baby presents by the breech, however it may be due to maternal reasons such as:

- Uterine malformation e.g. bicornuate uterus (a uterus with a division down the middle), fibroids or tumours
- Placenta praevia (when the placenta is situated in the lower uterine segment)

- Oligohydramnious (reduced amount of amniotic fluid) – restricting movement
- Polyhydramnious (increased amount of amniotic fluid) – providing plenty of space for movement
- Multiple pregnancy
- Contracted pelvis
- Primigravid woman (expecting her first baby) with firm uterine and abdominal muscles
- Grand multiparous woman (expecting her fifth or subsequent baby) with lax uterine and abdominal muscles

Or for fetal reasons such as:

- Anomalies, such as anencephaly (partially formed brain)
- Short umbilical cord
- Prematurity
- Lack of tone such as fetal death in utero

A breech is defined when the fetus is lying in a longitudinal position with the buttocks presenting. It may described as:

- *Flexed or complete breech.* The legs are bent at the hips and knees so the baby is sitting cross-legged. This is more common in a multiparous woman or when there is polyhydramnious
- *Extended or frank breech.* The hips are flexed and the knees extended so that the feet are near the head. This is more common in primigravid women with firm uterine and abdominal tone. It is also the most difficult to diagnose as the buttocks may be deeply engaged on abdominal palpation
- *Footling breech.* The foot or feet present before the buttocks. This is rare, but more common in premature gestations
- *Kneeling breech.* This is very uncommon, but occurs when the baby is in a kneeling position

A breech is identified by:

- *Abdominal palpation.* The presenting part will be firm, but not hard and smooth, although this might be difficult to identify if it is deeply engaged. The head may be ballotable (moveable) in the fundus, and the fetal heart may be auscultated above the level of the umbilicus, but again, this may be lower if the breech is deeply engaged
- *Vaginal examination.* The presenting part if breech may be higher in the pelvis prior to labour than when cephalic (head down). If the legs are in the extended position, the breech may be mistaken for the head, especially while the cervix is partially closed

- *Ultrasound scan.* This is conclusive and should screen for anomalies in the fetus and mother at the same time

If a baby is known to be presenting by the breech prior to labour, there are a variety of methods to try to turn the baby, including visualisation techniques, breech tilt exercises, massage, homeopathy, hypnosis, acupuncture, acupressure, moxibustion, chiropractic adjustments and external cephalic version (Banks 1998). However, discussion concerning these are beyond the scope of this chapter.

It is important to remember that if labour proceeds spontaneously and easily, the breech presenting baby should be born without problem. The baby should be born by propulsion, not traction. If labour is not progressing, a caesarean section may be advised. However, it is important to understand that the use of oxytocic drugs to augment labour, or forceful traction by the birth attendant, leads to an increase in poor outcomes such as brain and spinal injuries, particularly if the baby is preterm (Banks 1998; Cronk 1998).

It is commonly thought that the baby's bottom is smaller than the diameter of the head and may pass through a cervix that is not fully dilated. The concern is that the larger head may become trapped behind the cervix. However, this is more likely with preterm infants. For a term infant presenting in a frank breech position, the bottom will be the same size as the head (Banks 1998).

If a woman presents in established labour and a breech presentation is diagnosed, the following procedures will help to promote a safe outcome:

- If ultrasound facilities are available, they should be used to confirm the presentation of the baby and to identify if any obstruction is present such as placenta praevia or a fibroid
- The woman should be enabled to assume whatever position she is comfortable to labour in. Lying prone or semi-recumbent works against the normal physiology of birth. Hands and knees is a good posture to adopt (Cronk 1998). There is a concern that if an upright position is used in the second stage, the placenta may separate from the uterus too quickly because of traction on the cord/placenta just after the birth due to gravity and in the absence of a contraction (Cronk 1998)
- If the woman is semi-recumbent, her legs should be in a lithotomy position and an episiotomy is generally recommended when the buttocks distend the perineum, especially if it is the woman's first birth. If she is upright, this should not be necessary
- Hands should be kept off the breech that is birthing spontaneously. Excessive handling may cause the baby to extend its arm above its head and lead to more complications

- The fetal back needs to rotate anteriorly to the woman. If it is necessary to assist this process, the baby should be supported by the hips. It is not advised to hold the abdomen as damage can occur to the kidneys and adrenal glands
- If required, a finger may be used to flex the knee and abduct the thigh to deliver the legs. They should not be pulled out
- The umbilical cord should not be handled as it may go into spasm
- If necessary, once the tip of the scapulae is visible, the attendant can splint the baby's upper arm between the index and middle finger, then flex it and bring it down over its face, like a cat washing its face. If the arms are extended or nuchal (around the nape of the neck), it may help to undertake a modified Lovsett's manoeuvre. For this, the baby is first rotated by holding the hips and using downward traction, so the posterior arm is brought into an anterior position and then released as described above. If necessary the procedure can be repeated for the second arm by rotating the baby back through a semicircle, ensuring the back remains anterior. This manoeuvre is more likely to be required if the woman is lying on her back. It is rarely needed when an upright position is adopted (Banks 1998)
- Once the nape of the neck is visible, the woman should lean forward if she has been upright. A modified Mauriceau-Smellie-Veit grip may be used to assist the birth of the head, which should be born slowly (see Figure 6.4). The procedure is as follows:
  - Rest the baby with its face and body over your hand and arm with legs either side

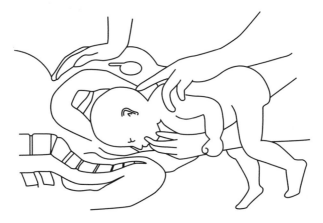

Figure 6.4 Breech presentation

- – Place the first and third fingers of this hand on the baby's cheekbones to encourage flexion of the head. Current advice is to avoid placing a finger in the baby's mouth as this can damage the jaw. An assistant could be asked to push above the mother's pubic bone as the head delivers, to keep the head flexed
- – Use the other hand to grasp the baby's shoulders and flex the baby's head towards its chest, while applying downward pressure to gently deliver the head (WHO 2003)
- Some breech babies will be slow to breathe spontaneously at birth, usually due to shock. It is important to have resuscitation equipment available and ready, and that the parents are aware that this may be required (Cronk 1998)
- As with any event, good communication with the parents is important as well as the maintenance of contemporaneous records

Manual removal of the placenta

Incidence: If delivery of the placenta is delayed beyond 30 minutes, more complications are observed in both physiological and active management. It becomes highest if the delay is over 75 minutes and occurs in approximately 3 per cent of all births (Combs and Laros 1991).

If the third stage is managed physiologically, up to one hour may pass before considering the procedure to be prolonged. With active management it is expected that the placenta and membranes should be expelled by controlled cord traction within 30 minutes. If the placenta is not delivered within an hour, it should be removed manually. Forceful cord traction and fundal pressure should be avoided as they may cause uterine inversion.

If a placenta is retained, it may either be separated or partially separated but trapped; or it may be morbidly adherent (see below) to the uterine wall.

Risk factors: If the placenta is separated or partially separated but trapped, bleeding is more likely as the uterus cannot contract adequately to seal the vessels from the placental site. Risk factors include:

- The cervix reforming
- Full bladder
- Mismanagement of third stage, i.e. performing controlled cord traction or fundal pressure without giving oxytocin

- Formation of a constriction ring or spasm between the upper and lower uterine segment
- Uterine abnormality, e.g. bicornuate uterus

If the placenta is morbidly adherent and there is no separation, bleeding may not occur. Risk factors for this include:

- Previous caesarean section
- Previous placenta praevia
- Previous retained placenta
- High parity

An adherent placenta occurs when there is a scanty or absent layer of decidua basalis (the maternal part of the placenta) at the site of implantation. Types of adherent placenta are:

- *Placenta accreta.* The chorionic villi have adhered to the myometrium
- *Placenta increta.* The chorionic villi invade the myometrium
- *Placenta percreta.* The chorionic villi have penetrated through the myometrium either to or beyond the serosa (outer layer of the uterine wall)

As with any emergency procedure, referral should be made to an appropriately qualified professional, in this case an obstetrician, to undertake a manual removal of the placenta (NMC 2004a). However, it is a procedure all midwives should be familiar with in case of emergency and there is no appropriate assistance available. The following actions will help to promote a safe outcome:

- Call for help. If at home this will be a paramedic ambulance
- If the bladder is not empty, catheterisation will be required
- Oxytocin 10 iu can be given by intramuscular injection if it has not already done for active management of third stage. Do not give ergometrine as it can cause a tonic uterine contraction, which may delay expulsion
- An intravenous infusion should be commenced as soon as possible to provide intravenous access and replace fluid loss
- Analgesia must be given as available. Shock may occur due to pain from the procedure if analgesia is not adequate
- Full aseptic precautions must be taken to minimise risk of infection
- The umbilical cord should be made taut and the attendant's leading hand inserted into the vagina and uterus following the direction of the cord. If the cord has separated, this will still need to be done

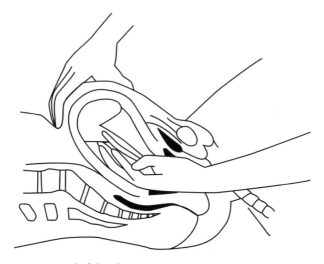

Figure 6.5 Removal of the placenta

- Once the placenta is located, the cord should be released and the fundus supported. This will provide counter-traction to prevent inversion of the uterus
- A separated edge of the placenta should be felt for and the edge of the attendant's hand should be eased between the placenta and the uterine wall (Figure 6.5). A careful slicing motion with the edge of the hand should be used to continue to separate the placenta until it is detached
- The fundus can then be massaged to assist the hand holding the placenta to be expelled from the uterus, still grasping the placenta

Following the procedure:

- The placenta must immediately be inspected for completeness. If any placental lobe or tissue is missing, the uterine cavity must be explored to remove it (see next section)
- An assistant should then massage the fundus of the uterus to encourage a tonic uterine contraction
- An intravenous bolus of oxytocin (10 iu) should be given after successful removal of the placenta, followed by an intravenous infusion of oxytocin
- Observations should be made for:
  - Vital signs (pulse, blood pressure, respirations) at least every 30 minutes for 6 hours or until the woman is stable

- Uterine contraction. The uterine fundus should be palpated and lochia should be monitored to ensure it is not excessive
- Signs of coagulopathy (the ability of the blood to clot), particularly if bleeding has been excessive
- Signs of infection, i.e. fever or foul-smelling vaginal discharge. Intravenous antibiotics should be given prophylactically, according to local protocols

- Intravenous fluid administration should be continued and a blood transfusion considered as necessary

(WHO 2003)

Problems

Tissue that is extremely adherent may be placenta accreta. If the placenta is unable to be separated easily, heavy bleeding or perforation of the uterus may result. There are two choices:

1. A hysterectomy
2. The placenta can be left in situ to be reabsorbed

If the placenta is retained due to a constriction ring, or if hours or days have passed since delivery, it may not be possible to get the entire hand into the uterus. The placenta should be removed in fragments using two fingers, ovum forceps or a wide curette. As with any event, good communication with the parents is important, as well as the maintenance of contemporaneous records.

Manual examination of the uterus

A manual examination of the uterus will be necessary following a manual removal of the placenta. This is because the placenta is likely to be evacuated in pieces and it may be very difficult to ensure it is complete. A careful examination of the uterus will ensure there are no remaining fragments of placental tissue left in situ. If placental fragments are retained, there may initially be minimal blood loss from the vagina. However, there is a high risk that bleeding will eventually occur as retained tissue will prevent the uterus from contracting effectively, and also the risk of infection will be increased.

The procedure for manual examination of the uterus is similar to the technique described for manual removal of the placenta. However, it is important to recognise that efforts to extract fragments of placental tissue that do not separate easily may result in heavy bleeding or uterine perforation, which usually requires hysterectomy. This procedure is carried out by a midwife in an emergency only when no obstetric help is available (NMC 2004a).

Management of postpartum haemorrhage

Incidence: Postpartum haemorrhage (PPH) was the second highest cause of maternal death in the United Kingdom in 2000–2002 (CEMACH 2004) (Figure 6.6). The rate of PPH has not dropped significantly in the last 25 years. Substandard obstetric care was reported in 80 per cent of women who sought treatment.

The definition of a PPH is a blood loss of 500 ml or more of from the genital tract following birth. However, calculation of blood loss is very subjective and is usually underestimated. Emergency treatment should be initiated if the woman becomes symptomatic, or if the blood loss is estimated to be over 1000 ml. The ability of a woman to cope with blood loss depends on her general health status. A primary PPH occurs within 24 hours of birth, and secondary PPH occurs after this time (WHO 2003). Table 6.1 outlines risk factors for a PPH.

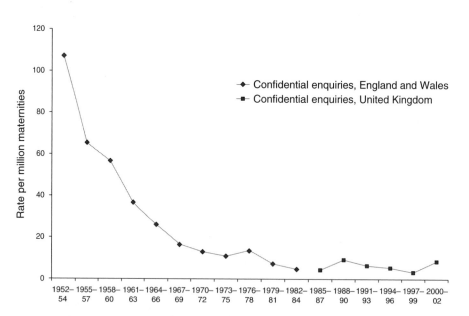

Figure 6.6 Maternal mortality for deaths due to haemorrhage; England and Wales 1952–84; United Kingdom 1984–2002 (CEMACH, 2004)

Table 6.1 Risk Factors for PPH

Antepartum	Intrapartum
Proven abruptio placentae	Delivery by emergency caesarean section
Known placenta praevia	Delivery by elective caesarean section
Multiple pregnancy	Retained placenta
Pre-eclampsia/gestational hypertension	Episiotomy
Nulliparity	Assisted delivery (forceps/vacuum)
Previous PPH	Prolonged third stage (>30 minutes)
Asian ethnicity	Prolonged labour (>12 hours)
Obesity	Big baby (>4 kg)
Previous caesarean section	Pyrexia in labour
	Augmented labour
	Arrest of descent
	Lacerations (cervical/vaginal/perineal)

Source: Combs et al. 1991; AAFP 2000

Management

Once a PPH has been identified, four actions need to occur *simultaneously*, but will be addressed individually. They are: communication; resuscitation; monitoring and investigation; and arresting the haemorrhage.

Communication
- The following should be called for: senior midwife, senior obstetric staff, senior anaesthetic staff. The midwife should alert the haematologist, and a scribe and portering staff should be called for note-taking and the delivery of specimens/blood to appropriate laboratories. If out of hospital, paramedic support will be required. Substandard care frequently relates to failure to involve appropriate senior professionals at an early stage. The consultant obstetrician and anaesthetist must be alerted if not present.

Resuscitation
- Airway, breathing, circulation as discussed in maternal resuscitation above.
- Oxygen by mask at 8 l/min
- Intravenous access with *two* large bore (14–16 G) cannulae
- Commence crystalloid infusion (e.g. Hartmann's solution) (maximum 2 l)

- Alternate with colloid (e.g. Gelofusine, Haemaccel, human albumin 4.5 per cent) (maximum 1.5 l)
- Lie flat/head-down tilt
- Transfuse blood as soon as available (if cross-matched blood is unavailable by the time 3.5 l of clear fluid have been infused, group 'O' Rhesus negative or uncross-matched, own group blood may be used).

Monitoring and investigation

Blood is taken from the woman and various tests performed. Blood should be sent immediately to the laboratory for:

- Cross-matching of 4–6 units
- Full blood count
- Clotting screen

A member of the team observes frequent pulse and blood pressure measurements to monitor the woman's condition. Oxygen saturations are observed; an indwelling urinary catheter is passed in order to monitor urine output; and central venous pressure monitoring is carried out to guide fluid volume replacement.

Arresting the haemorrhage

A haemorrhage may occur as a result of one or more of four causes. The AAFP (2000) identify them as the four Ts, listed in order of frequency, and they all must be considered as the potential cause:

Tone (70%) – Uterine atony is the most common cause of a PPH and should be perceived to be the cause of the bleeding, unless proven otherwise

Trauma (20%) – Cervical, vaginal and perineal lacerations; ruptured uterus; pelvic haematoma; uterine inversion

Tissue (10%) – Retained products (placenta, membranes, clots)

Thrombin (1%) – Coagulopathies

Tone

- Rub up a contraction by rubbing up the fundus: this will stimulate the uterus to contract
- Ensure bladder is empty. Insert an indwelling catheter and leave in situ
- Bimanual compression of the uterus if atony persists. This is done by inserting one hand into the vagina, then making a fist against the body of the uterus inside. The other hand is placed above the uterus and squeezes it against the first hand.

- Give drugs as appropriate:
  - Syntocinon 10 units by slow IV injection or IM if not already given by this route
  - Ergometrine 0.5 mg by slow IV injection
  - Syntocinon infusion at 10 iu per hour (e.g. 40 units in 500 ml Hartmann's at 125 ml/h)
  - Carboprost (Haemabate) 0.25 mg IM (repeated at intervals of not less than 15 minutes to a maximum of eight doses)
- If bleeding persists, transfer to operating theatre and consider the other Ts.

Trauma
If bleeding continues, consider the possibility of lacerations, a ruptured or inverted uterus. Continue bimanual compression until appropriate help is available.

Tissue
- If the placenta is delivered, ensure it is complete
- If the placenta is not delivered, a manual removal of placenta or manual examination of the uterus may be indicated as described previously

Thrombin
Coagulation disorders are very rare and are usually identified in the antenatal period. However, a large blood loss from one of the above causes may lead to the blood clotting mechanisms to become deranged. This is identified through blood clotting studies.

As with any event, documentation is vital, particularly fluid input and output, drugs given, who was present and what was done in what order, with timings. A scribe has a very important role in emergency scenarios and enables accurate, contemporaneous record keeping.

Following the event, it is helpful to use the documentation to debrief the woman and her family, as well as the staff.

Management of an eclamptic seizure

Eclampsia is defined as one or more convulsions occurring during or immediately after pregnancy, as a complication of pre-eclampsia (APEC 2005).

Before effective management of an eclamptic seizure can be undertaken, it is important that the signs and risk factors of severe pre-eclampsia/eclampsia are discussed, because rapid recognition may prevent progression to eclampsia.

Incidence: Severe pre-eclampsia/eclampsia is a major factor in maternal and fetal mortality and morbidity, and if not detected and monitored at the earliest opportunity can sometimes progress to eclampsia extremely rapidly.

- Five in 1000 women in the UK will suffer severe pre-eclampsia in pregnancy and for five in 10,000 women this will lead to eclampsia
- The mortality rate from severe pre-eclampsia/eclampsia is 1.8 per cent whilst those who will suffer from major complications the rate is 35 per cent (RCOG 2006)
- Eclampsia remains the second leading cause of maternal deaths in the UK and substandard care is constantly stated as being a major factor in a number of deaths (CEMACH 2004)
- In 2000–2002, CEMACH (2004) reported 14 maternal deaths due to pre-eclampsia or eclampsia
- Pre-eclampsia/eclampsia is the single leading identifiable risk factor in pregnancy associated with stillbirth. Twenty per cent of stillbirths are due to this cause in otherwise viable babies (Confidential Enquiry into Stillbirths and Deaths in Infancy 1997)
- Serious morbidity associated with pre-eclampsia/eclampsia can occur from 20 weeks' gestation to after delivery. It should be noted that the earlier pre-eclampsia presents, the more serious it can be. Onset prior to 32 weeks' gestation has the most serious outcome, with many women needing delivery within 72 hours (Sibai et al. 1994)

The midwife is usually the first professional in a position to detect pre-eclampsia and it is vital that she involves the obstetricians immediately so a management plan can be put in place and attempt to prevent progression to eclampsia.

Risk factors:
- First pregnancy
- Age 40 years or above
- History of pre-eclampsia in a mother or sister
- History of previous pre-eclampsia/eclampsia
- Body mass index >35 at booking
- Multiple pregnancies
- Pre-existing vascular disease, for example diabetes, hypertension or renal disease (PRECOG 2004)

Signs and symptoms

It is important to note that some women who present with eclampsia will have *no* pre-existing signs or symptoms. Therefore, the midwife must be aware of the risk factors of developing pre-eclampsia at booking and refer and monitor closely throughout the pregnancy. Women also need to be informed of symptoms of worsening disease so they are able to alert the midwife if they have any concerns.

Hypertension

Hypertension is said to occur when the diastolic blood pressure (BP) is 90 mm/HG or more on two occasions and the systolic BP is above 140 mm/Hg or above. The CEMACH Report (2004) has highlighted that whilst diastolic BP is one of the important indices of the severity of pre-eclampsia it is thought that it is the systolic BP which causes intracerebral haemorrhage. It therefore recommended that antihypertensive treatment should be considered for a systolic BP of 160 mmHG or above. However, if signs of severe disease are present, medication should be commenced at lower levels (RCOG 2006).

It should also be noted that eclampsia is not always preceded by severe hypertension, with 34 per cent of eclamptic women having a maximum diastolic BP of 100 mm/Hg or below (PRECOG 2004). Automatic BP devices will measure BP lower than a conventional sphygmomanometer (CEMD 2002). Therefore, a baseline reading with an automatic device should be compared with a conventional device so accurate comparisons can be made. The mercury sphygmomanometer remains the gold standard against which new BP monitor accuracy is judged (MHRA, 2005).

Proteinuria

A dipstick analysis of urine that reveals a 2+ of proteinuria or more should be confirmed by a 24-hour urine collection. A urine protein excretion of 300 mg or more over 24 hours is significant (PRECOG 2004).

NB Whenever BP is measured in pregnancy a urine sample should be tested for proteinuria at the same time. The CEMD Report (2002) highlighted that midwives had failed to test for proteinuria in women who went on to develop severe pre-eclampsia.

Severe headaches

These could be a sign of cerebral involvement.

Visual disturbances

Due to papilloedema, this is a swelling of the optic nerve and a sign of increased intracranial pressure.

Vomiting
One of the signs of increased intracranial pressure is vomiting.

Epigastric Pain
This is of particular concern if severe and may be associated with vomiting. It will be described by the woman as severe and there will be tenderness on palpation (PRECOG 2004).

Signs of clonus
Clonus is rapid rhythmic movements and is described as alternate muscle relaxation and contraction resulting in brisk reflexes.

Small for gestational age fetus
This could be one of the first signs of pre-eclampsia and occurs in 30 per cent of pre-eclamptic pregnancies (RCOG 2006). It is important that fundal height is measured, any abnormalities reported and a growth scan arranged if indicated.

Reduced fetal movements
This may indicate fetal compromise due to placental insufficiency.

Analysis of blood

Blood tests can provide important information about the severity of the disease and to what extent the maternal system has been affected. It is recommended that these are repeated *daily* when the results are normal, but more frequently if the clinical condition changes (RCOG 2006). Full blood counts, urea and electrolytes and liver function tests should be obtained to detect worsening disease, possible renal failure and HELLP (haemolysis, elevated liver enzymes, low platelets) syndrome.

Platelets
A falling platelet count is associated with worsening disease. Below 100 may mean there is an associated coagulation abnormality and clotting studies are indicated (RCOG 2006).

Alanine Aminotransferase (ALT) / Aspartate Aminotransferase (AST)
Above 75 iu/l is significant and above 150 iu/l is associated with increased morbidity to the mother (RCOG 2006).

Urates
Rising urate rates can indicate worsening disease. Normal rates are between 0.149 and 0.369 mmol/l.

Creatinine
Rising level can indicate renal involvement with risk of renal failure. Normal rates are between 62 and 106 umol/l.

Management of an eclamptic seizure

It should be noted that 44 per cent of women will have their first fit within 48 hours following delivery, 38 per cent in the antenatal period and 18 per cent during labour (APEC 2005). Almost 2 per cent of women suffering eclamptic seizures will die, 23 per cent will require ventilation and 35 per cent will have at least one major complication, including pulmonary oedema, renal failure, disseminated intravascular coagulation, HELLP syndrome, acute respiratory distress syndrome, stroke or cardiac arrest. Stillbirth or neonatal death occurs in approximately 1 in 14 cases of eclampsia (Munro 2000).

Help from a senior obstetrician and anaesthetist should be summoned. If in the community an emergency ambulance manned by paramedics must always be summoned and the woman should be protected from injury during the convulsion. Following convulsion the woman should be placed in a left lateral position and given oxygen. Assessment of the airway, breathing and circulation is required as well as measurement of blood pressure, pulse, temperature and oxygen saturation.

If not already instigated, intravenous access is required. In the treatment of eclampsia and pre-eclampsia magnesium sulphate is the anticonvulsant of choice (CEMACH 2004). A loading dose of magnesium sulphate 4 g should be given by infusion pump over 5–10 minutes, followed by a maintainence dose of 1 g/hr for 24 hours after the last seizure. (RCOG 2006).

Antihypertensive therapy is required to reduce the BP and this is provided according to local protocol. Blood is taken from the woman and is sent for grouping and saved. A full blood count, analysis of urea and electrolytes along with tests for liver function and clotting are also required.

If the woman is suffering breathing problems as a result of laryngeal oedema or if she is presenting with status eclampticus (continuous convulsions) she will require intubation and ventilation (Arulkumaran et al. 1997).

Fetal monitoring is required to assess fetal wellbeing if the baby is not already delivered. Delivery should be undertaken as soon as the maternal condition is stable as this is the only definite way to resolve the crisis (Arulkumaran et al. 1997).

An accurate fluid balance must be maintained. This is important as another cause of maternal death from pre-eclampsia/eclampsia is pulmonary oedema which can be attributed to fluid overload. Strict and vigilant fluid balance is essential. Fluids should be restricted to 85 ml/hr and hourly urine output measured using an indwelling urinary catheter (CEMD 2002). Urinary output of <30 ml/h is significant and must always be reported to an obstetrician/anaesthetist.

Pre-eclampsia/eclampsia remains one of the leading causes of maternal deaths in the UK. Therefore, the midwife needs to be aware of the risk factors and signs of the disease and ensure that women are screened regularly throughout pregnancy. Women who are high risk must be referred early for specialist care. If pre-eclampsia is detected, prompt referral must be made so the woman can be assessed and monitored appropriately. This will ensure that she receives optimum care and in some cases progression to eclampsia may be prevented.

Conclusion

Emergency scenarios occur both in and out of hospital. Fortunately, they are relatively uncommon in the community setting where midwives are more likely to be working without close access to obstetric support. However, it is midwives in these settings who will have to be prepared to carry out these procedures should the need arise.

When faced with an emergency situation, the key points are to:

- Call for appropriate help – paramedic assistance out of the hospital setting
- Deal with the emergency
- Work effectively as a team – good communication required
- Document the events and action taken clearly – this is a professional requirement (NMC 2004) and helpful for analysis of the event. Remember that if it's not written it didn't happen!
- Report the incident through the incident reporting system
- Debrief after the event with colleagues and a Supervisor of Midwives
- Reflect on the event

If possible, a member of the team should be allocated to remain with the woman and her partner to ensure communication and offer support throughout the emergency situation (NICE 2006).

References

Action on Pre-Eclampsia/Eclampsia (2005) www.apec.org.uk (accessed January 2007).

American Acadamy of Family Physicians (2000) *Advanced Life Saving in Obstetrics (ALSO) Provider Manual*, 4th edition. Kansas: AAFP.

Arulkumaran, S., Ratnam, S. S. and Bhasker Rao, K. (1997) *The Management of Labour*. India: Orient Longman.

Banks, M. (1998) *Breech Birth Woman-wise*. New Zealand: Birthspirit Books.

Clinical Negligence Scheme for Trusts (2006) *Maternity Clinical Risk Management Standards* (April). London: NHS Litigation Authority.

Coates, T. (2004) Shoulder dystocia. In *Mayes Midwifery*, 13th edition. London: Baillière Tindall.

Combs, C. A. and Laros, R. K. (1991) Prolonged third stage of labor: morbidity and risk factors. *Obstetrics and Gynecology* 77: 863–7.

Combs, C. A., Murphy, E. L. and Laros, R. K. (1991) Factors associated with postpartum hemorrhage with vaginal birth. *Obstetrics and Gynecology* 77: 69.

Confidential Enquiries into Maternal Deaths in the United Kingdom (2002) *Why Mothers Die 1997–1999*. London: RCOG Press.

Confidential Enquiry into Maternal and Child Health (2004) *Why Mothers Die 2000–2002. The Sixth Report*. London: RCOG Press.

Confidential Enquiry into Stillbirths and Deaths in Infancy (1997) *6th Annual Report*. London: Maternal and Child Health Research Consortium.

Cronk, M. (1998) Midwifery skills needed for breech birth. *Midwifery Matters* 78 (Autumn).

Eden, R., Siefert, L., Winegar, A. and Spellacy, W. N. (1987) Perinatal characteristics of uncomplicated post-dates pregnancy. *Obstetrics and Gynacology* 69 (3, pt 1): 296–9.

Enkin, M., Keirse, M., Neilson, J. et al. (2000) *A Guide to Effective Care in Pregnancy and Childbirth*, 3rd edition. Oxford: Oxford University Press.

Gibb, D. (1995) Clinical focus: shoulder dystocia. *The Obstetrics. Clinical Risk* 1(2): 49–54.

Lee, R., Rodgers, B. and White, L. (1986) Cardiopulmonary resuscitation of pregnant women. *American Journal of Medicine* 81: 311–18.

Luria, S., Ben-Arie, A. and Hagay, Z. (1994) The ABC of shoulder dystocia management. *Asia-Oceania Journal of Obstetrics and Gynaecology* 20(2): 195–7.

Medicines and Healthcare Products Regulatory Agency (2005) *Report of the Independent Advisory Group on Blood Pressure Monitoring in Clinical Practice*. London: MHRA.

Morris, S. and Stacey, M. (2003) ABC of resuscitation. Resuscitation in pregnancy. *British Medical Journal* 327(7426): 1277–9.

Munro, P. T. (2000) Management of eclampsia in the accident and emergency department. *Journal Accident and Emergency Medicine* 17(1): 7–11.

National Institute for Health and Clinical Excellence (2006) *Intrapartum Care: Care of Healthy Women and Their Babies during Childbirth.* Draft guideline for consultation. London: NICE.

Nursing and Midwifery Council (2004a) *Midwives Rules and Standards.* London: NMC.

Nursing and Midwifery Council (2004b) *Standards of Proficiency for Pre-registration Midwifery Education.* London: NMC.

Palme-Kilander, C. (1992) Methods of resuscitation in low Apgar score in newborn infants – a national survey. *Acta Paediatrica* 81: 739–44.

Pre-Eclampsia Community Guideline (2004) www.apec.org.uk (accessed January 2007).

Resuscitation Council (UK) (2005) *Resuscitation Guidelines.* London: Resuscitation Council.

Royal College Obstetricians and Gynaecologists (2006) *The Management of Severe Pre-eclampsia/Eclampsia.* Guideline No. 10A. London: RCOG.

Sibai, B. M., Mercer, B. M., Schiff, E. and Friedman, S. A. (1994) Aggressive versus expectant management of severe pre-eclampsia at 28 to 32 weeks' gestation: a randomised controlled trial. *American Journal Obstetrics and Gynaecology* 171(3): 818–22.

Smith, R. B., Lane, C. and Pearson, J. F. (1994) Shoulder dystocia: What happens at the next delivery? *British Journal of Obstetrics and Gynaecology* 101: 713–15.

Stables, D. (1999) *Physiology in Childbearing with Anatomy and Related Biosciences.* Edinburgh: Baillière Tindall.

Ueland, K., Akamatsu, T. J., Eng, M. et al. (1972) Maternal cardiovascular dynamics: caesarean section under epidural anaesthesia without epinephrine. *American Journal of Obstetrics and Gynecology* 114(6): 775–80.

Webster's New World Medical Dictionary (2003) 2nd edition. New York: Wiley.

World Health Organisation (2003) *Managing Complications in Pregnancy and Childbirth: A Guide for Midwives and Doctors.* Geneva: WHO.

Initial Assessment and Examination of the Newborn Baby

Lyn Dolby

Introduction

The *Midwives Rules and Standards* (NMC 2004a) clearly highlight a midwife's responsibility. Contained within this document is an extract from the EU Second Midwifery Directive 80/155/EEC Article 4 – activities of a midwife, which midwives within the EU member states are entitled to take up and pursue. Some of the responsibilities and activities from both documents are directly related to the recognition of neonatal normality and abnormality; the need to take emergency action and referral to the paediatric team. Both documents highlight the midwife's role in aiding the mother to care for her baby; observe and record normal progress; and offer information on health issues that may directly or indirectly affect the health of mother and baby These key responsibilities are also stated in Standard 15 as set out in the Standards of Proficiency for Pre-registration Midwifery Education (NMC 2004b). Therefore, by fulfilling the requirements expected within a midwifery programme of study, each student midwife should have achieved the agreed standard of competence, which qualified practice will further refine.

This chapter focuses on the immediate care and assessment of the baby at birth. The primary role of the midwife and key areas of the initial neonatal assessment and examination are highlighted.

The midwife's immediate role

The birth of a baby is a significant event in the life of its parents. For many mothers the minutes after birth are filled with emotions, including concern about the baby's condition. At birth the midwife's immediate concern is usually related to the baby's ability to accomplish the initial changes that are required in order to adapt and survive outside the uterus, such as the initial physiological changes in heart function. A midwife's ability and attitude at this time are extremely important in providing information the mother can understand.

Conversely, the baby's condition may not be good at birth or there may be an obvious physical abnormality. Occasionally, an abnormality that was not detected antenatally presents at birth. This may be due to a number of factors, for example:

- Some conditions cannot be screened for
- The mother declined any form of screening
- A comprehensive ultrasound scan was not possible in a multiple pregnancy

It is the midwife's sensitivity, professional experience and the actions that she takes which enable the parents to cope once the initial impact sinks in. However, it is paramount that the midwife voices her concerns to the parents followed by an explanation regarding the action that she is going to take.

The immediate care and handling of the baby should provide the parents with a professional and appropriate role model at all times – for example, limbs are not handles with which to turn a baby. Good support to the baby's body and an explanation of the baby's immature muscle and nervous system control may help parents understand how to avoid causing trauma to their baby's shoulder girdle or hip joints. Information should be appropriate to the individuals concerned.

The midwife is responsible for assessing and recording the initial vital signs of the baby (see later in this chapter), thus providing a comprehensive record of the baby's condition at birth and during the first few hours of life.

The initial introduction of the baby to his parents and, when appropriate, how the midwife assists the mother with the baby's first feed are important landmarks for the baby and his parents. Both events link with the need to observe the initial parent–baby attachment process. Factors arising prior to and during pregnancy can affect these processes, for example, maternal abuse, domestic violence, environmental and social concerns (for example, housing and sanitation) or the circumstances under which the pregnancy was conceived. If this initial attachment process is affected, good communication, both verbal and written, with members of the midwifery team and other health care providers is paramount, as it enables all professionals involved to be well informed of the situation.

Comprehensive record keeping is essential if the midwife is to demonstrate that she has acted in accordance with her professional responsibility, local guidelines/procedures and parental wishes (NMC 2005). The woman's record should provide information regarding an agreed plan of care, midwifery/obstetric and paediatric involvement including actions taken and why, any changes required and the rationale for so doing, maternal consent when required, observations performed and any other information as it arises. Information about the antenatal and intrapartum period may relate to the condition of the baby at or soon after birth. Reading notes made by other staff and providing comprehensive notes at the time of giving care is not a luxury but a professional requirement.

The initial assessment and examination at birth

Assessment

Assessing the condition of the baby at birth is, in the first instance, by means of the Apgar scoring system (Table 7.1), followed by a complete physical examination in order to confirm normality or detect any anomalies.

Dr Virginia Apgar devised this scoring system in the 1950s. It consists of a systematic assessment of five key factors, each significant in determining the health status of the baby. Each factor is given a score of 0–2, thus the overall condition of the baby can be determined by calculating the score out of a total of 10. The Apgar score is usually calculated at 1 minute and again at 10 minutes. A score of 0–3 at 1 minute indicates a baby that is in poor condition, requires

Table 7.1 The Apgar scoring system

Sign	0	1	2
Appearance (colour)	Blue, pale	Body pink, limbs blue	All pink
Apex beat	Absent	Below 100	Above 100
Grimace (response to stimuli)	None	Grimace	Cry
Activity (muscle tone)	Limp	Some limb flexion	Active movements, limbs well flexed
Respiratory effort	None	Slow, irregular	Good, strong cry

resuscitation and possibly ventilation, whereas a score of 7–10 at 1 minute indicates a baby that is in good condition and is able to make the adaptations necessary for extrauterine life. A good account of the Apgar scoring system can be found in Johnson and Taylor (2006).

Examination of the newborn baby

In the United Kingdom, each baby is given a neonatal discharge examination within a few days of birth (usually within 24 hours) by a midwife (who holds an additional qualification in Examination of the Newborn), paediatrician, GP or neonatal nurse specialist. This examination is more extensive than the initial assessment and examination performed by the midwife immediately after birth.

However, although the above examination will usually be performed, it is still the responsibility of the midwife to conduct a *comprehensive* physical examination of the newborn immediately following birth. This initial examination provides information regarding the initial parameters of health and well-being of the baby at birth.

Preparation

Under normal circumstances the initial examination can be performed within the first hour of birth after the parents have had time to look at and cuddle their baby. The process of the examination should be explained to the parents and their consent obtained. Make sure that the parents can easily see the examination process and that the lighting is good – natural daylight is excellent but not always available. Hands should be washed and dried prior to the examination and everything required should be close at hand – for example, scales and baby clothes. The examination itself should be performed quickly and comprehensively, only uncovering the part of the baby to be examined and re-covering the baby as soon as is practicable.

Prior to commencing the examination, look at:

- The baby generally
- Its posture
- Activity
- Respiratory effort
- Cry and colour

With these factors in mind, you can address any urgent requirements. However, continued observation of these five key points will aid ongoing assessment and detection of any negative changes that may occur during the physical examination itself.

Thermoregulation

A baby emerges from the warm uterine environment (37 °C+) to a much lower temperature of approximately 21 °C. Loss of body heat (particularly from the head) can occur quickly as the baby's skin is wet and the baby has a large ratio of surface area to body mass and a relatively thin layer of insulating subcutaneous fat. A drop of 1–2 °C can occur during the immediate post-birth period. Failure to recognise this can lead to a baby not being able to regain a normal body temperature for 4–8 hours (Black and Rose 2000).

The risk of the baby becoming hypothermic (low body temperature) will increase if the baby has not been dried adequately, is pre-term or is less than the expected weight for its gestational age This is because small and/or pre-term babies have less brown fat to utilise for energy/heat production. Brown fat (also known as brown adipose tissue) is present in the body of newborn babies and is used to generate body heat. In terms of the baby's body temperature one must be aware that the presence of infection may cause the baby's temperature to rise as well as fall.

As the need to prevent hypothermia is important, the room and cot in which the baby is to be examined needs to be warm (turn fans off) with no draughts (close windows/doors). It is also good practice to assess the temperature of the baby before commencing the examination and maintain awareness of the baby's temperature during the examination. In some practice sites, checking the temperature of the baby may not be routine, but assessing the warmth of the baby's chest and upper back with the hand during the examination is good practice. It must also be borne in mind that when using thermometers to measure temperature, their accuracy depends on the site and technique used (Scanga et al. 2000).

The head

Observe the shape and symmetry of the head, bearing in mind that these may be influenced by the presence of moulding (see below) or caput succedaneum (see below). The whole head needs to be examined for the presence of trauma (e.g. forceps marks, fetal scalp electrode or amnihook lacerations) or bruising (e.g. ventouse cup). In the event of any bruising, the parents should be told that the baby is likely to demonstrate physiological jaundice due to the increased breakdown of red blood cells.

The suture lines on the skull should be easily palpable and may be found to be overriding due to the pressures exerted during labour – a process known as moulding. The parents should be reassured and made aware that this will resolve over the next 24–48 hours.

The oedematous area on the fetal scalp in the vicinity of the presenting part of the head, is known as caput succedaneum. The oedema can cross suture lines and is more obvious after prolonged labour, but will usually only remain evident for a short while, usually disappearing within 48 hours.

Sometimes a soft, bruised-looking swelling is visible, which is restricted by the bone margins over which it is localised (usually the parietal bones). This is known as a cephalhaematoma. It is due to a localised subperiosteal haemorrhage, often occurring as the result of no apparent trauma except for the usual pressure that occurs on the presenting part of the fetal head. Parents will need to be reassured that the cephalhaematoma will gradually reabsorb, usually over a period of three months. If bilateral cephalhaematomas are present, they may take longer to disappear. In an extremely small proportion of cases, a fracture may be suspected and if present will be seen on an x-ray.

The cranial fontanelles should be observed for normality. The posterior fontanelle located at the junction of the lambdoid and sagittal sutures is usually triangular and measures approximately 0.5 cm at birth, closing shortly afterwards.

The anterior fontanelle measures approximately 3–4 cm at the largest diameter. It usually closes between 18 months and 2 years of age. A large fontanelle may be found in the premature baby or due to hydrocephalus, a small one may indicate microcephaly. If the fontanelle appears raised or tense, this may be associated with hydrocephalus or indicate raised intracranial pressure or infection. However, a depressed fontanelle may suggest that the baby is dehydrated. This is very rarely seen at birth and tends to be a late sign of dehydration.

Occasionally, a third fontanelle is found between the anterior and posterior fontanelles, the size of which can be variable. It can be indicative of congenital abnormalities (e.g. trisomy 21).

The occipital-frontal circumference is noted and provides a record, for example, in the event of hydrocephalus occurring. Place the centimetre scale of the tape measure 1 cm above the nasal bridge, encircle the largest diameter and note the measurement in the Neonatal Record. The measurement tends to be more accurate if the baby's head is lifted off the mattress (caput can distort the measurement); alternatively, the measurement can be taken when the baby is being held. The degree of moulding can affect the measurement noted. To prevent paper cuts, the tape measure should be shortened and the tape itself not dragged round the head when the measurement has been completed.

The face

The face should appear relatively symmetrical, with the eyes, nose and mouth lying in a normal relationship to each other. Observation of the face assesses normality and for signs of any dysmorphic features, such as low set ears (see below). However, make sure that you see both parents before assuming that a certain feature is part of a syndrome – it may just familial.

Eyes

Check that two eyes are actually present, assessing their size and shape. If the eye sits at a slight angle, this may be a racial characteristic (e.g. Chinese) or due to a genetic anomaly (e.g. trisomy 21). Eyelashes should turn outwards and there should be very little discharge. The features around them such as the epicanthic folds, eyelids and eyebrows should appear normal. The pupil should be round and not cloudy or silvery in appearance – often indicative of neonatal cataracts. Both eyes usually can be seen to move normally, but it is normal for a squint to be seen at this stage due to the immaturity of the muscles controlling the eyeball. The sclera should be white and clear, whereas a yellow discolouration points to jaundice and a blue sclera can be found in babies with osteogenesis imperfecta (brittle bones). Occasionally, a subconjunctival haemorrhage is present due to pressure exerted during the birth, so reassure the parents that this will disappear over time. A baby of even a few hours old is able to fix its eyes (an ability known as fixation) on an object or face and follow it if it moves.

Ears

Correct positioning of the ear can be determined by tracing an imaginary line horizontally across the eyes – and when looking straight down at the baby – and noting if the top of the pinna is positioned above this line. To produce a reasonably true horizontal line, you need to draw an imaginary line from the inner canthus of the eyes. Do not use the outer canthus as your point of reference, as these can change according to the slant of the eye due to race or anomalies.

Examine the ear and behind it for any skin tags, dimples or peri-auricular sinuses. At term, the ears should contain enough cartilage to allow them to 'spring' back into position if they are folded over slightly. The pinna should be of normal appearance with well-defined curves in the upper part, and the ear lobe should be a normal size and shape. Check that the orifice of each ear is not obviously blocked. Babies often have ears just like one of its parents or a grand-parent so always ask – 'sensitively'!

Nose

Note the shape of the nose and width of the bridge. It is not unusual to find a nose that has been squashed at birth and may not appear straight. However, if the baby is able to breathe easily, it is usually not a problem and it will revert to normal fairly soon. Babies are obligatory nose breathers, thus anything obstructing inhalation and exhalation will cause a problem. In respiratory illness, flaring of the nostrils is often observed. Quite often a baby may sneeze and the parents will need to be reassured that a sneeze is nature's way of blowing their baby's nose.

Lips

The lips should be complete and symmetrical, as asymmetry may indicate the presence of a facial palsy. The mouth should look in proportion to the face. A small mouth can be due to micrognathia (underdevelopment of the jaw), which is often associated with underlying abnormality.

The presence of a cleft (unilateral or bilateral) in the upper lip should be noted and referred. Internally, the hard and soft palate should be felt with a finger (noting if the suckle reflex is normal) and by visualising with a light source. Encourage the baby to open its mouth so that you can see and feel for any natal teeth round the alveolar ridges (gums) or other anomalies, and inspect the colour of the mucous membranes. Natal teeth are often removed as they can become loose and if so could be inhaled, obstructing the airway, so referral to the paediatric team is required.

The presence of one or two harmless white spots (Epstein's pearls) may be seen, usually on the soft palate. As the baby moves its tongue in the mouth, observe its condition, position, presence of cysts or dimples and the length of the frenulum as a short frenulum may interfere with feeding.

Neck

Babies tend to have short necks in proportion to their bodies. Observe both physically and visually if there are any swellings that may indicate, for example, a sternomastoid tumour or cystic hygroma (caused by a blockage in the lymphatic system). Any signs of webbing or thick/loose skin at the back of the neck should be noted. The former may be associated with Turner's syndrome and the latter may indicate a chromosomal abnormality such as trisomy 21.

Clavicles

The clavicles (the bones that run from either side of the sternum [breastbone] to the shoulder) should be examined with the index finger to check that there are no indentations or crepitus to be felt and that they are intact. Babies that may be more at risk of clavicular fracture include those who have had an assisted breech delivery, where there was shoulder dystocia at birth or if a palsy (for example, Erb's palsy) is suspected. Do not presume that a baby with a clavicular fracture cannot move its arm or that it will not elicit a Moro reflex (see reflexes) – some can.

Arms and hands

Both arms should be gently straightened and compared for equality of length. Any signs of fracture or bruising should be recorded and referred. The arms should move freely and demonstrate good muscle tone. A baby in the first week of life will exhibit flexed arms and closed fists. As the baby gets older, a more open posture will be adopted.

Encourage the baby to open his hand by gently tapping on the back of his hand or the inner aspect of the associated wrist. If this does not work, encourage the baby to grasp your fingers with the opposite hand and let go of the hand that you want him to open. You need to be able to visualise the palm for the number of palmer creases, as a single crease can suggest a chromosomal abnormality (for example, trisomy 21). An open palm also enables you to detect any anomalies such as extra digits that may be hidden by a closed fist. How many creases should there be?

The digits of the hand should be counted and the nails visualised for any sign of paronychia (inflammation of the folds of skin surrounding the fingernail) as infection may occur as a consequence. Any polydactyly (extra digits) or syndactyly (webbed digits) should be noted and referred. Both of these conditions can be associated with particular syndromes (for example, trisomy 21) or be familial in origin.

The chest

The general appearance of the chest should be noted for colour, shape and birthmarks or skin tags.

Movement on respiration should be symmetrical and the heart-beat should not be clearly visible on the skin surface. The respiratory rate can be easily counted and should be approximately 20 breaths per minute during sleep and 30–60 breaths per minute when awake. Any signs of respiratory distress, characterised by intercostal and sternal recession (where the chest wall is pulled inwards), tachypnoea (rapid breathing), grunting on expiration, cyanosis (where the baby's colour changes), nasal flaring or periods of apnoea (greater that 20 seconds) should be referred to a paediatrician immediately. These factors can be indicative of respiratory disease. It is not unusual for the baby born by caesarean section to demonstrate a transient tachypnoea, as the pressure exerted on the baby that aids removal of excess fluids during a vaginal delivery has not occurred.

If necessary the apex beat can be counted by putting a stethoscope over the heart – fourth intercostal space, midclavicular line – noting the rate and rhythm. Normal heart rate usually falls within the range of 110–160 beats per minute, but can be extremely variable over the first 48 hours of life. During sleep the heart rate will slow (sometimes to 90 beats per minute) but will rise in direct relation to an increase in the level of consciousness and activity.

In the term baby the nipples and areolae should be well formed and aligned symmetrically on the chest. If the nipples are wide spaced (distance between is greater than 25 per cent of the chest circumference), this may indicate the presence of a congenital disorder such as Turner's syndrome. Accessory (or supernumerary) nipples should be noted and the parents made aware of them. Accessory nipples can be found anywhere from the breast to the groin. Usually there is little or no breast tissue underlying the accessory nipple, particularly the further away from the breast that they are found.

The abdomen

The abdomen should appear relatively smooth and rounded, slightly pot-bellied and move in synchrony with respiratory effort. Refer to the paediatrician if there are any birthmarks or obvious swellings.

Check that the umbilical cord is securely clamped and that the clamp itself is not too near to the skin at the base of the cord as this can cause abrasion and encourage infection. It must be remembered that the cord if not properly cared for can provide an entry site for bacteria, straight to some of the major organs of the body. Therefore, assessing the base of the cord for inflammation, haemorrhage and signs of infection and discussing how to cleanse the area (during the daily examination) with the parents is a necessary part of care.

Male genitalia

Overall appearance should be assessed, noting any general deviations from the normal. The penis should be at least 2.5 cm in length (a micro-penis of less than 2.5 cm requires referral). Sometimes the penis may appear short due to a swollen scrotum in which case the base of the penis will need to be felt for.

The urethral meatus should lie centrally at the tip of the penis and when the baby passes urine, a good flow should be seen. Referral to a paediatrician should be made if hypospadias (urethral opening on the underside of the penis) or epispadias (urethral opening on the upper side of the penis) is found as a malpositioned meatus may be associated with abnormalities of the urethra and kidneys.

The foreskin is adherent to the glans penis until the child is between 3–10 years of age. Therefore, no attempt should be made to make the foreskin retract as this can lead to phimosis, inflammation and infection.

The scrotal sac should be palpated on both sides in order to palpate each individual testis. The testes in most newborn babies will have descended by 40 weeks' gestation. However, in a small number of babies one testis may not have yet descended and in only a few cases, both may remain undescended. Referral to the paediatrician must be made in the latter case as further investigation may be required in relation to ambiguous genitalia and prevention of torsion and later sterility. The colour of the scrotal sac may be darker depending on cultural heredity (e.g. Asian or black parents). The scrotal sac may also appear bruised or swollen due to trauma during delivery. However, a hydrocele (collection of fluid around the scrotum) or a scrotum that appears very swollen and/or discoloured needs referral for further assessment in case of hernia, haematoma or torsion of the testis.

Female genitalia

Parents often ask if the genitalia of their baby girl is normal. This is because in relation to a woman, the labia majora are relatively large, covering the labia minora.

As with the male infant, the labia can appear bruised or swollen due to the pressures exerted during birth. The labia can also be pigmented if the child is born to parents who are not Caucasian, but it can also be an early finding in congenital adrenal hyperplasia.

The vaginal orifice should be clearly visualised and the hymen may be clearly present. Occasionally it may be perceived that the hymen is imperforate as it may bulge slightly. It is also possible to mistake a bulging hymen for an enlarged Bartholin gland. Vaginal skin tags may be present. Most will disappear but some may require treatment so their presence should be discussed with a paediatrician.

Soon after birth a slightly blood-stained or creamy white discharge from the baby's vagina may be noted. This is a normal occurrence due to the withdrawal of maternal hormones after birth. The parents need to be reassured that all is normal, as sometimes this 'pseudo-menstruation' can, in rare cases, present as a mini-period. However, the duration of the blood loss should not be overly prolonged or excessive.

The clitoris can appear large in small-for-dates and preterm babies, but its size needs to be assessed in comparison to other associated structures. However, if the size of the clitoris arouses concern, paediatric referral to explore the possibility of indeterminate sex is required.

The urethral meatus is more difficult to locate in the female baby, but it should lie in a normal position between the clitoris and the vaginal orifice. When the urinary stream is observed, the flow should be good.

Anus

The position of the anal opening is best assessed in relation to its distance from the coccyx and other structures such as the base of the scrotum in males and the posterior fourchette in females. An anteriorly positioned anus may be associated with conditions such as malformation of the rectum and constipation in later life. It is necessary to visualise the anus clearly, as it is possible to mistake a large fistula for the anal opening.

The first stool to be passed from the bowel is known as meconium. On close inspection it can be observed that meconium is actually a dark green colour and not black as it is often perceived. The anus cannot be deemed patent until meconium has actually been seen to pass through the anal orifice, as it is possible that it may emerge from the urethral of vaginal orifice instead due to a fistula.

Legs and feet

As with the arms, the legs should be assessed for symmetry, equality of length, muscle tone and flexion. It should be remembered that newborns have a natural stricture behind the knees and therefore forcibly straightening them causes discomfort. Putting knees together with the feet placed flat on the cot mattress usually provides a good method for assessing leg length. Run the fingers down the major bones of the legs in order to assess for fractures or malformations.

The dorsal (upper) part of the foot should easily line up with the anterior (front) aspect of the shin. Sometimes the line of the foot is offset, a condition known as talipes, where the foot lies in an inwards, outwards, upwards or downwards position. If the foot can be easily moved into alignment with the shin, the condition is known as 'positional talipes' and occurs due to the squashed position of the feet in utero. However, in 'fixed talipes' the foot cannot easily be manipulated into alignment and referral for treatment is required.

An abnormal shape (e.g. 'rocker bottom', an abnormality of the foot in which the soles curve outwards, rather than inward, giving them the appearance of a rocker) or signs of oedema should be noted and the baby referred to a paediatrician. The number of toes must be counted and separated to check for the presence of webbing. Polydactyly and syndactyly should be noted and referred.

Spine

The spine is best examined by turning the baby over so it straddles your hand. In this position the baby curls comfortably over your hand, opening the vertebrae slightly so that they can be more easily seen. Examine the back making sure that you can see both sides adequately. Run your finger down the spine from just into the hairline at the back of the head, all the way down to the sacral area, checking for integrity. The presence of hair tufts, dimples or sinuses may indicate involvement with the spinal cord and referral to a paediatrician is paramount. Gently part the cleft of the buttocks, checking the anal sphincter (this time from a different angle) and the presence of any hidden dimples or sinuses. Quite often you may find a dimple just where the cleft of the buttocks begins and you need to ascertain if you can easily see the end of it. If you cannot, refer to a paediatrician.

Skin

Throughout the examination the condition of the skin needs to be examined. Observe for colour, birthmarks and where they are placed, rashes (not usually common at birth), bruising, cuts and abrasions, referring as necessary. The most common birthmarks that do not require referral to a paediatrician include salmon patch naevus and the Mongolian blue spot.

Salmon patches usually appear as a reddened 'patch' on the brow between the eyes and/or within the hairline at the back of the head. The former gradually fade over time and the latter may fade, but heat and anger may make them appear more prominent again.

The Mongolian blue spot usually appear as a bruised-looking area over one or both buttocks. It can also appear on the legs and arms. It is important that the size and position of each one should be documented to prevent confusion with cases of non-accidental injury.

Weight and length

The baby should be weighed at the beginning or end of the examination as long as the baby remains warm. The weight should be recorded in kilograms. Many units do not routinely measure the baby's length due the logistics of ensuring the accuracy of the measurement. However, it may be prudent for those babies that are small for gestational age, have obvious skeletal dysplasias or may have a possible thyroid instability (due to maternal history), to note the length measurement for future follow up (Hall and Elliman 2006).

Completion of the initial examination

Once the physical examination is completed, any drugs (e.g. Vitamin K) can be given if parental consent has been obtained. The baby can then be dressed or given to the mother for skin-to-skin contact.

The findings, if not already explained during the examination, should be discussed with the parents and they should be asked if they have any questions. Make sure that the baby is still warm and content or give the mother assistance if the baby wishes to feed.

Appropriate paediatric referrals can be made if necessary and the examination completed by documenting the findings in the baby's notes.

Conclusion

This chapter has highlighted the role and responsibilities of the midwife in the assessment and examination of the newborn baby within a very short time of birth. The midwife can help to facilitate the bonding process between the parents and their baby by answering their questions and giving them support and guidance as they start to get to know each other. The examination at birth also acts as a baseline so that the initial assessment of the baby can inform future care and management, particularly if deviations from the normal are noticed. In this case, referral to the appropriate health care professional (usually the paediatrician) is required as stipulated in the

Midwives Rules and Standards (NMC 2004a). Appropriate communication with the parents and accurate and contemporaneous record keeping are also highlighted as important elements in the examination of the newborn baby.

References

Black, J. and Rose, P. (2000) Temperature measurement in the preterm infant: a literature review. *Journal of Neonatal Nursing* 6(1): 28–32.

Hall, D. and Elliman, D. (2006) *Health for All Children*, 4th edition. Oxford: Oxford University Press.

Johnson, R. and Taylor, W. (2006) *Skills for Midwifery Practice*, 2nd edition. London: Churchill Livingstone.

Nursing and Midwifery Council (2004a) *Midwives Rules and Standards*. London: NMC.

Nursing and Midwifery Council (2004b) *Standards of Proficiency for Pre-registration Midwifery Education*. London: NMC.

Nursing and Midwifery Council (2005) *Guidelines for Records and Record Keeping*. London: NMC.

Scanga, A., Wallace, R., Kiehl, E. et al. (2000) A comparison of four methods of normal newborn temperature measurement. *MCN* 25(2): 76–9.

Effective Postnatal Care

Annabel Jay

Introduction

The puerperium (time following birth) is traditionally defined as the period from the delivery of the placenta, cord and membranes until the end of the sixth week postnatally.

Until very recently, the traditional pattern of postnatal care involved regular visits to each woman up to day 10, and thereafter as necessary until day 28, which marked the end of the midwife's involvement in the postnatal period. However, The National Service Framework (NSF) for children, young people and maternity services (DH 2004) recommends that midwifery-led services should continue to be provided for at least one month *and longer if needed*. The *Midwives Rules and Standards* (NMC 2004) therefore describes the postnatal period as:

> 'the period after the end of labour during which the attendance of a midwife upon a woman and baby is required, being not less than 10 days and for such longer period as the midwife considers necessary.'

This chapter focuses on the essential care that each woman and her baby should receive from the midwife during the postnatal period. Particular reference will be made to current guidelines issued by the National Institute for Health and Clinical Excellence (NICE) on postnatal care of women and babies (NICE 2006). In this chapter the baby will be assumed to be male, to reduce confusion when referring to both woman and baby.

Principles of postnatal care

The postnatal period is a time of change and adjustment for the woman and those close to her. The focus of attention is no longer on the woman alone, but on her baby too. The midwife's role, however, is essentially to care for the *mother* (NMC 2004) and to *enable* her to care for her baby, rather than to undertake the role of primary carer herself.

Individualised care

The NICE guidelines on postnatal care (NICE 2006) stress that women should at all times be treated with dignity, kindness and respect, regardless of their social status, age or culture. Furthermore, women should be encouraged to become fully involved in the planning of their postnatal care, which should centre on their individual needs rather than on routine patterns of care. There are many factors which influence the decision on how to plan the woman's postnatal care. These include the state of the mother and baby's health, the woman's parity (sometimes shortened to 'para') – this refers to the number of live infants that a woman has had; a woman expecting her first baby is described as 'para 0' until she has actually given birth – her chosen method of infant feeding, her ability to understand and assimilate information, her domestic background and her psychological state.

The woman's cultural and family background should always be taken into consideration when planning postnatal care (NICE 2006). Midwives working in culturally diverse areas should consider it part of their role to familiarise themselves with the postnatal norms of their clients (Baston 2004a) and avoid making judgements based on the prevailing norms of the majority population.

All information and advice should be given in a form that women and their families can understand (NICE 2006). An interpreter may be needed if the woman does not speak English. Information leaflets to back up verbal advice should be available in the language that the woman is most comfortable with; however, it should be remembered that some women may be unable to read in any language. Baston (2004a) emphasises that the woman's existing knowledge should be used as a starting point when giving advice and information. It is important to avoid making assumptions about a woman's need for knowledge (Baston 2004a). It is better practice to find out from her what she needs and/or wishes to know.

Advice and support can be given in ways other than a straightforward list of 'dos and don'ts'. For example, a midwife can act as a good role model in the way she handles the baby, dresses him, talks to him, etc. (Baston 2004a). Praising the woman as she learns baby care skills not only provides positive reinforcement but also boosts the woman's confidence.

Case Notes

Judy and her husband, Deepak, arrived home from hospital yesterday with their two-day-old son, Harry. Judy has two teenage daughters from a former marriage, but Harry is Deepak's first child. Deepak's mother is visiting from India and speaks very little English. Judy bottlefed her older children, but has decided to breastfeed Harry. The community midwife who visited the family today first ensured that Judy was making a good physical recovery and that Harry was feeding well. Then, as she had a lot of visits to make, she left Judy some information leaflets and a helpline number and told her that she would call again on day 6. As Judy is a 'multip' with good family support, the midwife assumed that she would not need much help or advice.

- Why might the midwife's assumption be wrong?
- List three suggestions for ways in which Judy's postnatal care could be individualised.

Record keeping and communication

The NICE guidelines on postnatal care (NICE 2006) set out key priorities. These state that each woman should have 'a documented, individualised care plan', which should be reviewed regularly. The usual place to document this is the woman's hand-held maternity notes. This allows the woman to read it whenever she wishes to and to add to or alter it as necessary. She should be advised to discuss any changes with her community midwife. The NICE (2006) guidelines recommend that the postnatal care plan should take into account:

'Relevant factors from the antenatal, intrapartum and immediate postnatal period. Details of the healthcare professionals involved in her care and that of her baby. Plans for the postnatal period.'

The aim is to promote good continuity of care, even if continuity of *carer* cannot be achieved. It is vital that information, advice and care given to women and their babies in the postnatal period are consistent, as a woman may be cared for by many people. Detailed record keeping in the woman's hand-held notes will facilitate continuity of care between carers. Any symptoms, tests performed, deviations from the norm or referral to other professionals should be meticulously followed up and documented so that the woman's and baby's progress can be continuously mapped (NICE 2006). (See Chapter 10 for further discussion regarding the importance of records and record keeping.)

Listening

Women should be offered an opportunity to discuss their birth experiences (Baston 2004a; NICE 2006). It is thought that in some cases powerful emotions generated by events during the birth may trigger long-term mental health problems such as depression and anxiety (Gamble et al. 2005). The midwife should make time to listen and allow the woman to talk about the birth as she wishes. This is *not* the same as a formal 'debriefing' which is a structured process (Gamble et al. 2005) requiring counselling skills which midwives may not possess.

Immediate post-birth care of the woman

This section focuses on the immediate care of the woman following a normal vaginal birth. Care of a woman after caesarean section will be addressed later.

Following the birth, the new parents may welcome some time to spend alone with their baby as they get to know each other. This is an important part of the bonding/attachment process. However, before leaving the room, the midwife must undertake some basic observations to ensure that the woman is not at immediate risk.

Observation of blood loss

The volume of blood loss should be estimated following delivery of the placenta and then observed frequently in the early postnatal period. The midwife will be observing for any signs of postpartum haemorrhage (PPH), a potentially life-threatening condition which is more common if the woman has had a prolonged or complicated labour or birth.

Assessing blood loss is notoriously difficult (Baston 2004b): it is soaked up by pads, bedding and clothing; it is often clotted or mixed with liquor. It is recognised that midwives generally underestimate actual blood loss (Razvi et al. 1996; cited in Baston 2004b) so great care must be taken.

A blood loss of 500 ml or more at or around the time of birth is classed as a 'primary PPH'. However, this figure is not a good indicator of maternal well-being: some woman can withstand a blood loss of 500 ml or more with little or no detriment to their health, whilst others will show symptoms of hypovolaemia well before 500 ml has been lost. The midwife must call for urgent medical assistance if PPH occurs or is suspected (NMC 2006) of if the woman showing signs of hypovolaemia regardless of the volume of blood lost.

Activity

Fill a 2 litre container with water and colour it red using food dye. Gather several plastic bowls of varying sizes and place inside them an assortment of sanitary pads, gauze swabs, incontinence pads and draw sheets. To each bowl, add a measured amount of liquid and allow the contents to soak it up. Ask colleagues to estimate the volume of liquid in each bowl.

How many got every one correct?

Observation of the fundus

Poor uterine tone following delivery may lead to excessive bleeding. The midwife should gently palpate the fundus, which should feel very firm and central, just below the level of the umbilicus. If the uterus feels soft and broad it will be necessary to 'rub up' a contraction until the uterus feels firm (Baston 2004b). If the uterus feels unexpectedly high or deviated to one side of the abdomen, it is most likely that the woman has a full bladder, in which case she should be encouraged to pass urine (Baston 2004b). A full bladder may impede involution (contraction and shrinking) of the uterus.

Other observations

The midwife will change any soiled bedding and pads, assist the woman into a comfortable position and offer her something to eat and drink. The woman should be encouraged to have uninterrupted skin-to-skin contact with her baby and given assistance (if needed) to offer him a feed.

The basic postnatal observations are listed below:

- Estimation of blood loss
- Observation of the lochia (discharge from the vagina)
- Temperature, pulse and blood pressure
- Observation of the perineum
- General well-being of the woman

These observations may be repeated on a regular basis according to local policy, or at the discretion of the midwife. Women whose blood pressure has been raised in pregnancy or labour should be monitored more frequently until their condition stabilises within normal limits (Baston 2004a). Raised temperature (pyrexia) which does not quickly return to normal should be reported to the duty registrar and the cause investigated. A raised pulse may be an indication of excessive blood loss (see above). If the lochia are excessively heavy but the uterus remains well contracted, the genital tract should be examined for trauma (see below).

If the woman has an intravenous infusion, the midwife must observe to see that it is running at the prescribed rate. Any medical condition, such as diabetes, must be continuously managed. Only when the midwife is satisfied that there is no immediate risk to woman or baby and that neither has any immediate care needs should she leave the delivery room to examine the placenta and complete her record keeping. The woman should have a call-bell to hand at all times and know how to use it.

In the homebirth setting, the midwife may carry out her documentation and examination of the placenta in the birthing room, if the parents do not object.

On returning to the delivery room, the midwife will repeat her earlier observations and offer the woman a bath or shower. If she is unable to walk, the woman should be offered a bowl of warm water to wash and helped to cleanse her perineal area.

Examination of the placenta

This should be undertaken as soon as possible after the birth to enable the midwife to assess whether any part has been retained. Retained placental products are a potential cause of PPH, as their presence may prevent full involution of the uterus. The midwife will examine the membranes to check that both amnion and chorion are present and can be pieced together. Both placental surfaces should be inspected. The midwife will be checking for evidence that the placenta has been expelled in its entirety. Evidence to the contrary includes:

- Blood vessels on the fetal side that extend beyond the placental edge, indicating a succenturiate lobe that had not been passed
- On the maternal side, any suspicious gaps which may indicate a retained cotyledon (placental lobe)
- An irregular outline, suggesting that a portion of the placenta is missing

In addition, the midwife will note any infarctions – gritty, discoloured plaques of calcification. These may not be of any significance, but may provide evidence to confirm a suspected intrauterine problem (McDonald 2003). All findings should be documented in the woman's notes and any abnormality reported to an obstetrician.

Activity

On examination of the placenta and membranes, the latter are sometimes found to be 'ragged'.

- What is the implication of this for the woman?
- What should the midwife do with regard to the woman's ongoing care?

Bladder care

The woman should be encouraged to pass urine at the earliest opportunity – ideally, she should not be transferred to the postnatal ward until she has passed urine. Reference should be made in the woman's notes of the time that urine was passed and, if measured, the volume passed.

Some women find that bladder tone is temporarily impaired immediately following childbirth and may not notice a full bladder. The latter is more likely if an epidural block has been used in labour (McDonald 2003). If left undetected, this may lead to distension and subsequent longer-term problems. NICE guidelines on postnatal care (NICE 2006) recommend that if the woman is unable to pass urine within six hours of labour, she should be encouraged to empty her bladder in a warm bath or shower. However, some women find this aesthetically unacceptable. If all else fails, the midwife should gently palpate the woman's lower abdomen to assess whether the bladder is full and if so, consider catheterisation to empty the bladder and prevent future complications.

Perineal repair

The repair of any perineal trauma is normally the responsibility of the person who assists at the birth. Following a normal vaginal birth the midwife will inspect the woman's perineum and vagina to assess the following:

- The presence of any trauma to the tissues
- The extent of any trauma
- Whether or not suturing is required
- Whether or not referral to an obstetrician is required

The procedure should be explained to the woman and verbal consent obtained prior to commencing. Inhalational analgesia (Entonox) may be offered if necessary. Some women prefer their partners not to be present whilst they are being sutured, and this wish should be tactfully supported.

Degrees of perineal trauma

Downe (2003) suggests that perineal trauma is usually classified in four degrees:

- First degree: involves the skin of the fourchette or vaginal wall mucosa only
- Second degree: includes fourchette and the muscle layers of the perineum
- Third degree:
  3a – <50% of the thickness of the external anal sphincter is damaged
  3b – >50% of the external anal sphincter is damaged
  3c – the internal anal sphincter is damaged
  (NICE 2007b)
- Fourth degree: trauma to the anal sphincter extending to the anal epithelium

Suitably trained and practised midwives may repair first and second degree tears and episiotomies if they feel it is within their competence to do so, but third and fourth degree trauma must *always* be repaired by an obstetrician. Women may also suffer trauma to the anterior aspect of the perineum: this may include damage to the clitoris, labia, urethra or anterior vaginal wall (Baston 2004c). Whilst the repair of labial tears is usually straightforward and within the midwife's role, other anterior tears require referral. Any bilateral labial grazes that are in apposition during normal postures should be sutured to avoid the risk of the labia healing together (Johnson and Taylor 2005).

Indications for repair of first and second degree trauma

It is usual practice to suture all episiotomies, regardless of their extent. If there is an obvious bleeding point, it will need to be repaired quickly before too much blood is lost. Current evidence suggests that the repair of second degree tears leads to better wound alignment and healing (Fleming et al. 2003; Kenyon and Ford 2004), therefore many maternity units have a policy of repairing all second degree tears unless the woman requests otherwise. In the case of a simple, first degree tear, the midwife's discretion is usually relied upon: if there is no excessive bleeding and the sides of the tear are in close apposition, it may be safely left to heal naturally (see the 'Ipswich Trial'; Gordon et al. 1998). Whatever the midwife's professional opinion, the final decision as to whether or not to suture is *always* the woman's.

Case Notes

Gemma has just given birth to a healthy baby in hospital. On examining her perineum, you discover a second degree tear. The tear is not bleeding excessively and the two sides appear well aligned. Gemma expresses a preference not to be sutured.

- How would you advise Gemma?
- Where could you find evidence to support your advice?

Perineal infiltration and repair

Unless the woman has an epidural block which is still fully effective, her perineum should be infiltrated with lidocaine according to local protocol. The procedure for infiltration and perineal repair is explained clearly in Johnson and Taylor (2005). Perineal repair caries a high risk of needlestick injury, so great care is needed. Prior to commencing the repair, a digital examination of the rectum should be carried out to exclude third degree tears (NICE 2007b).

The vaginal wall is sutured using a continuous stitch from apex to fourchette. The muscle layers of the perineal body are also brought together using a continuous stitch from the fourchette to the anal end of the tear. If the perineal skin on either side of the tear is in close apposition, it may be left unsutured. If not, it will be closed using a continuous subcuticular technique beginning at the anal end and finishing at the fourchette with a subcuticular knot (Johnson and Taylor 2005).

Once the repair is complete and haemostatis is achieved, the rectum must be examined to ensure no suture has passed through to the mucosa. The woman should be informed of this in advance. Analgesia such as diclofenac 100 mg (Kenyon and Ford 2004) may then be administered. The woman can be made comfortable again and the bedding changed. The woman will need to be advised on perineal hygiene, pelvic floor exercises and the need for further analgesia if necessary.

Initiating breastfeeding

Prior to the birth, the midwife will have established from the woman whether she wants her baby to be given straight to her for immediate skin-to-skin contact. This is generally recommended (Wallace and Marshall 2001) for the following reasons:

- It helps the baby to maintain his body temperature
- It promotes bonding and attachment
- It facilitates early breastfeeding

As long as both woman and baby are well, skin-to-skin contact should be initiated within 30 minutes of birth (Royal College of Midwives 2002) and continue uninterrupted for as long as is desired. This applies regardless of the chosen method of infant feeding (Wallace and Marshall 2001). It is quite possible for the midwife to undertake most if not all the necessary observations and procedures without separating the pair.

This is a good time to initiate the first feed, especially if the mother has chosen to breastfeed. Babies are usually alert and receptive to feeding in the first hour following birth. It is generally recognised that early and unrestricted feeding is an indicator of long-term successful breastfeeding (Inch 2003). The woman may need help to attach her baby to the breast, especially if she has not breastfed before, and the midwife should oversee the pair to advise and support as needed. Wherever possible, the midwife should adopt a hands-off approach and should never handle the woman's breasts or her baby without permission.

Many hospitals and NHS Trusts use the '10 Steps to Successful Breastfeeding' devised by the Baby Friendly Initiative (BFI) to underpin their breastfeeding policy. Full information about the '10 Steps' can be found on www.babyfriendly.co.uk. NICE (2006) sets out clear guidelines for NHS providers of breastfeeding support. These are:

- Women should be advised on the benefits of breastfeeding and colostrum within 24 hours of giving birth
- Initiation of breastfeeding should be encouraged within 1 hour of birth if possible
- Support for breastfeeding should be appropriate to the woman's culture
- Woman and baby should not be separated in the first hour after birth except at the woman's request or when medically necessary
- Skin-to-skin contact should be encouraged as soon as possible after birth

- Women should not be asked about their proposed method of infant feeding until *after* skin-to-skin contact has been commenced
- Women should be offered skilled breastfeeding support from the first feed to ensure correct positioning and attachment and to establish effective feeding
- Women who have had a caesarean section or narcotic drugs should be offered additional support with positioning and attachment

Activity

List the benefits of a successful early breastfeed to both the baby and mother.

Care following caesarean section

Rising rates of caesarean section across the UK mean that the post-operative care of women is becoming an increasingly larger proportion of the hospital midwife's workload. The woman recovering from a caesarean section requires particular care and attention, not just to her physical well-being but also her state of mind: she has undergone major surgery as well as the birth of her baby, both of which are major life events (Baston 2005a).

Care in the recovery area

The immediate post-operative care takes place in the recovery area of the operating theatre, where emergency equipment is on hand. The anaesthetist will hand over care to a midwife, who should remain constantly with the woman until she is fit to be moved to the postnatal ward. The timing of this will depend on the type of anaesthesia used: if a general anaesthetic has been used, the woman must remain in the recovery area until she is fully conscious, can maintain her own airway and any pain or nausea is under control (Baston 2005a).

The woman will have in intravenous (IV) infusion running and an indwelling catheter in situ. Observation of vital signs should be undertaken at five-minute intervals initially until the woman's condition stabilises, then less frequently as per local protocol. The NICE guidelines on caesarean section (NICE 2004) recommend that vital sign observations should be undertaken half-hourly for at least two hours and thereafter hourly until within satisfactory parameters. As

Table 8.1 Observations required post-caesarean section in the recovery area

- Oxygen saturation levels, using pulse oxymetry
- Care of pressure areas
- Assessment of returning sensation in lower abdomen and legs
- Pain assessment
- Care of intravenous infusion
- Fluid balance
- Urine output/catheter care
- Care of wound and dressing (and drain if used)
- Assessment of lochia
- Assessment of posture and general comfort
- Maintenance of dignity, i.e. ensuring that woman is suitably covered with bedding/clothing

If general anaesthetic has been used:

- Maintenance of airway
- Assessment of consciousness

Source: Adapted Johnson and Taylor 2005

well as the vital signs, observations listed in Table 8.1 should be undertaken.

All observations should be carefully documented. The fluid balance chart must be strictly maintained to spot any early signs of reduced urine output. Any cause for concern should be reported immediately to the anaesthetist.

Following caesarean under epidural or spinal block, most women are able to sit up in the recovery bed and take sips of water within an hour of surgery (Johnson and Taylor 2005). However, large volumes of fluid or solid food may increase the likelihood of vomiting, due to reduced gut motility caused by the epidural block.

A woman who has had general anaesthesia will be unable to sit up until fully conscious, but her partner should be encouraged to talk to her and tell her about the baby, as she is likely to be able to hear before she can respond and will be reassured by the sound of his voice (Baston 2005a). If the partner is not present, the midwife should do this.

The woman should not be separated from her partner and her baby for any longer than is strictly necessary. As long as she is fully conscious and feels well enough to do so, she should be facilitated to begin skin-to-skin contact with her baby and to feed him. She will need assistance to put her baby to the breast initially, and her partner or the midwife may need to help support the baby's body. Recovery areas may be quite cool, so the midwife should ensure that the baby does not become chilled.

Case Notes

Sian, a midwife, is caring for a woman alone in the recovery area. The woman's partner is present. What should Sian do in the event of the following?

- Her pen runs out of ink while completing her records
- The woman complains of increasing pain
- The intravenous infusion appears to have stopped running
- The woman asks to be helped to sit up

Care of the woman on the postnatal ward

The midwife who has cared for the woman in the recovery area should give a detailed handover to the midwife taking over her care. Once the woman and baby have been made comfortable in the ward, all observations listed in Table 8.1 (except oxygen saturation, which should have been normal long before the woman left the recovery area) should be repeated before she is left alone. She should be given a call-bell and encouraged to use it if she feels unwell or uncomfortable.

Psychologically, the early postnatal period is a difficult time for many women, especially if their caesarean was the result of an emergency (Johnson and Taylor 2005). As well as discomfort, they may feel frustrated at their lack of mobility or their need for help with baby care. Seeing other women around them who need no assistance may increase their sense of inadequacy. The midwife will need to reassure the woman that such feelings are normal, and give her the care and support needed, whilst enabling her to develop independence and autonomy in caring for herself and her baby.

Pain relief

Many women will have patient-controlled analgesia in situ on leaving the recovery area. Local protocol will dictate when this is discontinued and oral analgesia commences. The woman should be encouraged to report any returning pain as soon as it occurs (Baston 2005a). If necessary, the anaesthetist may need to be contacted to review the woman's drug regime.

Mobility

Early mobility should be encouraged where possible, as it improves venous circulation, thus reducing the risk of thrombosis and thromboembolism, one of the greatest causes of maternal death in the UK (CEMACH 2004). It also empowers the woman to regain control of caring for her baby and herself. A woman will need to be closely supervised when taking her first steps out of bed in case she stumbles or falls.

Prevention of thromboembolism

The Royal College of Obstetricians and Gynaecologists (1995) recommends that each woman undergoing caesarean section should be risk-assessed for thromboembolic disorders. The risk is increased by the following factors:

- Age over 35 years
- Obesity
- Parity above 4
- Gross varicosities
- Infection
- Personal or family history of thromboembolic disorders
- Emergency caesarean section

(Johnson and Taylor 2005)

Graduated compression stockings are generally worn by all women undergoing caesarean section to promote venous return from the lower limbs. Women who are considered to be at high risk of thromboembolic disorders will be given prophylactic anticoagulants according to local protocol.

Case Notes

Marie gave birth yesterday by emergency caesarean section for undiagnosed breech presentation. Marie is 38 years old and had a body mass index of 33 before becoming pregnant. She feels well, but does not want to get out of bed. She has refused a shower. Marie is eating and drinking normally and her urine output is good. Her catheter is still in situ.

Activity

- What might be the cause of Marie's reluctance to get up?
- What risks does Marie face by refusing to mobilise?
- How would a midwife explain these risks to Marie in a sensitive manner?
- What might the midwife do to reduce these risks if Marie continues to stay in bed?

Postnatal exercises

Teaching women to perform leg exercises will improve venous circulation until full mobility is regained, thus reducing the risk of DVT. Breathing exercises help clear secretions from the lungs following surgery and improve circulation (Baston 2005a). Pelvic floor exercises should also be encouraged as the pelvic floor muscles will have been weakened by pregnancy.

Fluid balance and diet

Intravenous infusion of crystalloids may continue and the urinary catheter may be left in situ until the day following surgery, or discontinued once the woman is tolerating a light diet and fluids and passing an adequate amount of urine (Baston 2005a). Local protocol should be followed. Once the catheter is removed, the woman should be encouraged to pass urine frequently. The effects of epidural anaesthesia on the urinary bladder are mentioned above.

Hygiene and wound care

The day after her operation the woman should be offered assistance to take a shower, following which the midwife should help her to remove her wound dressing. The wound site should be inspected to ensure that there is no bleeding or signs of infection and that the suture or staples remain intact. The wound is usually left uncovered by dressings and if non-dissolving sutures or staples have been used, these will be removed by the midwife when local policy dictates. The midwife may take this opportunity to outline the healing process and what to expect in the coming weeks. She can also remind the woman about wearing appropriate clothing to reduce discomfort.

Breastfeeding

After a caesarean section, a woman will require help initially with all baby care. A breastfeeding woman may have difficulty finding a comfortable position and should be helped to experiment with different ways of holding her baby. Many women find it easier to breastfeed lying on one side, or while holding the baby in the underarm position, with a pillow supporting his body. These positions avoid placing a weight on the woman's scar. Women who have undergone caesarean section may require more reassurance, time and support to breastfeed than women who have given birth vaginally. It may be desirable to arrange for support from a suitably trained health care assistant or lay support worker.

Daily care in hospital

Case Notes

Laura had an uncomplicated birth of a healthy baby girl yesterday. She breastfed her daughter twice during the night, with much help from the midwives. At 9 o'clock this morning Laura's husband arrives on the ward. When the midwife draws back the curtains, expecting to find Laura still in bed, she sees that she is up and dressed and wanting to go home right away.

How should the midwife respond?

During her stay on the postnatal ward, the woman will be encouraged to undertake all of her baby's care needs herself. It is disempowering for the midwife or care assistant to do this for her unless she is physically unable. However, this does not mean that women should simply be 'left to get on with it'. The midwife caring for her will check on the woman's progress as often as time allows and need dictates, offering advice and support as necessary.

It is no longer considered necessary to complete a daily 'tick-box' list of observations in healthy women unless there is a clear need to do so. One of the essential skills of a midwife is to decide which observations are appropriate (Marchant 2003a). If the woman's health gives cause for concern, the midwife should respond appropriately and refer to the appropriate professional. Analgesia should be offered as necessary and reassurance given that some degree of pain is normal and will pass. The midwife must be able to recognise pain which is *not* normal and act appropriately.

The length of a woman's stay in hospital will depend on many factors, such as her physical recovery, her baby's health and her confidence in her ability to cope at home. If there is cause for concern, the woman should be encouraged to remain in hospital. The midwife should refer to senior colleagues and her Supervisor of Midwives if a woman expresses an intention to leave hospital against medical advice.

A woman who has had surgery should have an opportunity to speak with the doctor who performed the operation, and he or she should be satisfied with her recovery. The midwife must follow up any blood tests or other samples sent for analysis and ensure that any prescribed drugs, including analgesics, are available for the woman to take home.

Prior to discharge from hospital, the midwife has a duty to ensure that she has discussed the following with the woman and, if appropriate, her partner:

- The woman's continuing pattern of postnatal care
- Routes of referral in case of illness of mother or baby
- Contact details of local support groups if breastfeeding or if there are special needs
- Contraception and the return of fertility
- Safe sleeping for the baby and how to reduce the risk of sudden infant death syndrome
- Postnatal exercises, including pelvic floor exercises
- Information on registering the birth
- Information on sterilising bottles and making up feeds if the mother is bottle-feeding
- Details of any follow-up appointments for mother or baby which may be required

Individual hospitals or Trusts may issue a 'discharge pack' of information leaflets for each woman. This should not be used as a substitute for a full verbal explanation and the chance for the woman and her partner to ask questions.

Continuing successful breastfeeding

The NICE clinical guidelines on postnatal care (NICE 2006) make clear recommendations to health professionals who support breast-feeding women. These are:

- Women's experience of breastfeeding should be discussed and assessed at each postnatal contact. Findings should be documented in the relevant notes
- Any needs for support should be identified
- If a woman believes she has insufficient milk, the baby's positioning and attachment should be reviewed
- If the baby is unable to take sufficient milk from the breast, he should be offered expressed milk via a cup or bottle
- Additional fluid supplements (including formula milk) should be avoided unless medically indicated

The NICE guidelines further recommend that all breastfeeding women be shown how to hand-express and advised on the safe storage and usage of expressed milk. If a breast pump is required, women should be shown how to use it, including how to cleanse and sterilise the removable parts.

Women should also be advised on the following:

- The importance of unrestricted duration and frequency of breastfeeds
- The need to offer the second breast if the baby appears hungry after feeding from the first breast
- The fact that transient discomfort at the start of each feed is not abnormal in the early days
- Ways to encourage their baby to open his mouth widely
- How to recognise good attachment and effective feeding from the breast
- Means of contacting local breastfeeding support networks

(NICE 2006)

The Royal College of Midwives book *Successful Breastfeeding* (RCM 2002) provides full information, including positioning, attachment and ways of recognising an effective breastfeed.

Case Notes

Tessa gave birth to baby Tom following a normal labour and delivery yesterday. They are both on the postnatal ward. Tom is Tessa's first baby and she is keen to breastfeed him. Tom has had two feeds so far and on both occasions the midwifery assistant attached him to the breast as Tessa was unsure what to do. Tessa now wants to do this for herself, but asks for your assistance as she is not sure where to start.

- How would you set about empowering Tessa to breastfeed Tom?
- What signs should Tessa look out for to tell whether Tom is feeding effectively?
- What follow-up care would you give to Tessa?

Supporting women who choose to bottle feed

The midwife has a duty to support all women in their chosen method of infant feeding. Although midwives should advise women of the benefits of breastfeeding for both mother and baby, the woman is free to make her own decision and should not be made to feel guilty or inferior if, for whatever reason, she chooses not to breastfeed. Parents who use formula milk should receive advice tailored to their needs and understanding to ensure that they have the knowledge and skills to feed their baby safely and in accordance with his nutritional needs (NICE 2006). The woman or couple should also be shown how to clean and sterilise feeding equipment in line with the manufacturers' instructions. Ideally, this should be done using the family's own sterilising equipment rather than hospital equipment. The Department of Health leaflet *Bottle Feeding* (DH 2005) gives clear, simple instructions, and this, or an equivalent, should be given to women to reinforce verbal information.

Other methods of infant feeding

If a baby is unable to take the breast for any reason, his mother can be shown how to feed him expressed milk using a cup, spoon or syringe. The latter is ideal in the first 2–3 days when the woman is producing colostrum. The very small volume makes it difficult to collect in a pump; therefore, the midwife should show the woman how to hand-express her colostrum while the midwife or the woman's partner collects it in a small, sterile syringe. This can then be fed directly to the baby.

The cup or spoon method is more suitable once the woman's milk has 'come in'. In either case equipment must be sterilised before use and strict hand hygiene observed. All methods of expressing and feeding expressed milk are time-consuming, require skill and patience and may not be acceptable for long-term use, in which case a feeding bottle may be preferable (RCM 2002). Parents in this situation may require additional support and encouragement.

Midwifery care in the community

Once the new family have returned to their home, the community midwife will visit. It is usual to visit the woman on the day after her discharge from hospital and thereafter according to her and her baby's needs (see 'Principles of postnatal care'). If the baby was born at home, the midwife may visit later the same day and then the following day. The visit will include an assessment of the woman's physical recovery from the birth, the baby's progress, the woman's psychological state and her adaptation to life with a new baby. The midwife will also take into account the role of the woman's partner and other family members and their impact on the dynamics of the family.

If the visiting midwife has not met the woman before, she will need to take some time building a rapport with her and gaining her trust. The first visit is especially important as the midwife's findings will set the pattern of her subsequent care (Baston 2005b).

Case Notes

Helen came home from hospital two days ago with baby Matthew, who is now four days old. Matthew is Helen and Tom's first baby. When you visited the family yesterday, all seemed well. This morning, Tom answers the door in his dressing gown, looking dishevelled. Last night's supper dishes are still on the table and there is a pile of laundry on the kitchen floor. The milk bottles are still on the doorstep and the post has not been picked up. Baby Matthew is on Tom's shoulder, crying. Tom is worried that Matthew seems hungry all the time and cries a lot. Helen is still in bed at 11.30, awake, but tired. She bursts into tears when she sees you.

Activity

- List the midwife's priorities in this situation.
- What information and advice might the midwife give Helen and Tom about Matthew's crying?

Prior to visiting a woman at home or in the postnatal ward for the first time, the midwife should have had an opportunity to read the relevant notes or receive a personal handover from the previous midwife. This enables good continuity of care. It also guides the midwife to any sensitive issues or causes for concern. On the first visit, the community midwife should ensure that the woman has received a copy of the Department of Health booklet *Birth to Five* and her child's personal health record (the 'Red Book'). These should be explained to the woman and her partner, if this has not already been done.

Physical assessment of the woman

Before any physical contact with the woman, the midwife will assess her general health and well-being by asking how she is feeling. This may give further clues to any problems or unexpected needs. Any examination of the woman or her baby should only take place following full verbal consent and thorough hand-washing. The midwife must assess whether it is appropriate to conduct any physical examination in a communal area of the home where friends and family may be present, or whether she and the woman should move to a more private area, such as a bedroom. Full account should be taken of the woman's cultural and religious background.

Vital signs observations

Providing that there is no history of abnormal vital signs in the postnatal period and the woman is generally well, vital signs need not be repeated unless her condition gives rise to concern.

If the woman's blood pressure is taken for any reason and found to be raised (diastolic >90 mm hg) it should be repeated four hours later provided there are no other symptoms (NICE 2006). If other signs of pre-eclampsia are present, or if the woman's blood pressure has not returned to normal within four hours, urgent referral is required (NICE 2006).

If a woman is found to have a raised temperature above 38 °C on two successive occasions 4–6 hours apart *or* she has other symptoms of infection, urgent medical referral is indicated (NICE 2006). These may be indications of genital tract sepsis, which is a potentially life-threatening condition. Less serious conditions such as mastitis or cystitis may also present with a raised temperature. These warrant referral to the woman's GP.

Breasts and breastfeeding

Activity

A midwife visits a woman in her home on day 3. The woman complains that her breasts feel uncomfortable.
   What information and advice would the midwife offer?

Regardless of whether or not the woman has chosen to breastfeed her baby, the midwife should enquire about the comfort of the woman's breasts at every visit. Women should be warned about what to expect when the milk 'comes in' on day 3 or thereabouts and that milk may leak from their nipples between feeds. Women should be advised on appropriate clothing, and, if they have chosen not to breastfeed, should be given appropriate advice on suppressing lactation.

Breast engorgement around day 3 is not uncommon whether or not the woman is breastfeeding, so appropriate, evidence-based advice should be given. The midwife should show the woman how to hand-express her milk to relieve engorgement around the areola which may prevent the baby from attaching to the breast.

Breastfeeding women should be asked whether they are experiencing any nipple pain and if so, the midwife should ask to examine the nipples. If trauma is evident, appropriate advice should be offered and the breasts re-examined the following day and thereafter until they are healing satisfactorily. In most cases, sore or cracked nipples are the result of incorrect positioning of the baby at the breast, therefore the midwife must make time to support and advise on correct positioning and attachment. She may refer the mother to a local breastfeeding support group for further assistance.

The woman should be advised on current evidence about nipple preparations to treat or prevent soreness and on the use of nipple shields (these are not recommended except as an emergency, short-term measure once the milk has 'come in') (RCM 2002).

Women should be advised on signs of mastitis and to report this to the visiting midwife (NICE 2006). Mastitis is most likely to be caused by a blocked milk duct. The midwife should show the woman how to relieve it by massaging from the affected area towards the nipple during feeding or hand expression. If there is no improvement after a few hours, the woman should be advised to contact her midwife again and may need to be referred to her GP for antibiotic treatment (NICE 2006). Advice on continuing to feed the baby and the use of simple analgesia should also be given.

There are still many examples of incorrect or outdated remedies for breastfeeding problems which persist in the community. The midwife must be alert to these practices and be able to give sound, evidence-based advice to counteract unsafe or ineffective remedies.

Activity

- What strategies can a midwife adopt to enable a woman to successfully *position* her baby at the breast?
- How can a woman tell that her baby is *well attached* to her breast?
- How can a woman tell whether or not her baby is actually *taking milk* from her breast?

The lochia and uterine involution

The midwife will need to enquire about the woman's lochia. This is a subject some women would rather discuss in private and the midwife needs to be aware of cultural and individual sensitivities when raising this subject.

The woman should be informed of the changing colour and volume of the lochia during the postnatal period. She should be alerted to the fact that the lochia may temporarily increase once she becomes more active, but the overall trend should be a general decrease in volume. Women may worry if they pass the occasional clot, but providing there are no other symptoms, they can be reassured that this is normal. The midwife should, however, advise the woman and her partner to be alert to any sudden or profuse loss, especially if accompanied by symptoms of shock. This requires emergency action (NICE 2006).

The process of involution, by which the uterus returns to its pre-pregnant shape and position, continues until the end of the puerperium. However, most of the reduction in size will have occurred by day 10 postnatally (Johnson and Taylor 2005). The rate of involution varies from woman to woman (Johnson and Taylor 2005). Until recently, it was common practice to palpate the woman's abdomen to monitor involution at every postnatal contact. However, current guidelines state that this is unnecessary unless the lochia is abnormal (NICE 2006).

If the woman reports excessive or offensive-smelling blood loss, large clots, abdominal tenderness or fever, the midwife should gently palpate her uterus. Any abnormalities in the size, tone or position need urgent investigation. However, simple explanations such as a full bladder or rectum should first be ruled out. Unless the woman has recently had a caesarean section, the uterus should not feel tender when palpated (Johnson and Taylor 2005). If infection is suspected, urgent medical referral is required.

Case Notes

You are working on the postnatal ward. A woman who was discharged home yesterday rings the ward in a state of panic. It is day 3 and she has just passed a large clot of blood. The woman had a normal vaginal delivery with no apparent complications.

Activity

- What questions do you need to ask the woman?
- Assuming there is no immediate cause for concern, what would you advise the woman?

Perineal care

At each visit, the woman should be asked how her perineum feels and, where there has been any degree of perineal trauma, whether she has any concerns about the healing process (NICE 2006). If the woman reports any pain, discomfort, offensive odour or dysuria (pain on urinating) the midwife should offer to look at her perineum and assess any changes. Any signs of infection or wound breakdown should be reported urgently (NICE 2006) to the appropriate doctor and treatment commenced. Otherwise, the midwife may advise paracetamol and/or cool gel pads to relieve discomfort while healing occurs (NICE 2006). The woman can be advised about perineal hygiene and pelvic floor exercises to promote wound healing and be reminded about appropriate clothing to reduce the risk of infection and discomfort.

The midwife should also note any history of haemorrhoids in the ante- or postnatal period, or she may observe them for the first time if inspecting the woman's perineum. This is often an embarrassing subject for women and should be treated with sensitivity. Dietary advice should be offered and a gentle laxative may be indicated if constipation is a contributing factor. Over-the-counter haemorrhoid creams are readily available and may be suggested if the haemorrhoids are uncomfortable. If the problem does not resolve, the woman should be referred to her GP.

Elimination

The midwife will ask the woman whether her bowel and bladder functions have returned to normal or whether she is experiencing any difficulties. It is not uncommon for women to experience minor stress incontinence postnatally, especially following an assisted delivery or prolonged labour. Pelvic floor exercises should be taught to help regain the tone of the perineal muscles (NICE 2006). If incontinence persists, the woman should be referred for specialist investigation.

Women should be advised on the treatment of constipation through dietary means and, if necessary the use of a gentle laxative. Faecal incontinence sometimes occurs following a third of fourth degree tear, but is not necessarily associated with this (Marchant 2003b). The midwife should raise this topic sensitively and if symptoms do not resolve, refer the woman for specialist evaluation (NICE 2006).

Headache

The current NICE guidelines on postnatal care recommend that all women should be asked about headache symptoms at each postnatal contact (NICE 2006). Special vigilance is needed when women who have a history of pre-eclampsia report a severe headache in the first 72 hours after giving birth, especially if accompanied by visual disturbances, nausea or vomiting. These may be symptoms of worsening pre-eclampsia or an impending eclamptic seizure and warrant urgent referral plus blood pressure monitoring. Even where there is no history of pre-eclampsia, women with a severe or persistent headache should be evaluated and referred for urgent medical attention (NICE 2006).

Legs

At every visit, the midwife will ask the woman whether she has any leg pains. This is due to the increased risk of thromboembolic disorders following childbirth. The risk is higher in women who have had a caesarean section (see above) or who suffer reduced mobility for other reasons. Women should be encouraged to mobilise, building up their physical activity gradually without becoming too tired. Any unilateral calf pain, redness or swelling should be treated as suspicious and evaluated for deep vein thrombosis (DVT) (NICE 2006). This requires immediate medical attention. If the woman complains of shortness of breath or chests pains, she should be evaluated for pulmonary embolism: this demands emergency action (NICE 2006).

Fatigue

It is normal for women to feel tired following the birth of a baby. Her partner may also be exhausted in the early days. The midwife should not expect either of them to be dressed and organised when she calls, nor should she expect a tidy house or the offer of refreshments. A woman who is persistently tired, however, warrants further investigation (NICE 2006). It is worth asking whether her fatigue is affecting her well-being and her ability to cope with her new role. It may be that she had simply not anticipated the demands of a new baby and just needs reassuring: however, she may be anaemic, in which case she may need to have a blood sample taken for Hb analysis. On the other hand, there may be a psychological cause, such as postnatal depression.

Sexual health and contraception

At some point the midwife must introduce the subject of resuming sexual intercourse: it is a topic which is sometimes avoided for fear of causing embarrassment or offence. Although this might be furthest from the woman's mind in the first few days after giving birth, it may eventually become a source of anxiety if not previously addressed. The midwife must carefully choose the moment to raise this subject, preferably when the woman is alone, and address any worries fully and honestly.

Activity

Fatima has recently given birth to her fourth baby. She speaks little English, but her husband, Mahmood, and sister-in-law have been translating for her. Fatima is healthy and is due to be discharged from midwifery care shortly. Fatima is feeding her baby with both breast and formula milk. The subject of family planning has not yet been raised.

- What should the midwife consider when broaching this subject?
- What resources might the midwife draw upon for help?

The *Midwives Rules and Standards* state that the activities of a midwife include the provision of family planning information and advice (NMC 2004). The matter of fertility control should be raised with all women, regardless of age or social circumstances (Hall 2005). The woman should first be asked if she wishes to discuss contraception and her wishes respected (Hall 2005). All advice should be tailored to the couple's needs and, where possible, supported with written information leaflets in the couple's first language. The couple may appreciate having contact details for expert advice (NICE 2006).

Immunisations (NICE 2006)

Women who are rhesus negative should be offered anti-D immunoglobulin within 72 hours of the birth of a rhesus-positive baby. Due to early discharge from hospital, many women now receive their anti-D at home via the community midwife. Women who screened negative for rubella antibodies antenatally should be offered the MMR vaccination prior to leaving hospital. The person who gives the vaccination should advise the woman to avoid pregnancy for one month afterwards. Breastfeeding is not contraindicated.

Assessment of the woman's psychological well-being

The arrival of a new baby can be a time of major psychological upheaval for a woman and her family. Some women take this in their stride, but others, for a variety of reasons, have difficulty adjusting. By providing continuous support and care for a woman and her baby over a period of time, a trusting relationship should develop between the woman and her midwife which will encourage the woman to confide any anxieties. Emotional support is particularly valued at this vulnerable stage in a woman's life (Baston 2005b).

The NICE guidelines on postnatal care (NICE 2006) recommend that at each postnatal visit, the midwife should ask the woman about her emotional well-being and whether she has any family or social support network. Women and their partners should be encouraged to inform their midwife of any concerns about mood changes or uncharacteristic behaviour. Midwives should inform the woman's GP if they suspect a mental health disorder or if they uncover a previously unreported history of mental health problems.

Mental distress during or shortly after pregnancy is common and affects around one woman in six (Wooster 2007). Those who have a history of mental health problems are at greater risk. It is known that women who have suffered depression in the antenatal period are more likely to suffer this postnatally (Evan et al. 2001; Buist 2002; NICE 2003; all cited in Hammond and Crozier 2007), therefore the midwife should carefully read the woman's antenatal notes for any indications about previous mental health issues.

Some 50–80 per cent of women experience 'baby blues' on or around the third day postnatally. It is thought that this is due to changes in the levels of oestrogen, progesterone and prolactin, causing a temporary alteration in the woman's emotional well-being (Raynor and Oates 2003). This is often compounded by discomfort at the milk 'coming in' and possibly by the transition from hospital to home. 'Baby blues' are often characterised by unexpected tearfulness and anxiety, which may take both the woman and her partner by surprise. If the woman has been warned of this in the antenatal period, she may be better able to accept these feelings and await their natural passing. If not, the midwife should gently explain why she is feeling this way, advise her that it is quite normal and observe her carefully over the next day or so to ensure that her mood returns to normal. This transient period of low mood is not a predictor of future mental health problems. If the symptoms of the 'baby blues' have not resolved by day 10–14, the woman should be assessed for postnatal depression (NICE 2006).

Case Notes

Mike's partner, Sadie, gave birth to their first baby three weeks ago. At first, all seemed well, but today Mike rings the community midwife and asks her to visit Sadie. He is concerned that Sadie seems tired all the time and has little enthusiasm for anything. He has suggested getting a baby-sitter and going out for a meal, but Sadie is not interested. Sadie has refused visits and offers of help from her family and friends and is often tearful and moody.

Postnatal depression affects 10–15 per cent of mothers (NICE 2006). It is characterised by persistent low mood, loss of interest or pleasure in everyday life, persistent fatigue, loss of self-confidence, poor concentration, despair or even suicidal thoughts (Gutteridge 2007; Wooster 2007). Other mental health disorders can also complicate the puerperium, therefore the term 'postnatal depression' must be used with care (NICE 2007). Women can be encouraged to look after their mental health by taking exercise, getting sufficient rest, getting help with baby cares and talking to an understanding person about their feelings. Social isolation is a known risk factor for postnatal depression, therefore access to social support networks may be a lifeline (NICE 2006). Women and their partners should be given information on how to recognise the signs of postnatal depression and contact numbers of where to seek help.

Women with mental health problems, whether new or pre-existing, should be offered a continued period of midwifery support, in line with the *Midwives Rules and Standards* (NMC 2004) and the NICE Guidelines (2006, 2007a), which may go well beyond the period of physical recovery. If midwifery resources cannot stretch that far, the woman's support should be taken over by an appropriate professional, such as her health visitor.

Puerperal psychosis is an acute condition affecting women after childbirth which causes sudden and dramatic changes of behaviour (Wooster 2007). Although this condition is rare (McGowan et al. 2007) it is often associated with thoughts of suicide or suicide attempts. The CEMACH report for the period 2000–2004 found that suicide was the leading cause of death after childbirth (CEMACH 2004). The report recommends that midwives should make a priority of assessing suicide risk in mothers suffering from any mental health disorder and, if necessary, refer for urgent specialist care. It is anticipated that the maternity services will implement a risk assessment tool as part of standard midwifery care in the near future (McGowan et al. 2007).

Guidelines on Antenatal and Postnatal Mental Health from NICE were published in February 2007. Key points of the guidelines are detailed below. At the first contact in the postnatal period, the woman should be asked:

- Whether she has a history of severe mental illness
- Whether she has a history of psychiatric treatment
- Whether there is any family history of perinatal mental illness

At 4–6 weeks postnatally and again at 3–4 months, the woman should be asked these two questions:

- During the last month, have you often been bothered by feeling down, depressed or hopeless?

- During the last month have you often been bothered by having little interest or pleasure in doing things?

If the answer to either is 'yes', the woman should be asked:

- Is this something you feel you need or want help with?

If there are concerns, the woman should be referred to her GP for assessment. If the woman has a known mental illness or history of such, the midwife should ask about her mental health at each visit. Women with mild to moderate depression should be offered:

- Self-help strategies
- Listening visits at home
- Short-term cognitive behavioural therapy
(NICE 2007)

Care of the baby in the community

The purpose of examining the baby is to monitor daily changes and detect any signs of deviation from the expected norm. When visiting a woman in her home or meeting her at a postnatal clinic, the midwife will offer information (NICE 2006) and advice to enable her to:

- Assess her baby's general health
- Recognise signs of ill health
- Contact the relevant health professional or emergency service if necessary

Detailed and accurate records must be maintained to enable continuity of care.

It is important that the midwife sees both mother and baby at each postnatal contact so that emotional attachment can be assessed (NICE 2006) and any barriers to this detected as early as possible. This presents a good opportunity for the midwife to explain to both parents and/or other family members the baby's social capabilities and changing needs. Questions from the family should be actively encouraged and information or reassurance offered as required.

When assessing the baby's health and development, the midwife may begin by asking the woman about his well-being. It may not be necessary to undress and physically examine a baby at every visit. However, if the midwife has concerns about the baby's health or about his parents' ability to care for him, this might form part of the overall assessment. As part of the assessment of the baby, the midwife will ask about and observe the following:

- Feeding: interest in feeding, method, frequency and (if bottle-fed) volume
- Elimination: frequency of urination and defecation, changing stools, signs of constipation or diarrhoea
- Muscle tone, posture
- Behaviour: including ability to settle between feeds, sleep patterns, response to stimuli, response to handling
- Crying: pitch and duration, response to comforting
- Temperature: it is not necessary to measure temperature with a thermometer unless the baby appears unwell
- Skin: colour, condition, lesions or trauma, rashes, spots, signs of non-accidental injury
- Umbilicus: signs of separation of cord stump, signs of possible infection
- Resolution of any birth trauma such as caput and moulding
- Eyes: any discharge is noted
- Mouth: any signs of thrush are noted

The midwife will monitor and record any jaundice until it has resolved. Parents will be advised on how to recognise signs of worsening jaundice and related symptoms and of how to seek help (NICE 2006). A mother who is breastfeeding may need particular reassurance and support at this time.

Skin care

Parents should be advised on the daily hygiene needs of the baby and the avoidance of unnecessary cleaning agents and toiletries (NICE 2006). The nappy area may be inspected to observe for soreness, thrush or nappy rash and appropriate treatment recommended.

Colic

If the baby shows signs of colic he should first be assessed to rule out other underlying conditions. The midwife will need to take a detailed history from the parents about the nature, onset and duration of symptoms. There is no medical treatment for colic, but parents should be given sensitive reassurance and advice on ways to position and hold their baby to minimise his discomfort (NICE 2006).

Weighing

Most babies lose up to 10 per cent of their birth weight in the first few days of life and regain it by around day 10. Babies are routinely weighed on day 5 to detect any abnormal weight loss so that the underlying cause may be investigated and treated. Regular weighing of babies is not done routinely unless there is a particular cause for concern.

Blood spot test

The midwife will undertake the blood spot test (formally known as the 'Guthrie test') to screen for certain metabolic anomalies and haemoglobinopathies between day 5 and day 8. Fully informed parental consent is required, so the midwife must ensure that parents have had time to consider their options beforehand, preferably with access to written information. The midwife must ensure that parents know when and how the results of the test will be conveyed to them.

Activity

- Make brief notes about the metabolic disorders and haemoglobinopathies that are screened for with the blood spot test.
- Find out how the results of the blood spot test are given to parents in your area.
- Find out what happens when a baby screens positive for one of these conditions.

Safety issues

When conducting home visits, health professionals should take the opportunity to assess and advise on relevant safety issues such as baby equipment and the home environment (NICE 2006). Advice on safe sleeping for the baby should be given and repeated as necessary. Current guidelines from the Department of Health about avoiding sudden infant death syndrome should be explained and reinforced with written information in the appropriate language. This should be documented in the woman's postnatal notes. Particular attention should be paid to high-risk practices such as smoking around the baby or bed-sharing when either parent is under the influence of drugs or alcohol.

The midwife must remain alert to the signs and symptoms of child abuse and should know the route for referral according to local child protection policies.

Table 8.2 Sources of continuing advice, care and support for parents with a new baby

Service	How to access	Purpose
Health visitor	Home visit around day 10, thereafter as per need of the family. Usually contactable in office hours only. Contact number given in hospital.	Qualified nurse or midwife. Cares for family until child aged 5. Arranges baby's vaccinations and routine checks. Screens women for risk of PND. Valuable source of childcare advice and information on support groups, etc.
Midwives' drop-in clinic	Not universally available. Local practices vary. Usually office hours only.	May be a substitute for home visits if woman is well enough to attend.
GP	During set surgery hours	Most GPs do home visits if the woman is unable to access the surgery.
Out of hours GP service	When the surgery is closed. May be directly transferred on ringing GPs number or via 'NHS Direct'.	Home visits or central clinic. For urgent cases only. The patient cannot expect to see their regular GP.
NHS Direct	24-hour telephone service.	An advice line staffed by qualified nurses.
Accident and Emergency	24-hour service at general hospitals.	For emergencies only. Some hospitals have a specialist paediatric A & E service.
Local support groups	Vary according to area. Advertised through Yellow Pages, local papers, notice boards in doctors' surgeries, word of mouth, health visitors, websites etc.	For social support, friendship, etc. or for specialist advice, e.g. breastfeeding support. Some groups teach particular skills, e.g. baby massage.

Ongoing advice and care

During the course of her postnatal visits to the woman's home, the midwife will take the opportunity to inform women and their families about sources of continuing care and local support networks. These are important not just for the woman's and baby's physical well-being, but also to help the family adjust to their new role and access means of social support if necessary (NICE 2006). These sources are detailed in Table 8.2.

Activity

- Identify three local networks of support in your area for new parents.
- Make notes of the location, contact details and cost (if any).
- Make notes of the aims of these organisations, including any specific group of parents/mothers they are aimed at.

Conclusion

The birth of a baby is a life-changing event, having physical, social and psychological consequences for the woman. Most women adapt well to these changes and become happy and confident mothers. A few succumb to the physical or emotional stresses that this time brings and need ongoing support and care. The midwife has an important role not only in preparing women for birth and motherhood, but also in supporting them through this transition stage and identifying their changing needs. Both woman and baby deserve the best possible care at this crucial time.

References

Baston, H. (2004a) Midwifery basics: postnatal care – principles and practice. *The Practising Midwife* 7(11): 40–4.

Baston, H. (2004b) Midwifery basics: care during labour: third stage. *The Practising Midwife* 7(4): 31–6.

Baston, H. (2004c) Midwifery basics: postnatal care – perineal repair. *The Practising Midwife* 7(9): 12–15.

Baston, H. (2005a) Midwifery basics: postnatal care – post-operative care following caesarean. *The Practising Midwife* 8(2): 32–6.

Baston, H. (2005b) Midwifery basics: postnatal care – postnatal care in the community. *The Practising Midwife* 8(3): 35–40.

Buist, A. (2000) Managing depression in pregnancy. *Australian Family Physician* 29(7): 663–7.

CEMACH (2004) *Why Mothers Die 2000–2. Report on Confidential Enquiries into Maternal Deaths in the United Kingdom.* London: HMSO.

Department of Health (2004) *National Service Framework for Children, Young People and Maternity Services.* London: HMSO.

Department of Health (2005) *Bottle Feeding.* London: DH. www.dh.gov.uk/publications.

Downe, S. (2003) Transition and the second stage of labour. In D. Fraser and M. Cooper, *Myles Textbook for Midwives.* Edinburgh: Churchill Livingstone.

Evans, J., Heron, J., Francombe, H., Oke, S. and Golding, J. (2001) Cohort study of depressed mood during pregnancy and after childbirth. *British Medical Journal* 323: 257–60.

Fleming, E. M., Hagen, S. and Niven, C. (2003) Does perineal suturing make a difference? The SUNS trial. *British Journal of Obstetrics and Gynaecology* 110(7): 684–9.

Gamble, J. A., Creedy, D. K., Webster, J. and Moyle, W. (2005) A review of the literature on debriefing or non-directive counselling to prevent post-partum emotional distress. In S. Wickham (ed.), *Midwifery Best Practice*, Vol. 3. Edinburgh: Elsevier Butterworth-Heinemann.

Gordon, B., Mackrodt, C., Fern, E. et al. (1998) The Ipswich childbirth study: a randomised evaluation of two stage postpartum perineal repair leaving the skin unsutured. *British Journal of Obstetric and Gynaecology* 105(4): 441–5.

Gutteridge, K. (2007) Making a difference. *Midwives: The Official Journal of the Royal College of Midwives* 10(4): 173–5.

Hall, J. (2005) Midwifery basics: postnatal care – postnatal fertility control advice. *The Practising Midwife* 8(5): 39–43.

Hammond, S. and Crozier, K. (2007) Gloomy anticipation. *Midwives: The Official Journal of the Royal College of Midwives* 10(4): 164–6.

Inch, S. (2003) Feeding. In D. Fraser and M. Cooper (2003) *Myles Textbook for Midwives*. Edinburgh: Churchill Livingstone.

Johnson, R. and Taylor, W. (2005) *Skills for Midwifery Practice*, 2nd edition. Edinburgh: Elsevier Churchill Livingstone.

Kenyon, S. and Ford, F. (2004) How can we improve women's postbirth perineal health? *MIDIRS Midwifery Digest* 14(1): 7–12.

Marchant, S. (2003a) Physiology and care in the puerperium. In D. Fraser and M. Cooper, *Myles Textbook for Midwives*. Edinburgh: Churchill Livingstone.

Marchant, S. (2003b) Physical problems and complications in the puerperium. In D. Fraser and M. Cooper, *Myles Textbook for Midwives*. Edinburgh: Churchill Livingstone.

McDonald, S. (2003) Physiology and management of the third stage of labour. In D. Fraser and M. Cooper, *Myles Textbook for Midwives*. Edinburgh: Churchill Livingstone.

McGowan, I., Sinclair, M. and Owens, M. (2007) Maternal suicide: rates and trends. *Midwives: The Official Journal of the Royal College of Midwives* 10(4): 167–9.

National Institute for Health and Clinical Excellence (2004) *Caesarean Section*. Clinical Guideline 13. London: NICE.

National Institute for Health and Clinical Excellence (2006) *Routine Postnatal Care of Women and Their Babies*. Clinical Guideline 37. London: NICE.

National Institute for Health and Clinical Excellence (2007a) *Antenatal and Postnatal Mental Health*. Clinical Guideline 45. London: NICE.

National Institute for Health and Clinical Excellence (2007b) *Intrapartum Care: Care of Health Women and their Babies during Childbirth*. Clinical Guideline London: NICE.

Nursing and Midwifery Council (2004) *Midwives Rules and Standards*. London: NMC.

Raynor, M. D. and Oates, M. R. (2003) The psychology and psychopathology of pregnancy and childbirth. In D. Fraser and M. Cooper, *Myles Textbook for Midwives*. Edinburgh: Churchill Livingstone.

Ravzi, K., Chua, S., Arulkomaran, S. et al.(1996) A comparison between visual estimation and laboratory determination of blood loss during the 3rd stage of labour. *Australia ard New Zealand Journal of Obstetrics and Gynaecology* 36(2): 152–4.

Royal College of Obstetricians and Gynaecologists (1995) *Report of a Working Party on Prophylaxis against Thrombo-embolism in Gynaecology and Obstetrics*. London: RCOG.

Royal College of Midwives (1999) Transition to motherhood. In *Transition to Parenting: An Open Learning Resource for Midwives*. London: Royal College of Midwives Trust.

Royal College of Midwives (2002) *Successful Breastfeeding* 3rd edition. Edinburgh: Elsevier Churchill Livingstone.

Wallace, H. and Marshall, D. (2001) Skin-to-skin contact: benefits and difficulties. *Practising Midwife* 4(5): 30–2.

Wooster, E. (2007) *Supporting Mental Health Midwives* 10(4): 170–2.

Medication and the Midwife

Cathy Hamilton

Introduction

The practice of midwifery is concerned with supporting women and their families through the normal, physiological process of childbirth. However, women may complain of discomfort or minor disorders associated with childbirth, they may become unwell during pregnancy or labour or they may have a pre-existing medical condition. In these cases, the midwife may be required to administer medicine to relieve the discomfort or to treat the condition. Headley et al. (2004) have reported that 92.4 per cent of pregnant women in their research group had taken a medicinal product at least once during their pregnancies. At least a third of the women reported taking a pain-relieving medicine such as paracetamol, while 23 per cent reported using an antacid to relieve symptoms of indigestion. The use of medicinal products during pregnancy is such that it is important that midwives are competent to safely undertake all aspects of drug administration. They should have a sound knowledge of how drugs work and their usual dosages, side-effects and contraindications, as well as those drugs that may commonly be administered during childbirth. The midwife should be up to date with any changes in drug therapy which may impact on a woman's treatment. Midwives should also be fully conversant with the legislative framework governing the administration of drugs.

For the purposes of this chapter the following definitions will be used:

- Medicines: these include substances that are prescribed with a view to providing a remedy for a disease or ailment. Examples

of medicines are drugs, dressings, topical creams, ointments, blood products (but not blood), intravenous/subcutaneous fluids and oxygen.
- A drug is defined as any substance that can be used to modify a chemical process in the body with the intention of treating a disease, relieving a symptom, enhancing performance and altering a state of mind.

(NMC 2007)

Any drug which a midwife administers to a pregnant woman is liable to cross the placenta and could have a detrimental effect on the fetus. Similarly, for a woman who is breastfeeding any drug taken could be transmitted to the baby via her breast milk. For these reasons it is particular important that a midwife is aware of which drugs are safe to take during pregnancy and while breastfeeding, and if she is not sure, to find out and advise the woman accordingly.

In response to Headley et al. (2004), it is advised (British Medical Association and the Royal Pharmaceutical Society 2004) that the use of medicines should be avoided as much as possible during pregnancy. It is also recommended that drugs which have been extensively tested and found to be safe during pregnancy should be prescribed in preference to new or untried drugs.

This chapter aims to give an overview of issues relating to the use of medicines in the context of midwifery practice.

Legislation governing the administration of drugs

Midwifery practice in relation to the administration of drugs to women and babies is governed by several documents including *Guidelines for the Administration of Medicines* (NMC 2004b) and the *Midwives Rules and Standards* (NMC 2004a). The Nursing and Midwifery Council (NMC) guidance document (NMC 2004b) highlights the fact that the administration of medicines is an important aspect of the professional practice of all individuals registered with the Council. However, it is emphasised that it should not be viewed as a mechanical task which is performed exactly in accordance with the written prescription of a medical practitioner. This is where professional judgement and thought is important when each practitioner views the client as an individual, taking all aspects of her care into consideration (the holistic approach). This includes issues such as what other drugs the woman is taking, how they might interact with each other and what reactions she has had to a drug previously.

Rule 7 of the *Midwives Rules and Standards* (NMC 2004b) states that a practising midwife should only supply and administer those drugs for which she has received appropriate training. This includes being familiar with the dosage of the drug, any potential side-effects, restrictions to its use and method of administration.

Midwifery practice is further subject to medicines legislation. This enables qualified midwives to supply and administer on their own initiative any of the medicines which are specified as being under midwives exemptions (this term is discussed later), provided they are doing so as part of their professional midwifery practice. In other words, a midwife is entitled to administer certain medicines on her own responsibility without the need for them to be prescribed by a doctor.

The Medicines Act 1968

This legislation was introduced by the then Department of Health and Social Security following a review of legislation relating to medicines, prompted by the thalidomide tragedy of the early 1960s. During this time, many pregnant women took the drug thalidomide as treatment for morning sickness. It was not known at the time that this drug could have an adverse effect on the developing fetus as no testing on pregnant animals had been done prior to the drug being released to the public. This led to thousands of babies being born with severe and very distinctive limb deformities.

The Medicines Act 1968 brought together most of the previous laws relating to medicines and introduced other legal provisions for the control of medicines, including supply, possession and manufacture. It classifies medicinal drugs into three categories depending on the dangers they pose to the public and the risk of misuse. The categories are:

1. Prescription-only medicines
2. Pharmacy-only medicines
3. General sale list medicines

Prescription-only medicines (POM)
These are medicines that can only be supplied and given to a client on the instruction of an appropriate practitioner (for example, a doctor or dentist). Since the Medicinal Products Prescription by Nurses Act 1992, health visitors and district nurses who have recorded their nurse prescribing qualification with the NMC are also able to prescribe certain medicines from the approved nurse prescribers list.

Pharmacy-only medicines (P)
Pharmacy only medicine can only be bought from a registered pharmacy provided that the sale is supervised by the pharmacist, enabling

the pharmacist to confirm with the client that it is safe for them to take the medicine. For example, the client will be asked if they are taking any other types of medicine which might interact or interfere with the requested medicine, or if they have any other condition, such as pregnancy, high blood pressure or cardiac problems, which might be affected by the medicine.

Some medicines may only be sold once the pharmacist is satisfied that certain circumstances have been fulfilled. For example, emergency contraception (also known as the 'morning-after pill') may only be sold to the person who requires the contraception and she must be over the age of 16 years.

General sale list medicines (GSL)

These do not need a prescription or the supervision of a pharmacist and can be obtained by members of the public from supermarkets or other retail outlets. Usually only a small pack size of the medicine may be sold in these stores. For example, the largest pack size of paracetamol that may be sold from a shop is 16 tablets whereas packs of 32 tablets may be sold from a pharmacy. Similarly only low strengths of the medicine may be sold from a general store. For example, the highest strength of ibuprofen tablets that may be sold from a shop is 200 mg whereas tablets containing 400 mg may be sold from a pharmacy.

Some medicines may be reclassified from prescription only to pharmacy or from pharmacy to general sale list. This can happen once it is considered that the medicine is safe for most people to use. For example, acyclovir cream, which is used to treat cold sores, was initially available as prescription only. After a few years, it was reclassified to a pharmacy medicine, and recently it has been reclassified again to a general sale list medicine.

Midwives' exemptions and prescription-only medicines

Case Notes

Fay is a first-year student midwife and is undertaking her first placement on the delivery suite. The woman she is caring for is in the first stage of labour and requesting pethidine as a method of pain relief. Fay asks her mentor if she should ask the Senior House Officer to come to the ward to prescribe the drug. She is surprised when her mentor informs her that this is not necessary as pethidine is one of the drugs on the midwives exemption list.

Specific drugs, including those usually available only on prescription, may be supplied to midwives for use in their professional practice. In this case midwives are recognised as being exempt from certain restrictions on the sale or supply and administration of medicines under the Medicines Act 1968. Examples of drugs commonly used in midwifery practice include syntometrine, which is given during the third stage of labour to facilitate the delivery of the placenta, and pethidine, which may be administered as pain relief during labour. The midwife can administer both these drugs on her own responsibility without the need for a prescription.

These drugs may be obtained from a retail or hospital pharmacy by a registered midwife who has notified her intention to practise to the Local Supervisory Authority. She may use them only in her professional midwifery capacity. For example, she would not be permitted to administer the drug to a friend or family member unless she was caring for them during childbirth.

If, however, a medicine is not included in midwives exemptions then an appropriate prescription or Patient Group Direction (this term is defined later) will be required in order for the midwife to administer the drug to a woman or baby.

Preparations for use by midwives are shown below. They are included in Schedule 5 (parts I and III) of the Prescription Only Medicines (Human Use) Order 1997. By Statutory Instrument (SI) 1997, 1830, the midwife can supply:

1. All medicines that are not prescription only medicines and are included in the British National Formulary (see below for information about this resource).
2. Prescription only medicines containing any of the following substances but no other prescription only substances:
   - Choral hydrate (Welldorm) (this drug is no longer recommended for use during pregnancy because the chemical composition has changed)
   - Ergometrine maleate (but only when contained in a medicinal product which is not for administration via an injection)
   - Pentozocine hydrochloride
   - Phytomenadione: Vitamin K (SI 1998 2081)
   - Triclofos sodium (choral hydrate derivative)

The midwife can also administer via injection and in the course of her professional practice prescription only medicines containing any of the following substances (SI 1997 1830):

- Diamorphine* (heroin)
- Ergometrine maleate
- Lignocaine
- Lignocaine hydrochloride
- Morphine*
- Naloxone hydrochloride (Narcan)
- Oxytocins (natural and synthetic)
- Pentazocine hydrochloride (Fortral)
- Pethidine hydrochloride
- Phytomenadione (Vitamin K)
- Promazine hydrochloride (Sparine)

Lignocaine, lignocaine hydrochloride and promazine hydrochloride may only be given by a midwife while attending a woman in childbirth.

Examples of P and GSL medicines which a midwife may use in her practice are paracetamol, often used to relieve mild to moderate discomfort in the antenatal and postnatal period, oral iron preparations, laxatives and enemata and inhalational analgesia, such as entonox (RCM 2006).

A community-based midwife or independent midwife may need to carry antiseptics, sedatives, analgesics, oxytocic drugs, local anaesthetics and approved agents for neonatal resuscitation. The drugs a community midwife can use should be determined locally and a written policy available to stipulate what these medicines are (Dimond 2003).

Whatever drugs a midwife uses in her practice it is clearly stated in the *Midwives Rules and Standards* (NMC 2004b) that a midwife should not administer any drug unless she is familiar with its usage and has received appropriate training with regards to its use.

Activity

Find out what medicines a community midwife carries in your own local area.

- How does she obtain her supplies?
- How does she store them?

* An Amendment Order in 2004 added the two controlled drugs – diamorphine and morphine – to the midwives exemptions list.

The British National Formulary

The *British National Formulary* (BNF) is a joint publication of the British Medical Association and the Royal Pharmaceutical Society of Great Britain. It is published twice a year under the authority of a Joint Formulary Committee which comprises representatives of the two professional bodies and of the UK Health Departments. The BNF aims to provide all healthcare professionals with sound, up-to-date information about the use of medicines. It includes key information on the selection, prescribing, dispensing and administration of medicines. Medicines generally prescribed in the UK are covered and those considered less suitable for prescribing are clearly identified. It is available in hard copy or electronically (www.bnf.org).

Administering medication: principles

The midwife should ask herself the following questions before administering any medication to the women or babies in her care. These form the basic principles for the safe administration of medicines and are recommended by the NMC in its guidance document (NMC 2004a):

- Are you familiar with the drug? For example, do you know how it works, the normal dosage, any potential side-effects or possible reason why it should not be given to this particular woman (contraindications)?
- Are you aware of the woman's plan of care and do you know that there is actually a need for her to receive the medication?
- Has all the relevant information about the medication been given to the woman and has she made an informed decision to have the drug?
- Have you confirmed the identity of the woman to ensure that the correct drug is given to the correct client? In maternity care, most women are conscious and are able to confirm who they are, but if the woman is unconscious, then her identity will need to be confirmed by checking the name and hospital number on her identity band
- Does the woman have any known allergies?
- If appropriate, is the prescription chart clearly written and unambiguous?
- Does the prescription chart include the correct name of the drug, how it is to be administered (for example, orally or by injection into the muscle or vein), the amount to be given, how frequently

it is to be given, when treatment started and the date when it should be completed?

- Has the medication reached its expiry date and is therefore unsuitable to use?

Drug administration checklist

Immediately prior to administering the drug, the following questions should be asked:

- Is it the correct woman? (there may be other women on the ward with the same or similar name)
- Date?
- Time?
- Drug?
- Dosage?
- Route?
- Is the woman allergic to the drug?

Following administration of the drug:

- Record accurately in the woman's notes that the drug has been given as required by Rule 9 of the *Midwives Rules and Standards* (NMC 2004b)
- Record if the woman declines to take the medication as prescribed
- Sign and date the prescription chart to show that the drug has been given
- Inform the doctor who prescribed the drug or another authorised prescriber if the woman has any contraindications to the use of that particular drug or develops an adverse reaction to the drug
- Inform a doctor if assessment of the woman suggests that the medication is no longer needed
- Rule 7 of the *Midwives Rules and Standards* (NMC 2004b) highlights the fact that midwives should expect their records in relation to drug administration to be checked by a Supervisor of Midwives every so often

Checking of drugs

In some cases, a midwife may be required to supply and administer drugs on her own responsibility (Siney 2004). However, in the interest of preventing drug errors, it is considered good practice for a registered midwife to check the drug that she is going to give with a second practitioner. This is particularly important if the drug is to be given intravenously or if a complex calculation is required (NMC 2004a). A student midwife, on the other hand, must always be supervised when giving any medication and the registered midwife should countersign the student's signature (NMC 2004a).

In order to reduce the number of drug errors, the NMC (2004a) considers that it is unacceptable for a drug to be prepared before it is needed. An example of this in midwifery practice would be when a midwife draws up an injection of syntometrine into a syringe and leaves it by the bedside of the woman in labour ready for the third stage of labour. If labour does not proceed as expected and there is a delay, then there is the potential for this drug to be given in error during rather than following labour. If syntometrine is given during labour, this would lead to the potentially disastrous situation of the uterus undergoing a strong, sustained contraction with the fetus still inside.

With the same principle in mind, a midwife should not administer a drug which has been prepared by a colleague unless she was present while it was being prepared and is satisfied with the checking procedure (NMC 2004b). An exception to this is when a woman already has an intravenous infusion in place which was prepared by a midwife and another midwife then takes over her care.

Controlled drugs

Certain POM are further classified as controlled drugs. Examples which a midwife might use are pethidine and diamorphine. In some cases, these medicines may be misused or sold illegally, so for this reason there are stricter legal controls on their supply – hence the term 'controlled drugs'.

There are controls on:

- Who may prescribe these medicines
- How the prescription is written
- How much may be prescribed
- How the medicines are stored

However, a registered midwife is able to administer certain controlled drugs on her own responsibility without a prescription from a medical practitioner.

Misuse of Drugs Act 1971

This Act prevents the possession, supply and manufacture of medicinal and other products, except where this has been made legal by the Misuse of Drugs Regulations 1985. This was amended by the Misuse of Drugs Regulations 2001.

These regulations further divide the controlled drugs into five categories or schedules. The Schedules are as follows.

Schedule 1: Drugs which may be used illegally and for social enjoyment such as drugs which stimulate hallucinations and a sense of euphoria. These drugs currently have no recognised medicinal uses. They include cannabis, coca leaf, LSD (lysergic acid diethylamide – 'acid'), and mescaline. Only individuals with a Home Office licence may legally possess schedule 1 drugs for use in medical research.

Schedule 2: Drugs which may become addictive, for example, pethidine, diamorphine and morphine.

Schedule 3: Some barbiturates and pentazocine.

Schedule 4: The benzodiazepine tranquilisers, for example, diazepam, nitrazepam and temazepam. Midwives may administer these drugs to help women sleep or relax during pregnancy or following childbirth.

Schedule 5: Medicines which may contain a small amount of a controlled drug. For example, certain pain-relieving drugs and cough mixtures.

Activity

Jenny is planning to deliver her baby at home. She informs her community midwife that if the pain gets very severe she would like to use pethidine as pain relief.

How can the midwife ensure that Jenny has a supply of the drug for use during labour?

Issues in the handling of controlled drugs

Supply

Community midwives or independent midwives may sometimes want to obtain a supply of a controlled drug such as pethidine for use at a homebirth. Legislation surrounding this is in accordance with the Prescription Only Medicine (Human Use) Order of 1997. The midwife will need to obtain a Midwives Supply Order form from a Supervisor of Midwives. This order must be in writing, including the full name and occupation of the individual requesting the drug; it must state the purpose for which the drug is intended and include the total quantity of the drug to be obtained. As well as these details it might be helpful for audit purposes for the midwife's NMC personal identification number (PIN) to be included as well as the contact details of the Supervisor of Midwives and the name of the woman for whom the drug is to be administered.

The controlled drug is then supplied to the midwife by a pharmacist for use in her own professional practice only. In other words, it can not be given to another midwife or health care practitioner to administer (NMC 2005b). The pharmacist should have a prior agreement with the midwife to supply the drug and should have a record of the midwife's signature.

On providing the drug, the name and amount of the drug supplied and name and address of the supplier should be recorded in the midwife's drugs book. This should also contain information about the dates the drug was given, the woman's name and the amount used.

The procedure as described above is intended for use by community-based midwives or independent midwives attending home-births. Midwives working in NHS hospitals need to comply with local policies and procedures when administering controlled drugs, although it may be decided that they will follow the same procedures as community-based midwives (RCM 2006). In some NHS Trusts, a standing order (see below) may be signed by a consultant obstetrician and the Head of Midwifery authorising the administration of controlled drugs by midwives based in the hospital.

For a homebirth, rather than the midwife obtaining a supply of controlled drugs, the woman may obtain a prescription for pethidine from her general practitioner. In this case, the drugs are owned by the woman and she becomes responsible for the destruction or return of any unwanted ampoules.

Storage of controlled drugs

Controlled drugs on Schedules 1 and 2 must be kept in a locked cupboard within another non-moveable locked cupboard. Drugs on schedules 3, 4 and 5 do not need to be kept in the controlled drug cupboard (i.e. double-locked), but should still be locked away.

Administration of a controlled drug

Two people, one of whom is a registered midwife or nurse, are required to check the drug, observe it being given and then sign the controlled drug register.

The recommended procedure is as follows:

- Confirm that the stock of the drug in the cupboard tallies with the drug register total
- Record the woman's name, amount of drug to be given, date of administration and amount of stock remaining in the drug register

- Check the name, amount and expiry date of the drug
- Draw up the drug if being given by injection and take to the woman
- Confirm her identity by checking her name band or asking her name and date of birth
- Give the drug in the appropriate way and dispose of all equipment
- Sign the drug register, including the time that the drug was actually administered
- Record the name of drug, amount, route, time and date of administration in the appropriate documentation – for example, the prescription sheet and the woman's notes

Destruction of unused controlled drugs

If a midwife has obtained a supply of controlled drugs which are no longer needed then she must destroy them, but only in the presence of an authorised person. This procedure is stipulated in the Misuse of Drugs Regulations 1985. An authorised person varies slightly throughout the UK but includes the following:

- A Supervisor of Midwives
- A regional pharmaceutical officer (England)
- A pharmaceutical officer of the Welsh Office
- A chief administrative pharmaceutical officer of the Health Boards (Scotland)
- An inspector appointed by the Department of Health and Social Services (Northern Ireland)
- Medical officers (England, Scotland, Wales)
- An Inspector of the Royal Pharmaceutical Society of Great Britain
- A police officer
- An Inspector of the Home Office drugs branch

A midwife is also permitted to take any unused controlled drugs back to the pharmacist who originally supplied them or to an appropriate medical officer but not to a Supervisor of Midwives.

If a woman has obtained her own prescription for pethidine, then by law these drugs are her property and she is responsible for destroying any which are not used. She should be advised to destroy the unused drugs, preferably with the midwife in attendance. Alternatively they can be returned to the pharmacist but this must be done by the woman and not by the midwife acting on her behalf.

Regardless of the way in which the drug is disposed of, it is important that the midwife includes in the woman's records what advice she gave and what action was taken including the type and quantity of the drug.

Controlled drugs: The legacy of Harold Shipman

Harold Shipman was the notorious Hyde GP, who in the 1990s was convicted of killing 15 of his patients by injecting them with a fatal dose of controlled drugs. It is believed that he was almost certainly responsible for the deaths of many more using the same method. He was able to do this by stockpiling a large quantity of controlled drugs, which he obtained from local pharmacies for use in his medical practice. As a result of this the focus of the Shipman Inquiry 4th Report (2004) was on the regulation of controlled drugs in the community setting. The government response to this report (DH 2004) agreed that there needed to be a strengthening of current systems of control. As midwives use controlled drugs in the community they will be subject to any forthcoming legislative changes. If any of the changes impact on current midwifery practice, this will need to be reflected in an updated *Midwives Rules and Standards* (RCM 2006).

Activity

Familiarise yourself with the procedures surrounding the supply, storage and administration of controlled drugs within your own maternity unit.

Patient group directions

Patient group directions (PGDs) are documents which make it legal for medicines to be given to groups of patients without individual prescriptions having to be written for each person (Dimond 2005). They are useful for providing treatment for a clearly defined condition where there is a proven advantage for care without compromising the patient's safety. PGDs are drawn up locally by doctors, dentists, pharmacists and other health care professionals. They must be signed by a doctor and a pharmacist, both of whom should have been involved in developing the direction, and it must be approved by the appropriate health care body.

If a medicine to be supplied or administered is on the midwives exemption list, no PGD is needed. To date, none of the midwives exemptions contained within the medicines legislation has been replaced by the PGD legislation and there is no legal need to change existing locally agreed policies into PGDs (NMC 2005a).

In midwifery practice, a PGD might be an appropriate option to consider if a group of women require a prescription only drug on a regular basis which does not appear on the midwives exemption list (NMC 2005a).

Unlicensed medicines

Doctors are free to prescribe drugs without an appropriate UK licence, but they do so on their own responsibility and must accept full liability. However, the regulations state that a medicine can only be included in a PGD if it has a current UK marketing authorisation or a homeopathic certificate of registration (NMC 2005a). In addition, drugs usually have a UK product licence stating how they are to be used.

In certain exceptional circumstances, drugs with a marketing authorisation can be used outside the terms of their product licence (that means administered via a different route from that stated in the terms of the licence). In these cases any PGD must clearly state that the drug is being used outside the terms of its licence with the reasons as to why this is necessary. An example of this in midwifery practice is syntocinon. This drug is on the midwives exemption list and so does not need a PGD and is usually used via the intravenous route to increase uterine contractions during the first and second stages of labour. However, it is not currently licensed in the UK for *intramuscular use* during the third stage of labour. Intramuscular syntometrine is the drug normally used in the third stage of labour, but sometimes, particularly when a woman has high blood pressure, intramuscular syntocinon is the recommended drug as it does not have the side-effect of raising the blood pressure, which syntometrine has.

In this context, intramuscular use of syntocinon in the third stage of labour could be considered for a PGD so that midwives are able to administer it intramuscularly without needing a prescription from a doctor.

Patient-specific directions

A patient-specific direction (PSD) can be used once a patient has been assessed by the prescriber, who then asks another health care professional to give a drug to the patient. A PSD is a form of prescription and can be for a single dose of drug or a course of drugs to be given over several days. The PSD can be a written request in the medical notes or on the patient's drug chart (RCM 2006).

Standing orders or locally agreed policies

The term standing order is often used to refer to local guidelines for the administration of medicines. These may be used to supplement medicines legislation relating to midwives exemptions. For example, a midwife may say that there is a standing order for her to administer pethidine to women in labour. However, the term does not legally exist and there is no requirement in the law to use standing orders for those medicines which midwives exemptions legislation permits them to supply and administer anyway (RCM 2006).

The use of standing orders for hospital-based midwives began in 1972. The Aitken Report (1958) had recommended that midwives working in hospitals be subject to the same regulations for the administration of medicines and controlled drugs as nurses. This suggestion was made in order to ensure safe and secure handling of medicines (RCM 2006), but it meant that all medicines given by a midwife would need to be prescribed by a doctor before they could be administered. This created many difficulties for midwives and led to unacceptable delays in treatment as women were forced to wait for their pain relief and oxytocic drugs to control bleeding during the third stage of labour.

In response, the Department of Health and Social Security permitted doctors to authorise standing orders for the range of drugs used by midwives. Following this the use of standing orders became widespread in maternity units (RCM 2006). The current position is that whilst the NMC acknowledges that the term standing order does not exist in medicines legislation, many midwives do value them because they provide guidance on appropriate circumstances, the administration and dosages for medicines that midwives may supply and administer (NMC 2005a). There is, however, no legal requirement to replace these with PGDs (NMC 2004b).

Activity

Find out whether there are any standing orders and/or PGDs in your maternity unit.

- Which health care professionals have been involved in producing them?

Teratogenic drugs

Any drug taken during pregnancy will cross the placenta and may affect the growth and development of the fetus. For this reason, any drug administered during pregnancy must offer benefits to the woman which outweighs the risk to the baby. Drugs which may have a potentially adverse effect on the fetus resulting in malformation or death are called teratogens. This is more of an issue during the early part of pregnancy when the baby's organs are developing. Much of the fetal development occurs before the woman even knows that she is pregnant. Thalidomide has already been mentioned, but there are many others. Women with known medical conditions such as epilepsy and depression have difficult decisions to make. For example, women taking the antidepressant paroxetine have been warned to avoid taking it in the early part of pregnancy due to the association of heart defects in babies born to women who have taken the drug (MHRA 2006). Women with epilepsy who wish to conceive need to weigh up the benefits of reducing their anti-epileptic drugs (which are known teratogens) in order to protect their babies against the fact that they may experience more seizures as a result. It is recommended that women seek advice from the medical specialists overseeing the treatment of their condition before reducing doses or stopping their therapeutic drugs.

Drugs and breastfeeding

If a breastfeeding woman takes any drug, then there is a potential risk that the substance may enter the baby's blood stream via the breast milk and possibly cause an adverse reaction. For example, the antidepressant amfebutamone has been shown to cause seizures in babies (Chaudron and Schoenecker 2004). As highlighted in the previous section, the risk of taking any drug needs to be weighed against the benefit to the mother.

The age of the baby is an important factor in deciding what the risk of an adverse reaction is. For example, a premature baby whose kidneys and liver are not fully mature may not be able to detoxify the drug effectively and toxic levels may accumulate in the baby's body to levels which cause an adverse reaction. On the other hand, an older baby who is being weaned onto solid food will be taking less breast milk and as a consequence will not be exposed to such high levels of the ingested drug.

If the woman is given a drug by injection which is destroyed in the gut (for example, insulin and heparin), this will not pass into the baby's circulation and so is safe to take while breastfeeding.

Certain drugs affect lactation by reducing milk production. For example, oral contraceptives containing oestrogen (the combined pill) have this effect. Progesterone-only pills, however, do not adversely affect the milk supply (Siney 2004). Other drugs may have an effect on the taste of the milk, which may make the baby reject it. For example, the antibiotic metronidazole makes breast milk taste bitter.

Case Notes

Treatment for Thrush and Breastfeeding: A Practice Dilemma

Sarah has been breastfeeding her baby since his birth ten days ago. She has been experiencing shooting pains in both breasts after each feed and her nipples feel very itchy and sensitive. On looking in her baby's mouth she can see creamy white patches inside his cheeks. Her midwife suggests that this may be a case of thrush (Candida albicans), a fungal infection which can affect the breasts during breastfeeding. It is thought that the most effective treatment for this infection is fluconazole.

Sarah visits her GP and asks for a prescription of fluconazole. However, her doctor explains that it is not licensed for use in breastfeeding mothers and he is reluctant to prescribe it as he would need to take full liability for its use. Sarah is very upset and feels that she must give up breastfeeding her baby as the pains are so severe.

Despite the fact that fluconazole is not licensed for use in breastfeeding mothers, it is licensed to be given to babies and the amount which can be given to babies within the licence is 6 mg/kg/day (Hale 2002). The amount which gets through into the breast milk is only 0.6 mg/kg/day (Amir and Hoover 2002). Studies on its use in premature babies weighing less than 1000 g has demonstrated no ill effects (Kaufman et al. 2001) and the World Health Organisation (2002) suggests that its use is compatible with breastfeeding. However, it is unlikely that the manufacturers of fluconazole will apply for a licence due to the costs involved. It has been difficult to secure funding for clinical trials to research the most effective treatments for thrush due to the ethical implications of undertaking randomised controlled trials on babies (Jones 2003). For these reasons, treatment options are based on small trials, which are mainly anecdotal in nature. The Breastfeeding Network produces evidence-based leaflets for health care professionals which have been designed to reassure them regarding the safety of fluconazole, the aim being that doctors feel confident to prescribe the drug despite its being unlicensed.

Routes of administration

It is beyond the scope of this chapter to describe in detail the pharmacological actions of all drugs which may be given during pregnancy and childbirth. The reader is referred to other resources such as the BNF or *The Midwives Pocket Formulary* (Banister 2004). There are also resources online. The pharmacist is the most valuable source of expert advice and as such should be consulted as soon as possible if the midwife or woman has any concerns or questions about medicines which have been prescribed.

Activity

Go to www.medicines.org.uk. Type in a commonly used drug such as syntometrine and find out how much information can be obtained from this resource.

It is important that the midwife is familiar with and competent to administer drugs.

Orally

Medication taken by the mouth (orally) will be absorbed via the gastrointestinal tract. In order for a woman or baby to take a drug orally they must be wiling to take the medication, alert and capable of swallowing (Johnson and Taylor 2006). As oral medications can be affected by other constituents in the stomach, it is important that the manufacturer's instructions are followed and the drug taken as directed – for example, before, during or after eating.

Oral medications can be available in several different preparations:

- Tablets: usually should be swallowed whole. If scored, they can be cut in half using a tablet cutter. Some tablets are coated with an outer layer to protect the stomach lining or to make them easier to swallow. If they are bitten and chewed, this effect is lost
- Capsules: these should also be swallowed whole and not chewed
- Granules and powders: these should be dissolved thoroughly (usually in water) before being given. Certain drugs such as paracetamol are available in soluble form for women who have difficulty swallowing tablets
- Elixir: certain drugs are also available in liquid form. The midwife should ensure that she shakes the bottle several times before measuring out the required amount to ensure thorough mixing of the drug. If giving a drug in liquid form to a baby, then the required amount should be drawn up into a sterile syringe and

inserted into the baby's mouth, usually towards the cheek (Johnson and Taylor 2006). Some hospitals now use special oral syringes in order to administer liquid medication to babies. These look very similar to ordinary syringes but with the markings appearing in blue rather than black. They also come with a hub, which prevents any of the medication leaking out of the sides

- Lozenges: these should be sucked rather than swallowed. They are usually used to treat conditions in the mouth such as a fungal infection
- Sublingual medication: these are absorbed under the tongue

Injection

Drugs are given by injection if they cannot be absorbed or are absorbed too slowly when given orally. Drugs given by injection are given parenterally, that is, they are taken into the body in a manner other than through the digestive tract, by intravenous or intramuscular injection.

Intramuscular (IM) injection

The drug is given straight into a muscle. The midwife needs to have a good knowledge of anatomy when choosing the best site to give an IM injection to make sure that she avoids nerves, bone and blood vessels.

Popular sites for an IM injection include the deltoid muscle (upper, outer part of the arm), the quadriceps muscle (upper outer part of the leg) and the gluteus maximus muscle (the upper, outer quarter of the buttock).

Example of a drug given by IM injection in midwifery practice is syntometrine, the oxytocic agent which causes the uterus to contract following the delivery of the baby in order to facilitate delivery of the placenta. This is commonly given in the quadriceps muscle.

Subcutaneous (SC) injection

This injection is given into the area beneath the skin containing connective tissue and fat. As these tissues have a reduced blood supply absorption is slower. Examples of drugs given by SC injection are insulin and heparin.

Intradermal injection

This injection is given just below the skin and is often used to administer local anaesthetic (lignocaine) prior to repair of the perineum following childbirth.

Intravenous (IV) injection

Drugs given straight into the blood stream via a vein work very quickly. This is advantageous if a quick effect is needed, but not so good if the woman reacts badly to the drug or has an allergic reaction to it. Drugs can be given intravenously as a bolus or IV 'push' injection, as an intermittent infusion (via a drip) or a syringe driver (equipment which pushes a measured dose into the vein over a set period of time). Sometimes, women can control the amount of drug given via the syringe driver at the push of a button. This is known as patient-controlled analgesia and is used in some maternity units so that women can control their post-operative pain relief following a caesarean section.

The midwife must be fully trained and informed in all aspects of IV drug administration. In some areas it is considered an extended role of the midwife and extra training is required following initial registration as a midwife. Regular updating may also be required in order to maintain competence (Johnson and Taylor 2006). However, all midwives are able to give IV ergometrine maleate for the treatment of postpartum haemorrhage (severe bleeding following childbirth) in an emergency. This is in accordance with Rule 6 of the *Midwives Rules and Standards* (NMC 2004b), which states that only in an emergency situation can a midwife provide care which she has not been trained to give. IV ergometrine has the effect of causing a rapid, sustained contraction of the uterus which should lead to cessation of the excessive bleeding. Up to two doses of 500 mg can be given intravenously in these situations. The midwife should not on her own authority give any more than these two doses because ergometrine can cause extreme constriction of the blood vessels leading to a sharp increase in the woman's blood pressure (Siney 2004).

Complementary and alternative therapies

Case Notes

Trudy shows her midwife Sandra some bottles of homeopathic pills which she intends to take during her forthcoming labour. She asks Sandra if this will be all right. Sandra has no knowledge about homeopathy and is unfamiliar with the pills Trudy shows her.

What should she advise?

Complementary and alternative medicine can be defined as any form of health care which does not form part of the traditional, mainstream medical approach (Tiran 2004). Women are increasingly turning to natural remedies to help them cope with the discomforts associated with pregnancy, childbirth and the postnatal period as they are reluctant to use pharmacological preparations which may have adverse side-effects for themselves or the baby (Tiran 2004).

Examples of alternative treatments associated with pregnancy include:

- *Aromatherapy*: this involves the use of highly concentrated essential oils which have been taken from plants and have a wide range of therapeutic properties. During childbirth the oils may be massaged into the skin once they have been dissolved in carrier oil in order to induce a sense of relaxation and help to relieve the pain of labour
- *Homeopathy*: this involves the use of extremely tiny doses of certain substances which, if administered in large amounts, would actually cause the condition they are attempting to treat. Many women use homeopathic arnica tablets for perineal bruising after childbirth
- *Medical herbalism*: this involves the medicinal use of plants and plant extracts, acupuncture and the use of herbal medicines. During pregnancy and childbirth, camomile tea may be used for its sedative, antispasmodic and anti-inflammatory effect
- *Acupuncture*: this therapy has its origins in traditional Chinese medicine. It is based on the theory that the body has lines of energy running through it with various focal points where energy is concentrated. Insertion of acupuncture needles at these points will lead to a rebalancing of energy. Dried moxa sticks placed over various acupuncture sites is another form of this therapy and is known as moxibustion. Acupuncture has been found to be effective in turning a baby who is presenting by the breech into a head down (cephalic) presentation (Cardini and Weixin 1998)

A midwife who wishes to use any of these or other types of alternative therapies during the course of her midwifery practice must have successfully completed the required training and have been judged competent in its use (NMC 2004b). In addition, complementary therapies can only be administered if it is judged in the best interests of the woman and with her fully informed consent (Tiran 2006).

Midwives who are not fully qualified complementary therapists can use aspects of the treatment as long as they have received training in its correct usage (Tiran 2006). For example, there are a few essential oils specifically for labour which a midwife may use without being a fully qualified aromatherapist as long as she has received the appropriate training. For example, essential oils such as clary sage, lavender and jasmine can be massaged into the abdomen, used as a room spray or put into a warm bath (Tiran 2004). However, it is very important that midwives who wish to use such treatments are fully versed in their correct usage to avoid potential problems and incomplete advice. For example, it has been found that some midwives give insufficient information to women about the use of raspberry leaf tea during labour to enhance the contractions and others are unable to explain how cabbage leaves work to reduce breast engorgement (Tiran 2006).

If a midwife working in the NHS has qualified as a complementary therapist and wishes to incorporate aspects of treatment into her midwifery practice, she must obtain permission from the local NHS Trust, and policies will need to be put in place to support her in this work. If she has obtained this permission, she will be covered by her employer's (i.e. the Trust's) vicarious liability. This means that the Trust is responsible for the midwife's actions and will take responsibility if anything untoward happens to a woman in her care as a result of her treatment.

It should be remembered that many of these treatments have not been tested scientifically to ensure that they are completely safe to take during pregnancy and childbirth. The assumption of safety is based on word of mouth and anecdotal evidence. Homeopathic and herbal medicines are subject to the licensing rules of the Medicines Act 1968, although those on the market when the Act became law had already received product licences without undergoing a formal evaluation of their safety and effectiveness (Siney 2004).

If a woman wants to use natural remedies during childbirth and the midwife believes that the substances chosen might be detrimental to the woman or her baby or interfere with traditional treatment which has already been given, then the midwife must discuss this with the woman. For example, certain essential oils are known to raise blood pressure which could be dangerous for a woman who is already showing signs of a raised blood pressure. A full discussion of the possible risks should ensue and if possible the midwife should contact another practitioner who is an expert in the field of that particular treatment for further guidance and support. In accordance with the NMC *Code of Professional Conduct* (2004c), however, the midwife must respect the rights of the woman to make her own decisions in relation to her care. All the midwife can do in these circumstances is to ensure as far as she can that the woman's decisions are informed ones.

Drug errors

Case Notes

Alice is a newly qualified midwife working on a postnatal ward. She has just realised that by mistake she has given an antibiotic to one of the women in her care instead of the pain relief the woman had requested. The woman seems fine and is unaware of the error.
    What should Alice do?

In the event that the wrong drug or wrong dosage of drug is given to a woman or baby it is essential that this is reported to the senior midwifery staff and a doctor as soon as it has been recognised so that appropriate action can be taken to rectify the situation and hopefully cause less harm to the woman. For example, in the scenario cited above, the woman might be allergic to the antibiotic administered, in which case she may require urgent treatment.

A study by Stanhope et al. (1999) found drug errors in 18.4 per cent of obstetric cases with only about 4 per cent being reported appropriately. It has also been suggested that errors of omission (drugs not given at the time they should be) are usually not reported and so are underestimated (Goldstein 1982).

Following an audit of the administration of post-operative pain relief and heparin in a maternity unit, Birch and Culshaw (2003) suggested that drug errors in obstetrics are a common and hidden phenomenon and that multi-professional working is needed to ensure that safe working practices are put in place to reduce the numbers of errors.

It is suggested that an open, non-judgemental culture should exist within health care settings in order to encourage immediate reporting of such incidents (NMC 2004b). Where a blame culture exists the fear of disciplinary action will prevent midwives from owning up to mistakes which may put women's and babies lives at risk.

In the event of any kind of drug error occurring, a careful local investigation is required to look in detail at what occurred and why. Often drug errors are due to deficiencies in process, such as commonly mistaken drugs being stored together or midwives undertaking a particularly heavy work load at any particular time. The aim of such investigations is to learn from such errors, to educate all staff accordingly and to revise policies and procedures to prevent future incidents. It is suggested that the Supervisor of Midwives can play a crucial role in this kind of investigation as well as offering professional support to the midwife who has made the mistake. Any midwife who is involved in a drug error should inform a Supervisor of Midwives soon as possible (NMC 2004a).

A multidisciplinary approach is also recommended so that teams of health care professionals, including midwives, doctors and pharmacists, can work together to ensure that potential improvements in the administration of medicines are fully discussed and disseminated within the team (NMC 2004b).

Conclusion

This chapter has demonstrated how important it is for midwives to have sound knowledge of legislation related to medicines, the various routes of administration and the checking procedures. A multidisciplinary approach between midwives, doctors and pharmacists is recommended to ensure that safe and effective policies are put in place in terms of the prescribing, dispensing and administration of drugs. The role of the midwife also involves ensuring that women in her care are aware of risks and benefits associated with taking medicines during pregnancy and labour so that they can make informed choices about their treatment. If there is any doubt about the safety or suitability of a medicine, then the midwife should refer to another health care professional such as a pharmacist, who will have more detailed expert knowledge about the potential effect of the particular medicine.

Fundamental to the issue is the midwife following the *Midwives Rules and Standards* (NMC 2004a), which clearly state that she shall only use those medicines in her practice for which she has received appropriate training and is familiar with the dosage and method of administration.

The fact that the midwife is able to supply and administer a number of medicines on her own responsibility through the use of midwives exemptions, highlights her unique role as an autonomous practitioner able to provide a first-class, woman-centred service.

References

Aitkin Report, Standing Advisory Committee: Joint Sub-committee Ministry of Health (1958) *Control of dangerous drugs and poisons in hospitals.* London: HMSO.

Amir, L. and Hoover, K. (2002) *Candidiadis and Breastfeeding.* Schaumburg, USA: La Leche League International.

Banister, C. (2004) *The Midwife's Pocket Formulary Books for Midwives*. London: Elsevier.

Birch, L. and Culshaw, A. (2003) Drug error in maternity care: a multiprofessional issue. *British Journal of Midwifery* 11(3): 173–8.

BNF (2004) *British National Formulary Extra: News 6 October 2004. BNF response to new study on medication use during pregnancy*. London: British Medical Association and the Royal Pharmaceutical Society.

Cardini, F. and Weixin, H. (1998) Moxibustion for correction of breech presentation: a randomised controlled trial. *Journal of the American Medical Association* 280(18): 1580–4.

Chauldron, L. H. and Schoenecker, C. J. (2004) Bupropion and breast feeding: a case of a possible infant seizure (Letter). *Journal of Clinical Psychiatry* 65(6): 881–2.

Department of Health (2004) *Safer Management of Controlled Drugs: The Government's Response to the Fourth Report of the Shipman Inquiry*, London: HMSO.

Dimond, B. (2003) Midwives and the correct administration of medicines. *British Journal of Nursing* 12(17): 1048–51.

Dimond, B. (2005) *Legal Aspects of Medicine*. London: Quay Books.

Goldstein, M. S., Cohen, M.R. and Black, M. (1982) A method for monitoring medication omission error rates. *Hospital Pharmocology* 17(6): 310–2.

Hale, T. (2002) *Medications and Mothers Milk*, 10th edition. Texas: Pharmsoft.

Headley, J., Northstone, K., Simmons, H. and Golding, L. (2004) Medication use during pregnancy: data from the Avon longitudinal study of parents and children. *European Journal of Clinical Pharmacology* 60: 355–61.

Johnson, R. and Taylor, W. (2006) *Skills for Midwifery Practice*, 2nd edition. London: Elsevier.

Jones, W. (2003) *Thrush and Breastfeeding*. Paisley: Breastfeeding Network.

Kaufman, D. et al. (2001) Fluconazole prophylaxis against fungal colonisation and infection in pre-term infants. *New England Journal of Medicine* 345(23): 1660–6.

MHRA (2006) Update on Risks of Birth Defects in Babies Born to Mothers Taking Paroxetine. http://www.mhra.gov.home (accessed 10 March 2007).

Medicinal Products Prescription by Nurses Act (1992) London: HMSO.

Medicines Act (1968) London: HMSO.

Misuse of Drugs Act (1971) London: HMSO.

Nursing and Midwifery Council (2004a) *Guidelines for the Administration of Medicines*. London: NMC.

Nursing and Midwifery Council (2004b) *Midwives Rules and Standards*. London: NMC.

Nursing and Midwifery Council (2004c) *The NMC Code of Professional Conduct, Standards for Conduct, Performance and Ethics*. London: NMC.

Nursing and Midwifery Council (2005a) *1/2005 Medicines Legislation: What it Means for Midwives.* London: NMC.

Nursing and Midwifery Council (2005b) *25/2005 Midwives Supply Orders.* London: NMC.

Nursing and Midwifery Council (2007) *Essential Skills Clusters for Pre-Registration Nursing Students: Medicines Management.* Unpublished draft.

Prescriptions Only Medicines (Human Use) Order 1997 (IS 1997/1830 Schedule 5) London: HMSO.

Royal College of Midwives (2006) *Midwifery and Medicines Legislation: An Information Paper.* London: RCM.

Siney, C. (2004) Drugs and the midwife. In C. Henderson and S. McDonald (eds), *Mayes Midwifery.* London: Bailliere Tindall.

Stanhope, N., Crowley-Murphy, M., Vincent, C., O'Connor, A. M., and Taylor-Adams, S. E. (1999) An evaluation of adverse incident reporting. *Journal of Evaluation of Clinical Practice* 5(1): 5–12.

The Shipman Inquiry: Fourth Report (2004) *The Regulation of Controlled Drugs in the Community* (Cm 6249). London: HMSO.

Tiran, D. (2004) Complementary therapies in childbearing. In C. Henderson and S. McDonald (eds) *Mayes Midwifery.* London: BailliereTindall

Tiran, D. (2006) Midwives' responsibilities when caring for women using complementary therapies during labour. *Midirs Midwifery Digest* 16(1): 77–81.

WHO (2002) *Breastfeeding and Maternal Medication.* Geneva: WHO.

Effective Documentation

Carole Yearley, Celia Wildeman and Chandra Mehta

Introduction

This chapter discusses and analyses the legal and professional framework that governs midwifery practice and the accountability of the midwife in relation to the documentation of his or her records. Activities and practical exercises are included to help you to integrate the theory of the topic area with practice and to offer practical advice and guidance for how you can improve your personal standard of documentation.

The aim of the chapter is to explore the rules and guidance produced by the Nursing and Midwifery Council (NMC 2004a, 2005) concerning the role and responsibilities of the midwife in the context of effective documentation and professional practice. It is anticipated that having read the chapter the reader will be able to describe the various forms of record keeping in use in contemporary practice, and explore and analyse the rationale for keeping contemporaneous records in relation to the various documents produced by the NMC that inform the concept of record keeping. The reader will also be encouraged to analyse the meaning of ownership and collaboration within the multi-professional team with regards to record keeping, utilise reflection as a means to enhance record keeping skills, as well as being able to use a record keeping audit tool competently for monitoring personal and peer records to enhance professional development.

The importance of effective documentation

The NMC came into being on 1 April 2002. It succeeded the former professional body, the United Kingdom Central Council for Nursing, Midwifery and Health Visiting (UKCC). With the establishment of the NMC, new rules for midwives came into effect on 1 August 2004 (NMC 2004a). The rules state the requirements for practice and the accompanying standards provide additional guidance on what standard would reasonably be expected from a midwife's practise.

Rule 9 relates specially to records (NMC 2004a). The NMC (2005) states that:

> 'Record keeping is an integral part of nursing, midwifery and specialist community public health nursing practice. It is a tool of professional practice and one that should help the care process. It is not separate from this process and it is not an optional extra to be fitted in if circumstances allow.'

The *Midwives Rules and Standards* make it clear that midwives are accountable for the quality of their documentation (NMC 2004a): '*a practising midwife shall keep, as contemporaneously as is reasonable, continuous and detailed records of observations made, care given and medicine and any form of pain relief administered by her to a woman or baby*'. This ruling applies wherever the midwife carries out her/his duty, whether in a private, agency, independent or NHS context.

Effective documentation is part of the midwife's duty of care. Within this the midwife is expected to use professional judgement to make decisions that will enhance client care through her/his documentation. The NMC states that the *Guidelines for Records and Record Keeping* (NMC 2005) '*is not a rule book that will provide the answers to every question or issue that could ever arise*', however the intention is that it should be used for guidance together with the *Midwives Rules and Standards* (NMC 2005) to strive for excellence in record keeping.

Good record keeping equates with good care

'*Good record keeping helps to protect the welfare of patients and clients*' (NMC 2005). Its value has been consistently identified and highlighted in various professional guidelines (NMC 2004a, 2004b, 2005, 2006a, 2006b; DH 2006).

In summary, good record keeping promotes:

- High standards of clinical care
- Continuity of care

- Better communication and dissemination of information between members of the inter-professional health care team
- An accurate account of treatment and care planning and delivery
- The ability to detect problems, such as changes in the patient's or client's condition, at an early stage
- The professional duty to keep adequate and accurate records
- The midwife practitioner to meet legal requirements

The NMC asserts that '*the quality of your record keeping is also a reflection of the standard of your professional practice*' (NMC 2005).

Activity

Review a client's record that you have written during the previous six months and assess the quality of the content and style of your documentation. Now go to the feedback box below for guidance and suggestions.

Feedback

Your record keeping would be considered to be of a good standard if it included the following features:

- Factual, consistent and accurate
- Written as soon as possible after the event or an explanation given when written retrospectively, for example what, who and why the delay in writing the records became necessary
- Clear, concise and legible in black ink (it must be able to be photocopied if necessary) (Dimond 2005a)
- Signed and your name printed (follow the format for the Trust or other employer)
- Dated and the time included using a 24-hour clock
- Jargon, abbreviations, irrelevant speculation and offensive, subjective statements not included
- Any dialogue with the patient included in a form that provides evidence of client participation in their care
- Any alterations or additions dated, timed and signed in such a way that the original entry can still be clearly read
- Evidence that the client collaborated with the practitioner in the construction of the records – quotes or statements from the client are included in language that supported the client's involvement
- The tone and quality of the communication is such that the client's understanding was ensured

How did your records compare with the contents of the feedback section? Reflect on this exercise and identify areas for further development.

Documentation as good risk management strategy

Byrne (1999) asserts that the record keeping skills of health carers arose as a recurring theme in the risk management literature. Indeed, although no professional practitioner would like to become obsessed by the negative aspect of legal claims, increasingly medico-legal actions have become commonplace in obstetrics. The NMC has highlighted the rarity of midwives being referred with allegations of misconduct and incompetence. Although midwives make up only a small proportion of all registrants, numbers are still significant and poor record keeping remains the most common reason for midwives being referred to the NMC conduct committees.

Clinical audit is an aspect of clinical governance (Currie et al. 2004). It is a quality initiative that aims to improve the care and services to patients and clients. According to Rodden and Bell (2002), the clinical governance agenda should ensure that the evaluation of record keeping skills has the same level of importance as other clinical skills. Recognition by the midwife of her professional · accountability in the constructing, monitoring and reflexivity (i.e. being aware of one's thinking and learning processes) in relation to his or her record keeping abilities is essential and fundamental for her client's well-being. Strict criteria must be set to facilitate best practice which is not only related to record keeping skills but also includes practical issues to preserve effective documentation for the future – for example, how client records are stored, whether manually and/or electronically. It is now common practice for the majority of midwifery clients to carry their own notes. It is important that women understand the importance and significance of their hand-held case records and that appropriate policies are put in place to ensure the safe return of the notes once the woman has been discharged from the maternity service.

Documentation standards

As a registrant, the midwife is ultimately accountable for any delegated duties that she entrusts to a student midwife (NMC 2005). However, it is a dual responsibility of student and midwife to ensure that the delegatee is competent to carry out the allocated task. Any written records must be signed by the student and countersigned by the midwife. Entries in the client's records should be made with the assumption that they will be *'scrutinised at some point'* (NMC 2005).

The Clinical Negligence Scheme for Trusts (CNST) was established by the NHS Executives in 1994 to provide a way for Trusts to fund the cost of clinical negligence litigation and to encourage and support effective management of claims and risk (NHSLA 2005). Essentially, the key role of CNST is to promote good standards of documentation (Dimond 2005c). The effectiveness of quality documentation in the prevention and limitation of litigation is not disputed. Indeed, the enhancement of communication between client and practitioner through the making and sharing of recorded information can make a significant difference to whether a client will pursue litigious claims.

A key quality issue is the practitioner's knowledge of the rationale for constructing contemporaneous client records. Dimond (2005c) asserts that it is a basic principle that records are kept, not for the protection of the registered practitioner, but as part of the duty of care owed to the patient. It is essential that not only the writer of the record but also the multi-professional team input, through effective documentation, to become members of a documented communication system that appropriately maps the client's management and care, past, present and future. In this way, the client's records represents an historical account of the nature and quality of care decisions and treatment carried out in consultation with the client and others participating in the care.

The extent of the problem and common deficiencies in record keeping

In the year prior to the publication of the revised *Midwives Rules and Standards* (NMC 2004a), the NMC Fitness to Practise Rules were introduced. Part of the work of the NMC is to produce an annual *Fitness to Practise Report* (these are available to view and download from the NMC website, http://www.nmc-uk.org under the heading Fitness to Practise). The reports retrospectively review the nature of the complaints that have been reported to the NMC during the previous year, how they have been managed and the outcome of the hearings.

The number of allegations of misconduct against registered nurses, midwives and specialist community public health nurses from the most recent report for the period 2004–2005 was 1,389, a slight decrease from the previous report (NMC 2005). Of the practice-related charges 6 per cent concerned poor record keeping. Even though midwives make up only a small proportion of all registrants, this is a recurrent issue with scope for improvement. Midwives have the unique benefit of Statutory Supervision of Midwives which provides a mechanism for support and guidance for each midwife, the aim being to actively promote a safe standard of midwifery practice for the protection of mothers and babies (ENB 1999). However, poor record keeping still accounts for notable numbers of NMC referrals and generally reflects an overall poor standard of care. For more details on the purpose and function of Statutory Supervision of Midwives and the role of the Supervisor of Midwives, see Chapter 18.

Having reviewed the impact of the legislative framework for the profession, it is evident that practitioners employed within an NHS Trust who do not comply with the local trust policies and procedures, the *Midwives Rules and Standards* (NMC 2004a), the Local Supervisory Authority Standards (LSA 2005) and the professional legal and ethical requirements, risk sanctions, which may result in professional conduct proceedings and possible disciplinary action by an employer, or even civil action by a claimant.

There is consistent evidence that certain areas of practice incur repeated errors in the context of record keeping (Byrne 1999; Dimond 2005b; Jones 2006). One such aspect is documentation related to the use of cardiotocograph (CTG) recordings. These are regularly lacking, with common problems being the omission of information for the identification of the client and recordings which are not dated and timed (Byrne 1999). Although CTG machines now have automated date and time, it is still essential to check for accurate callibration with a 24-hour clock. It is also important that on completion the recording is securely filed and attached in the client's case notes in succeeding order and there is evidence of discussion with the client and the relevant multi-professional team member(s) relating to care management decisions.

Other problems include illegible handwriting. It is important to know your Trust or other work setting's policies regarding this matter. All practitioners should print their name at least once in the client's records. Abbreviations can be extremely confusing and misleading, therefore it is good professional practice to omit them unless they are approved and recognised by the local Trust. The standard could be enhanced by including the approved list in every client record. The activity below will help you apply some of these principles to a common practice situation.

Activity

You have been delegated the care of Cindy. She was admitted to the labour ward with a history of regular contractions since 1400 hours. It is now 1700 hours.

What would you record about her condition and midwifery care on admission to the labour ward?

Feedback

A good standard of record keeping would consist of the following documentation:

- The time she arrived on the labour ward
- The time you attended to her
- A clinical assessment, to include a full history, physical findings and observations
- The length, strength and frequency of the contractions, and how the client is coping
- Physical examination, including the status of the membranes
- Investigations and findings of urine testing
- Investigation results, e.g. blood results
- Discussion with client, e.g. birth plan and any changes decided by the client
- A recorded plan of care
- Companion – who this person is and their relationship to the client
- Evidence of reporting these findings to your midwife mentor if you are a student midwife

This information should be recorded and if you are a student midwife working under the supervision of your mentor, countersigned by your mentor.

Clearly, the quality of the student midwife's/midwife's record keeping protects the client's welfare by encouraging high standards of clinical care, continuity of care, better communication and dissemination of information between members of the inter-professional health care team. It provides an accurate account of treatment and care planning delivery. It also facilitates the mid-wifery practitioner's ability to detect problems early, such as changes in the client's condition. It is considered good practice to keep a professional journal to help you develop your reflective skills to enhance learning from your practice experiences. Recording, monitoring and auditing client records provide the student and practitioner with the potential for improvement and change.

Benchmark of best practice

The Department of Health (2001) has set guidelines that provide a patient-focused benchmark of good health care practice, in particular benchmarks for best record keeping practice. These criteria closely correlate to the clinical governance standards which provide guidelines for best practice. Indeed, it is strongly argued that the policy to involve clients in the assessment, planning, implementing and evaluating of their care improves the quality of health services (Currie et al. 2004). Table 10.1 highlights the Essence of Care in relation to patient-focused benchmarking for health care practitioners.

Table 10.1 The Essence of Care in relation to patient-focused benchmarking for health care practitioners

Factor	Benchmark of good practice
Access to current health care records	Patients/clients are able to access all their current records if and when they choose to, in a format that meets their individual needs
Integration of theory and practice was of patient/professional partnership	Patients/clients are actively involved continuously negotiating and influencing their care
Integration of theory and practice was of records across professional and organisational boundaries	Patients/clients have a single, structured, multi-professional/agency record which supports integrated care
Holding lifelong records	Patients/clients hold a single, lifelong multi-professional/agency record
High quality practice- and evidence-based guidance	Evidence-based guidance detailing best practice is available and has an active and timely review process
High quality practice	Patients'/clients' records demonstrate that their care follows evidence guidance or supporting documents describing best practice, or that there is an explanation of any variance
Security/confidentiality	Patients'/clients' records are safeguarded through explicit measures with an active and timely review process

Source: DH 2001

Activity

Having reviewed the Essence of Care benchmarks of good practice for record keeping, identify in your place of work the Essence of Care guidelines that inform the quality standards.

- How well are the guidelines achieved?
- Compare the written policies and procedures with the benchmarking criteria and best practice benchmark.
- Discuss your findings with your midwifery practice mentor. Reflect on this exercise and identify areas for further development.

Who owns midwifery records?

One could be forgiven for thinking that the NHS Trust employing the midwife owns the client's records or indeed that the woman herself does. After all, the records relate to the woman's care, much of the content is provided by the woman herself, and the majority of women now carry their own maternity records which contain all necessary information about their care. To clarify the situation, the NMC issued a circular to explain more about the ownership and sharing of midwifery records (NMC 2007).

In fact, it is the Secretary of State who owns the records made by midwives employed by the NHS. Where a midwife is employed in the private sector, the records are owned by her employers. In the case of self-employed midwives, the midwife owns the client's records. However, the principle that the Secretary of State has ultimate ownership applies to all midwives, regardless of where they practise. Should a midwife choose to withhold documentation relating to the care of a woman, this could place her in breach of her professional duty. For a self-employed midwife additionally this means breaking the contractual duty to the woman. According to the NMC it should be remembered that *'midwives have a duty to co-operate with internal and external investigations and their records can be used as evidence for this purpose'* (NMC 2005). In such cases, it is expected that all midwives, regardless of their employment status, comply with any request made to share their records for this purpose.

It has already been emphasised that records are made for the benefit of both the woman and the midwife. For the woman this means that she can be actively involved in planning and directing her care; for the midwife this ensures clear, written communication in participation with other health carers for the planning and delivery of care which demonstrates the midwife's decision-making and serves to protect her should any allegations be made against her practice. Should the woman require transfer from a midwifery-led unit to obstetric unit or from home to obstetric unit, her records must accompany her, including a detailed account of recent events, so that staff in the receiving unit can provide timely and appropriate care in accordance with the principle of sharing records with the multidisciplinary team (NMC 2004a).

Summary: Why keep records?

- It is the midwives' professional and legal duty of care
- It is an integral part of nursing and midwifery practice
- It is a tool of professional practice which helps the care process
- It helps to promote high standards of clinical care
- It promotes continuity of care
- It promotes better communication and dissemination of information between members of the inter-professional health care team
- It helps to give an accurate account of treatment and care planning and delivery
- It promotes detection of problems, such as changes in the patient's or client's condition, at an early stage
- It is a component of the risk management process
- For legal matters and complaints: records are called in evidence before a court

Developing your record keeping skills

Having reviewed the importance of effective documentation, why we must maintain records, the implications of poor record keeping and the extent of the problem, we shall now explore various strategies that could be used to develop your record keeping skills. Group guided reflection, the use of a self- and peer record keeping audit tool and an example of the content of a record keeping workshop are presented to give you some practical ideas that you can adopt in your own workplace. You may like to find out if similar initiatives for midwives and other members of the multidisciplinary team already exist. If so, go along and find out more!

Group guided reflection to support the development of record keeping skills

Reflection is a valuable learning resource (Schön 1991). Yearley (2003) argues that guided reflection, under the direction of practitioners who have reflective skills, strengthens professional learning and can be used constructively to develop knowledge and skills. This model can be used to focus on the development of record keeping skills. Such a forum provides an opportunity for student midwives to review their documentation together, share issues relating to practice and record keeping and identify areas for improvement. Thus examples of good record keeping can be shared and areas for development highlighted.

During the process, an experienced midwife practitioner with facilitation skills and knowledge of group guided reflection, such as a Supervisor of Midwives, link lecturer or consultant midwife, provides leadership and support for the group. The facilitator helps the group to understand the significance of effective documentation in their practice and is able to provide ongoing support to individual students. Additional strategies can be identified that will enable students to meet their professional development needs in relation to their record keeping skills (Yearley 2003). This kind of forum could be implemented in your clinical placement with the support of your link lecturer or placement facilitator and with the input of local Supervisor of Midwives.

Format and structure of sessions

Having some structure for the reflective session is useful as student midwives may need help, guidance and continuing support to develop their documentation skills and apply these in their daily record keeping activities. Meetings need to be planned in advance and dates and times of the sessions disseminated through a variety of communication channels such as the Learning Information Services – for example, StudyNet or Blackboard facilities which are an integral part of student communication within education programmes at university. Other means include Trust newsletters, student midwife notice-boards, etc. Through these channels, the value of the initiative as an essential learning opportunity to help the development of record keeping skills can be emphasised. As student midwives are supernumerary, the timings of the meetings may be flexible, somewhere between one and two hours. Additional ad hoc and opportunistic meetings could also be held during quieter times in the clinical placement areas with the support of mentor midwives. In this way both students and midwives benefit as the need to strive for effective documentation becomes a shared goal and remains a high priority on everyone's agenda.

Adopting a user-friendly reflective model, such as a framework based on the 'what?', 'so what?', 'now what?' series of questions (Boud and Walker 1991), or alternative familiar examples such as the Gibb's Reflective Cycle (1988), or Johns' Model for Structured Reflection (Johns 1994) can be useful in providing a structure for learning together, particularly if you are recalling the practice experience with the records to hand. This will enable student midwives to recognise and gain confidence in using their reflective skills when reviewing their own and others' documentation and apply them constructively to learn from past practice experiences and inform their future behaviour and practice.

Record keeping audit and a self- and peer record keeping audit tool

Having discussed the timing and structure of group guided record keeping sessions and argued that record keeping is a topic of such importance it should be an integral part of each session, it is useful to provide an overview of what is meant by the audit of record keeping. Following this, a record keeping audit tool will be introduced and an explanation given for how it can be used in practice to encourage the audit of self- and peer review of record keeping as a practical way to ensure your records meet the *NMC Guidance for Records and Record Keeping* (NMC 2005).

The NMC (2005) explains audit as one component of the risk management process, the purpose of which is to promote quality in health care for the benefit of patients. Through audit activity, areas for development are identified, and in response improvements are implemented with the aim of improving health care outcomes, reducing or minimising client risk and subsequent costs to the employer (NHS Trusts) are reduced. In the context of developing the quality of record keeping through audit, it can play a vital part in ensuring that quality of care is delivered to patients. From reviewing the records, the quality and standard of care are reflected and issues can be identified for improvement. If undertaken within a facilitated and supportive environment such as in a group or with peers, the audit record keeping emphasises the value of sharing and learning together and reduces a culture of fear and blame that predominates some practice areas (Leap 1997; Kirkham 1999) which may create a barrier to learning and skills development. The NMC (2005) supports the development and use of local audit tools '*to monitor the standard of the records produced and to form a basis both for discussion and measurement*' and encourages the use of peer review in the process.

Self-review encourages individuals to examine their performance in practice, thus promoting individual professional accountability (Malkin 1994), as the *Code of Professional Conduct* reminds us that '*as a registered nurse, midwife or specialist community public health nurse, you are personally accountable for your practice*' (NMC 2004b). The process of self-review is important as it is generally accurate and, as Meredith (1994) argues, no one knows our behavioural trends, strengths and weaknesses better than we do ourselves. In contrast, peer review involves an evaluation by colleagues of equal status based on prede-termined criteria the process of which helps individuals plan for future improvement (Meredith 1994). Peer review as a system is both efficient and effective, and democratises and shifts power towards the learner (Gopee 2001). Therefore, self- and peer review are thought to improve standards of care, increase awareness of personal profes-sional accountability in practice, help individuals identify personal areas of strength and weaknesses, and stimulate professional devel-opment that promotes mutual learning.

Record keeping in action

Having defined the term and explained the value of it in this context, we now need to examine the Self and Peer Tool for Review of Record Keeping. The development of the audit tool was based on the *Guide-lines for Records and Record Keeping* (NMC 2005). It has been adopted for use by the London Local Supervision Authority (LSA). It is shown in Table 10.2 and is also available for download from the LSA website, http://www.midwife.org.uk

Self-/peer review of record keeping tool

This audit form is designed to facilitate self- or peer review to monitor the quality of record keeping (NMC 2005). Each midwife should audit ten records a year. It is anticipated that this will provide a learning experience for all those involved and extend the sharing of good practice.

The tool is simple to use yet emphasises the content and style that contributes to effective record keeping, the notion being that the more it is used, the more you will become familiar with the identified criteria, thus improvements become an integral part of your record keeping practice with each documented entry. For the purposes of explaining its use, each criterion has been numbered. Criteria 1–7 are self-explanatory. For example, it is clear to see if the entries (criterion 1) have been made in anything other than black. If this has been achieved for every entry in the records, the score is 100 per cent. If this was mostly the case, the score would be 75 per cent, and so on, with the appropriate column being ticked accordingly. Table 10.3 provides further guidance and explanation on the expected standard required.

Record keeping in action – further guidance

A full assessment of client is recorded (criteria 8)

In order to meet this criterion, it is suggested that you return to the Activity on page 241 and review the kind of information recorded against it. Alongside the feedback given, review the content again; this time undertaking a self-evaluation using the record keeping tool for this criterion to ensure you have included all aspects required for a full client assessment.

There is a plan of care recorded (criteria 9)

Achieving a 100 per cent score on this criterion is an aspect that midwives tend to find difficult. In contrast, if you were to peer review a doctor's records, you would find this tends to be achieved at every entry. This may be because midwives are consistent at recording *what is happening* rather than planning *what could happen in the future*. In order to be able to recognise deviations from normality in accordance with rule 6 (NMC 2004a) and adjust management options accordingly, it is important that a plan of care is recorded and reviewed at regular, planned intervals and adjusted according to the findings.

The plan of care should include a summary of:

- Any relevant antenatal/medical or obstetric risk factors
- The onset and progress of labour to date
- The assessment of maternal and fetal well-being
- All existing plans and any obstetric involvement if applicable
- A new plan of care based on your analysis of the above
- A subsequent time to review the recorded plan

One would expect that provided the plan of care was being reviewed at regular intervals, the rationale for the decisions made

Table 10.2 Guidelines for records and record keeping

Criteria*	100%	75%	50%	25%	0%
1. Entries are written in black ink					
2. Writing is legible					
3. Entries are dated and timed					
4. Entries are signed					
5. Name is printed alongside first signature					
6. Records are factual					
7. Entries are consecutive					
8. Full assessment of client is recorded					
9. There is a plan of care recorded					
10. Recorded evidence plan of care delivered					
11. Rationale for decisions is recorded					
12. Client is involved in decision-making					
13. Frequency of entries is appropriate to client's condition					
14. Entries are jargon-free					
15. Entries could be understood by client					
16. There is evidence of appropriate communication with medical staff					
17. Communication with Supervisor of Midwives documented when appropriate					
18. Amendments are dated, timed and signed					

* If criteria are not applicable, you should write N/A
In ten years' time, would the record give a clear picture to the reader of the health and well-being of mother and baby (born or unborn) and the environment of care?

Comment:

Having undertaken this self/peer review, what changes do you consider should be made to enhance record keeping?

Comment:

Name: **Date:**

Table 10.3 Self-/peer review of record keeping tool: guidance and explanation on the expected record keeping standard required

Criteria	Guidance and explanation on the expected standard required
Entries are written in black ink	Black ink photocopies well. If records are required as evidence, the copies will be of good quality if written in black ink.
Writing is legible	If writing is legible it will be easy to understand the care and treatment provided.
Entries are dated and timed	A maternity record must be retained for 25 years and correct dates and times are essential in following the care process if complaints are lodged or investigations are required for any maternity episode. Every new page should be dated.
Entries are signed and name is printed alongside first signature	If entries are not signed or staff designation is not included, it is difficult to identify who was involved in any incident. It is difficult to track staff to request statements; this becomes even more complex if they leave the employment of the Trust. Every new page should have the name printed, designation and signature.
Records are factual	They must be a true account of the events that occurred.
Entries are consecutive	The entries must follow in the sequence in which they occurred.
Entries are jargon-free	Most maternity records will have an explanation of some of the words used in midwifery so that clients are aware what those words mean. Entries should be made in full in the initial text and the shortened version in brackets and then can be used in the rest of the notes, e.g. fetal heart heard (FHH).
Amendments are dated, timed and signed	If mistakes are made during writing, a line should be put through the error and the correction made, but it should be dated and signed either over the top of the text or to the side of the text. If notes are written retrospectively, it should be documented when they were written and the reason for this and should be dated and timed of this entry, as well as date and time of the actual events.

is recorded, in addition to documented evidence of communication with relevant members of the health care team, then criteria 10–18 would achieve 100 per cent.

The record keeping tool is intended for use in both low- and high-risk cases, hence the inclusion of the footnote: 'If criteria are not applicable, you should write N/A'. This tool encourages practitioners to strive for the same standards in record keeping for women categorised as 'high risk' as well as midwife-led care clients regardless of where the care is given be it in an obstetric unit, midwifery-led unit or at home.

Record keeping for practice

Following the introduction and exploration of the self- and peer tool for review of record keeping, try these activities to apply the tool in practice.

Activity

Use the tool to undertake a self-review on the standards of your record keeping on a client's records that you have written in during the previous six months and assess the quality of the content and style of your documentation against the criteria included in the tool

- How well did you score against each of the criteria?
- If you scored less than 100 per cent on any criterion, identify the changes you consider should be made to enhance your record keeping.

Activity

Ask a fellow student to use the tool to undertake peer review on the standards of your record keeping of a client's records you have written in during the previous six months and assess the quality of the content and style of your documentation against the criteria included in the tool

- How well did your colleague score your record keeping against each of the criteria?
- Together discuss and identify what changes could be made to enhance your record keeping.
- Ask him/her to complete the comments section on the tool. If your colleague gave you a score of less than 100 per cent on any criterion, discuss with him/her how you could enhance your record keeping skills.

Multidisciplinary record keeping workshops

Having reviewed a self- and peer review record keeping audit tool with the aim of achieving effective documentation, the final section of the chapter will consider a record keeping workshop as an initiative for improving a multidisciplinary record keeping and standards of client care. An example of a record keeping workshop teaching plan is included in Table 10.4, the intention being that an experienced midwife facilitator could use this for guidance for the preparation and delivery of the workshop in your local area. In addition, some case notes extracts are included. These can be copied or adapted to be incorporated in a similar kind of record keeping workshop in your workplace. Investigate locally to find out if your Trust runs a workshop for record keeping. If not, you may wish to discuss ideas for implementing and development one with the support of your local link lecturer, practice educator or Supervisor of Midwives.

All attending participants are invited to bring a set of client records that they have written in to the workshop. As Trust records cannot be removed from the Trust site, records may be photocopied or the workshop can be provided in the clinical workplace.

Facilitating a record keeping workshop

In this section, some guidance is offered to help apply the teaching plan in a practical situation. All participants who attend the record keeping workshop are invited to bring along a set of client records they have written previously if the workshop is to be held in the workplace/Trust. Trust records cannot be removed from the Trust site; therefore, records must be photocopied if the workshop is to be held away from the Trust.

Participants are encouraged to share their notes with peers, thus providing a forum to review each other's note keeping. This can be particularly helpful with members of different health professions as it creates mutual respect and understanding of professional responsibilities and boundaries. Byrne (1999) suggests that auditing each other's records helps to facilitate good communication between health professionals and helps to update and maintain record keeping standards. Frequently in the working environment, staff do not get the chance to read each other's notes, thus time to do this in a workshop setting helps to create a culture in which new ideas are welcomed. Participants give and receive constructive feedback and learn how to strengthen their record keeping skills as part of peer review and reflective learning (Hunt 1997).

Table 10.4 Example of a record keeping workshop teaching plan

Topic Activity	Time	What You Do (Facilitator)	What Group Members Do	Teaching Method/Activities
Introduction	5 minutes	Present session: aims and learning outcomes	Listen/observe	PowerPoint/OHP, handout
Exercise: How do you rate yourself in record keeping?	5 minutes	Ask each group members to write down how they rate/score their record keeping from 1–10, 1 being poor and 10 being excellent.	Group members will reflect and jot down how they rate their standard	On the paper provided each member will rate themselves
Self- and peer review of records in pairs. Share feedback with partner	15 minutes + 15 minutes	Provide photocopied examples of records to any members who have not brought notes to review	Self-review own notes and if comfortable swap to do peer review	Using records
In pairs, review examples of antenatal intrapartum and postnatal records provided by facilitator	15 minutes	Give each group photocopied notes to see for themselves what sort of standard they feel the notes are	Review the set of notes they are given and jot down what they feel is missing or compliment on the record keeping	Discussion and feedback in the group Facilitator to encourage discussion on consent, choice, care of plan and other issues
Optional. May introduce local maternity audit tool for record keeping and in small groups audit a set of records	40 minutes	Introduce the revised audit tool so midwives are aware what tool is used and its criteria	With the aid of the audit tool look at a set of notes and check the record keeping standards against the criteria given	Discussion and feedback in the group As the audit tool is lengthy just looking at small area will give them some idea of the criteria required
Summarise learning 1. Do the records meet the record keeping standard/criteria 2. Share examples of good records 3. Share examples of poor record keeping and how this could be improved	10 minutes	Invite each group to give feedback on the flip chart to note the key points	Discuss information	Flip chart feedback and facilitated discussion
Repeat exercise Having completed the workshop how do you rate yourself in record keeping now?	5 minutes	Invite members to share how they feel about their record keeping skills having completed the workshop	If the group members feel safe they may honestly share what they feel about their record keeping standards	General discussion Evaluation Close

Examples of good and poor records are shared in the workshop and the use of self- and peer review encourages discussion in relation to what should be included in the records. This provides an opportunity for practitioners to learn from each other's experience, identify difference of approach and the reasons for taking a particular course of action. Such a dialogue can be an excellent way of broadening horizons, deepening understanding and enhancing skills, all of which create an open and supportive working environment (Thompson 2002). One outcome from this was a compilation of a trigger reminder to act as a prompt for students and midwives to document their care at various stages in the woman's maternity journey. You may find this helpful in practice for developing your own record keeping skills (see Table 10.5).

Learning through sharing is emphasised during the workshop. Extracts from records are a useful way of illustrating particular aspects of record keeping and are useful to demonstrate examples of good and poor standards of record keeping and the variety of consequences and problems that can directly result from the quality of record keeping.

Activity

Included below are some extracts from maternity records. In each case, read the records as they appeared in the woman's notes, and then read the outcome. For each extract, identify the key record keeping issues and make suggestions, if any, for changes that might improve the standards of record keeping.

Case Notes

This extract provides a good example of the standard of record keeping during the management of shoulder dystocia at a homebirth.

Records as they appeared in the notes

Time recorded 'Head born, slow no restitution – asked client to push – no descent. Diagnosed shoulder dystocia and immediately asked client to stand (as she was in the pool). Tried to deliver baby standing, woodscrew attempted – unable to deliver baby'. Time recorded 'Client helped on her back and McRoberts performed – cord tight round baby's neck – not cut in view of shoulder dystocia. Suprapubic pressure applied by the other midwife, still no baby therefore woodscrew manoeuvre attempted again (no need for episiotomy) to free anterior shoulder'.

Time recorded 'Baby delivered (altogether 5 minutes from the delivery of head) Baby – heart beat above 100 but not breathing. Inflation breaths of oxygen given via mask and asked father to call for an ambulance. Baby's condition improved within 5 minutes.'

Comment on standard of record keeping

These records show appropriate times, the two midwives' clear printed names and signatures, the diagnosis of the problem, appropriate manoeuvres to free the shoulder, their rationale for decisions made and emergency services called to stand by in case transfer to hospital is necessary.

Midwives are advised to attach the Trust's guidelines for such events so that if cases that are brought up several years later, the investigators can see if the professionals acted according to the appropriate guidelines that were in place at the time of the incident.

Case Notes

These records were required for lawyers ten years after delivery as the child was diagnosed with Erb's palsy.

Records as they appeared in the notes

'Difficult delivery/poor maternal effort (second degree midline tear). Delivery performed by midwife with assistance by Dr X following no progress after crowning of the head'.

Comment on standard of record keeping

The notes were poor, very little information on the labour summary is included, midwife's and doctor's name were not recognisable. The Trust was advised to pay compensation for poor management of care.

Case Notes

A complaint was received from the client to the Trust, stating that she felt she did not receive appropriate care.

Records as they appeared in the notes

Date and time recorded 'Arrived at birth centre for antenatal check due to SROM [spontaneous rupture of membranes] at [date and time given].

Continued

Antenatal check carried out given information sheet and thermometer. Asked to phone as needed'.

Next day date and time recorded 'Arrived with h/o [history of] contractions 1 in every 5 mins. Antenatal assessment carried out and advised to go home to await events'.

Comment on standard of record keeping

It was this woman's first baby; she had transferred her care from another hospital at 36 weeks of pregnancy and the record does not demonstrate that she was given any guidance on what to do if she was not in labour after 48 hours after the rupture of her membranes. There was no plan of care recorded or implemented. She lost her confidence in the Trust and went to deliver in another local Trust.

Case Notes

A complaint was received by the Trust from this client stating that following delivery of her baby, her perineum had not been examined and that the presence of a perineal tear was not identified.

Records as they appeared in the notes

Time recorded 'Placenta seems to be visible at the vaginal entrance – encouraged to push down'.
Time recorded 'Third stage completed [physiologically] – trickling blood. Client helped to the bed to inspect the vagina. Uterus relaxed, rubbed up contraction while the other midwife went to get syntometrine. Client feeling well, pulse 88 uterus now well contracted, trickling of blood stopped – no need for syntometrine.'

Comment on standard of record keeping

The Trust was required to pay compensation as the records showed there was no documentation that the perineum had been examined. Although it was recorded that the client had sustained a second degree tear in the labour and delivery summary page in the notes, in the legal remit, what is not documented in the main notes means it was not done.

Table 10.5 Trigger reminder to aid documentation at various stages in maternity care

Initial Antenatal Booking Appointment
Social history – appropriate referral for smoking/and drug use
Medical and obstetric history
Document any history of depression and treatment
Discussion of health screening that is offered and documentation of that discussion
Document what tests/scans the woman has consented to and what she has declined
Determine if pregnancy is low- or high-risk
Documentation of referral if high-risk
Diet discussion and written information has been given
Information about parenthood education
A/N assessment to include and document BMI, BP, Urinalysis
Aware of due date
Document what written information packs have been given

Plan of care to include
Antenatal care – location? How often
Place of delivery (if decided)
Contact number of where to call if any queries
When to return to hospital/birth centre

Documentation in labour
Where the woman is, i.e. hospital, home, birth centre
Who is with her as her support?
Basic history – gestation, what has happened, contraction history, emotional state
General readings – consent – abdominal palpation

Care plan
Food and drink
Mobilisation
Pattern of auscultation of FH
When to reassess
Documentation of care discussed and agreed
Rational for any advice or treatment

Second stage and birth
Who is present in the room
Pattern of auscultation of FH recording every 5 minutes
Contraction history
Where the mother is, i.e. pool, bed, on all fours, stool
Time head delivered
Time of whole baby's delivery
Sex of baby
Estimated blood loss
Discussion and management of third stage
Examination of the perineum
Any laceration or tear noted, including intact perineum
Perineum sutured or not and reason for not suturing
Administration of Vitamin K for the baby
Examination of baby
Any other problems

Documentation at Every Antenatal Visit
Basic maternal assessment – BP, urinalysis, general health, fundal height measurement
Document findings and advice given
Appropriate referral if any problem

Plan of care to include
Screening tests are undertaken
Reason for test, and explanation has been given so woman is aware of reason for test
Consent and any other discussion and plans agreed with mother
Explanation for how she will find out results
Contact number if necessary
Discussion on breastfeeding, third stage management choices, vitamin K injection for baby, and any other relevant information

Documentation postnatally Mother's well-being:
Observations
Uterus – involution rate
Lochia
Passed urine

Care of plan included

Baby's well-being
Feeding – any help required
Cord site
Passed urine
Passed meconium
Care of plan included

Case Notes

A complaint was received by the Trust for this client some time after her delivery. Labour was induced and apparently all had gone well, but the client reported that she had not consented to her blood being taken during labour for blood grouping and to cross-match her blood should she need it during labour.

Records as they appeared in the notes

Time recorded 'Bloods sent urgently for FBC [full blood count], group and save'.

Comment on standard of record keeping

It is a normal practice within the hospital setting for high-risk women or those being induced to identify the client's blood group and save a small sample if blood should it be needed. However, as it was not recorded that the woman's consent had been obtained, the Trust subsequently met with the couple to apologise for not recording that client consent had been given for the procedure.

Conclusion

This chapter has discussed and analysed the legal and professional framework in relation to midwives' responsibilities for record keeping. The importance of effective documentation has been emphasised and contextualised within the clinical governance framework, which is a mechanism for reducing risk and improving the quality of care and services for women and their families. Common record keeping deficiencies have been identified, the extent and implications of the problem discussed and the issue of the ownership of clients' records has been clarified. Various strategies have been presented and discussed to enable readers to enhance their individual record keeping skills including: group guided reflection, the application of a tool for undertaking self- and peer audit of record keeping and a template for a multidisciplinary record keeping workshop that could be adapted for local use. Throughout the chapter, activities, exercises and examples have been used to encourage practical application and the ongoing development of proficiencies that enhance the skills for effective documentation.

Student midwives and midwives must remember that record keeping and documentation are an intrinsic part of the professional activity and that the onus for improving standards of records lies with individual health professionals (Mann and Williams 2003). All professionals should have a chance on regular basis to reflect on their standards of record keeping and identify whether their records are congruent with the guidance provided by the statutory bodies. Implementing strategies to improve record keeping standards will benefit health care professionals, organisations and mothers and babies.

References

Boud, D. and Walker, D. (1991) *Experience and Learning: Reflection at Work.* Geelong, Victoria: Deakin University Press.

Byrne, U. (1999) Record keeping – a risk management perspective. *British Journal of Midwifery* 7(7): 436–9.

Currie, L., Morrell, C. and Scrivener, R. (2004) Clinical governance: quality at centre of services. *British Journal of Midwifery* 12(5): 330–4.

Department of Health (2001) *The Essence of Care. Patient-focused Benchmarking for Health Care Practitioners.* London: DH.

Department of Health (2006) *Safer Management of Controlled Drugs: Changes to Record Keeping Requirements.* London: DH.

Dimond, B. (2005a) Exploring the principles of good record keeping in nursing. *British Journal of Nursing* 14(8): 460–2.

Dimond, B. (2005b) Exploring common deficiencies that occur in record keeping. *British Journal of Nursing* 14(10): 568–70.

Dimond, B. (2005c) Documentation standards set by the Clinical Negligence Scheme for Trusts. *British Journal of Nursing* 14(11): 610–12.

Dimond, B. (2005d) Abbreviations: the need for legibility and accuracy in documentation. *British Journal of Nursing* 14(12): 665–6.

English National Board for Nursing, Midwifery and Health Visiting (1999) *Supervision in Action. A Practical Guide for Midwives.* London: ENB.

Gibbs, G. (1988) *Learning by Doing: A Guide to Learning and Teaching Methods.* Oxford: Further Education Unit, Oxford Polytechnic.

Gopee, N. (2001) The role of peer assessment and peer review in nursing. *British Journal of Nursing* 10(2): 115–21.

Hunt, C. (1997) The challenge of change in the organisation of midwifery care. In I. Kargar and C. Hunt, *Challenges in Midwifery Care.* London: Macmillan.

Johns, C. (1994) Guided reflection. In A. Palmer, S. Burns and C. Bulman (eds), *Reflective Practice in Nursing.* Oxford: Blackwell Scientific.

Jones, S. (2006) Conflicting evidence: the importance of accurate record keeping. *British Journal of Midwifery* 14(11): 677.

Kirkham, M. (1999) The culture of midwifery in the National Health Service in England. *Journal of Advanced Nursing* 30(3): 732–9.

Leap, N. (1997) Making sense of 'horizontal violence' in midwifery. *British Journal of Midwifery* 5(11): 689.

Local Supervising Authority (2005) *Statutory Supervision of Midwives, LSA Standards for England 2005–2008*. London: Local Supervising Authority.

Malkin, K. F. (1994) A standard for professional development: the use of self and peer review; learning contracts and reflection in clinical practice. *Journal of Nursing Management* 2(3): 143–8.

Mann, R. and Williams, J. (2003) Standards in medical record keeping. *Journal of Nursing Management* 2(3): 329–32.

Meredith, S. (1994) Peer review: preparing the evaluator. *Canadian Journal of Nursing* 7(2): 69–91.

National Health Service Litigation Authority (2005) *CNST, General Clinical Risk Management Standards*. London: NHSLA.

Nursing and Midwifery Council (2004) *Fitness to Practise Annual Report 2004–2005*. London: NMC.

Nursing and Midwifery Council (2004a) *Midwives Rules and Standards*. London: NMC.

Nursing and Midwifery Council (2004b) *The NMC Code of Professional Conduct: Standards for Conduct, Performance and Ethics*. London: NMC.

Nursing and Midwifery Council (2005) *Guidelines for Records and Record Keeping*. London: NMC.

Nursing and Midwifery Council (2006a) *Confidentiality*. London: NMC.

Nursing and Midwifery Council (2006b) *The Prep Handbook*. London: NMC.

Nursing and Midwifery Council (2007) 03 January 02/NMC circular. *Ownership and Sharing of Midwifery Records*. London: NMC.

Rodden, C. and Bell, M. (2002) Record keeping: developing good practice. *Nursing Standard* 17(1): 40–2.

Schön, D. (1991) *The Reflective Practitioner*. San Francisco: Jossey-Bass.

Thompson, N. (2002) *People Skills*, 2nd edition. Great Britain: Creative, Print and Design.

Yearley, C. (2003) Guided reflection as a tool for continuing professional development. *British Journal of Midwifery* 11(4): 223–6.

Regulating the Midwifery Profession – Protecting Women or the Profession?

Christine Lawrence and Carole Yearley

Introduction

This chapter discusses the regulation of the midwifery profession. An historical perspective is taken first, to help determine why the British government passed a law in 1902 to establish the Central Midwives Board (CMB). This approach distinguishes in particular the special difficulties that women in the nineteenth century had in gaining public and political attention to the shocking state of affairs affecting women in childbirth. This review identifies in particular the importance of two key principles – education and self-regulation – which together brought about the changes desired to protect the public from unsafe midwifery practitioners. These two perspectives are retained to focus on how the midwifery profession is currently being affected by developments in these areas, with particular emphasis given to the impacts they are having for women's care and professional practice. The chapter concludes by looking forward to some of the issues that the profession will have to address over the coming decades regarding professional education and regulation. In particular, we consider current thinking about both the benefits and limitations of allowing a profession to monitor and control its own practitioners, and if it is now timely for midwives to move to a more all-embracing health care professions regulatory body.

There is a wealth of information about health carers' professional roles, professionalisation, professional self-regulation, professional monopolies and the control and policing of professionals (Johnson

1972; Seligman 1980; Shaked and Sutton 1981; Stevens 2002; Hilton 2005). These, together with the extensive literature available on medical history (Galt 1978; Donnison 1988; Lewis 1993; Fox 1995; Porter 1997) will further inform and expand the reader's understanding of this topic. In order to help apply and broaden thinking, however, the reader is asked to debate – with themselves or with others – what they think the impact of different situations would or could be for a variety of persons.

Students of midwifery and maternity care may already be forming ideas about what it means to have professional status, and what the implications of professional education and registration are upon qualifying. Further to this perspective, however, you are particularly asked to consider what the implications of the different issues could be for the 'public' – i.e. the government, the employers of midwives, the people in our communities and the pregnant women themselves. There are no definitive answers to these challenges; they serve more to help you reflect on the issues and possibly raise more questions that you may consider warrant further study.

Activity

Imagine it is 1871 and you are in labour. You have no idea what will happen to you during the next few hours. You and your husband are both orphans and have no family to support or inform you. He is at work. You only know that it is usual to call a woman in the next village to come and deliver babies, but you don't know her. You are aware that it is not uncommon for babies to die while being born, but you were a bit shocked when your neighbour two floors above died two months ago, the day after this midwife delivered her baby. You think it is normal to pay the midwife to attend but only have enough money to pay the rent and for food for the two of you – all other expenses are usually met through bartering or scrounging.

What is the likelihood of this woman surviving her delivery?

Why registration?

In the nineteenth century when the death of a woman during childbirth was common and the demise of the baby a familiar experience, it is not difficult to see why childbearing was entered into with much apprehension (Cowell and Wainwright 1981; Loudon 1991). Channelling this fear into pressure for change, however, required an immense amount of courage and determination on the part of those who started to pioneer safer childbirth.

The individual experience of women having a baby varied widely throughout the country and across the social classes. The care a woman received depended on social connections and how much money she had. At one end of the spectrum were the trained medical practitioners, some of whom had a good reputation for participating in the professionally high-risk business of delivering babies. Financially secure households might purchase the services of this type of practitioner, anticipating that their medical training and knowledge would inevitably be superior to that of others.

Those doctors who were able to achieve a safe birth outcome would increase their practice and hence the financial rewards, though this was more the result of clients' gratitude and their reputation than their skill or training in obstetrics, which only a minority had. Other doctors would be called because of their 'kind' or 'good' reputation, in the belief that they could help difficult childbirth and the high associated risk of deaths. Rarely called at the start of the labour, these doctors gained experience with difficult childbirth and would have direct knowledge of the skills and practices of the 'lying-in' nurses and midwives who attended most women in their area. The majority of women, however, relied on the local midwife. The local midwife presented with a standard of care ranging from the neglectful ignorance to some level of training and experiential development as an apprentice to a skilled midwife of good reputation. Which midwife a family employed was largely down to luck, where they lived or whether or not a 'good' midwife could be encouraged – financially – to attend a birth beyond her normal area of practice.

Education and instruction

This parlous situation underlines the importance of education and preparation to undertake midwifery. Most midwives in the more rural areas had little or no formal instruction and so had limited skills and ability in reading or accessing medical literature and texts. However, by the mid-nineteenth century an increasing number of women had attended school and this undoubtedly helped expand their views about their capabilities and role in society (Porter 1997). Women were better placed to confront the male-dominated institutions about their complacency over the welfare issues that so acutely affected women's well-being, homes and families. In particular they were able to direct their 'trained' thinking (Hudson 2001) to challenge the authorities about the care childbearing women received – a situation the majority might one day find themselves in. In addition, by the late nineteenth century the articulate single or widowed women could consider pursuing a career in nursing or midwifery (Cowell and Wainwright 1981). Hitherto these roles would not have been considered appropriate for a socially aware and self-respecting woman, but with changes being brought about by pioneers such as Ethel Bedford Fenwick (Donnison 1988) the caring professions became more reputable trades with which to be associated. Midwifery was becoming increasingly more acceptable for women in the growing middle classes who may have needed employment to satisfy their requirement for societal standing and financial security, however insignificant these particular rewards were at that time.

The education of girls and the need for respectable 'womens' work were undoubtedly key changes for women in the nineteenth century. But the development of skills required of a midwife was not a structured event. Women wanting to learn and understand about the process of childbearing could pay fees to gain admittance to some of the reputable training institutions found in the women's hospitals of the major cities. Here a certain amount of both formal and informal tuition could be gained from the medical profession. Although this training was not necessarily preparatory for the role, it did provide some direction on the topics around childbirth which could then be followed up by gaining experience and skill at 'poor law' and voluntary hospitals, or in the homes of women where the majority of midwives practised. The assistance available for women in childbirth therefore was highly dependent on their social status, financial background and access to practitioners who knew about childbirth, or had practical experience in the processes of labour. Where all of these factors were good, the outcomes of childbearing were seen to be superior. For those women who, for whatever reason, were excluded from accessing these predictors of better outcomes, their care could be overtly hazardous, the outcomes unpredictable and death not unexpected.

Safer childbirth

Midwifery in this era was an exclusively female occupation, a factor which may be have been one of its greatest contributing challenges as it needed intrepid and articulate women in the politically influential social classes to be interested – let alone able – to discuss the issue of childbirth in a sexuality-sensitive and male-dominated society (Donnison 1988; Porter 1997). Social mores meant discussion of issues around what was effectively an intimate 'female' health matter needed a great deal of tact and diplomacy. Gaining the interests of male policy-makers and other philanthropic entrepreneurs in a domestic, 'feminine' subject such as childbirth proved to be an uphill struggle and required a range of skills to engage the influential in a discussion on the subject and take it to parliament for legislative action. Indeed, anyone willing to engage in public discussion of the issues and challenge those who held power or influence in this domain required boldness of character and the fearlessness that came from conviction that change was vital. They may be considered to be the true pioneers for safer childbirth in the UK.

Women's issues

Informing and raising social awareness about the intricacies and perils of childbirth and then harnessing the public's interest and enthusiasm to produce action at government level were indeed challenges for women, midwives and the medical profession (Donnison 1988; Leap and Hunter 1993). However, it may be considered fortuitous or astute timing that women's issue were being advanced by an increasing, and seemingly unstoppable, number of women's societies and interest groups. Not least of these was the women's suffrage movement, which was bringing into sharp focus the role that women should be accorded in making legislation in the UK. These simultaneous events slowly but surely changed the environment to one where women's issues could be discussed – and more importantly supported – by the public. The polite debates which started in the mid-nineteenth century on the poor state of affairs for childbirth in England became a focus of increasing public interest, questions in Parliament and finally the subject of legislation at the beginning of the twentieth century.

Regulation and control

The battle to improve childbirth was fought on several fronts and from several different social and professional perspectives. However, it was the campaign for the regulation and control of midwives that captured the public's attention. Indeed, the keenest proponents for regulating midwives were the midwives themselves, with the lead being taken by members of the Midwives Institute (now the Royal College of Midwives). Those midwives who had some form of training and understanding about the progress of childbirth, and were successful in assisting the majority of their clients through the hazards of labour, were keen to ensure that midwives practising dangerously or who were associated with high mortality rates should be curtailed. The poor reputation of these 'practitioners' could at the very least undermine their own reputation. But more importantly it meant the mortality and morbidity so acutely associated with childbirth in this era was unlikely to be reversed if these people could not be prevented from practising. Although for some midwives the strategy to seek formal control over poor standards derived from self-interest, for the majority it enabled them to share their knowledge, enthusiasm and experiences about childbearing whilst supporting the drive to improve standards of care.

The struggle for legislation of the medical profession in 1834 and other associated health practices during the latter part of the nineteenth century is described in a range medical history texts (Donnison 1988; Porter 1997). These texts also discuss how the various White and Green Papers progressed through the committees and tiers of government legislation. The outcome – The Midwives Act 1902 – was an important landmark for those championing the cause of safer childbirth through having appropriately trained midwives. It was a significant moment in history as central government decided to protect, by law, its childbearing women from those who were not registered with the Central Midwives Board (CMB).

To summarise, midwifery became a profession with the passing of the Midwives Act 1902. The need to prepare and educate midwives for their role had been endorsed by government, which acknowledged the relationship between educated midwives and better outcomes for women and babies during childbirth. The title midwife became protected by law and along with this established the principle that only *trained* practitioners (midwives or doctors) could attend women during childbirth. The professionalisation of midwives became established through a self-regulating approach giving the profession wide-ranging powers and autonomy over its direction and protocols for care.

Activity

It is 1902. You have been practising successfully for nearly 18 years and have built up a business in both a rural and urban locality in the North-East. You are well respected, and the local doctors are pleased to have you to hand when they are attending a delivery. You learnt midwifery by watching and being corrected by an experienced midwife who seemed to have a great innate knowledge about what to do, which she shared with you. Many women now come to you to ensure you will be available when they go into labour.

You have heard that there is a Central Midwives Board with which you 'must register' to get a licence to practise as a midwife. If you don't, they could stop you practising. It is said it is about making childbirth safe – but you know you practise safely and have done so for years.

- How do you feel about this action imposed by midwives in London?
- Can you afford it anyway
- What benefits will it bring for you?

The professionalisation of midwifery

Now that is was charged with protecting the public, the CMB had to address the preparatory education of midwives entering the profession and establish systems to monitor the standards of care being delivered by its registrants. Its functions of preparing and guiding the care that midwives should provide was undoubtedly distinguishable from its other major function – protecting the public from poor practitioners and preventing them from registered practice and employment as a midwife. Concurrent with these two key functions was the need to address the ethical and moral dilemmas that professional regulation brought. These issues are now explored to help demonstrate how the profession evolved its stature, relationships and duty of care to the public.

Self-regulation

The status of self-regulation for midwives resulted in several significant and intrinsic qualities being afforded to the profession, most important of which was the power given to the CMB to select or appoint persons from within its own professionals to lead and implement its self-determined regulations (Maks and Philipsen 1999). The board of the CMB therefore was made up largely of representatives from within the profession, with a minority from other professions or interested allied organisations appointed or invited by the government to be members of the board. Whilst extending to these interested parties some entry to the board's business, debates and actions, it nevertheless was an organisation run by midwives, who took the requirement to police its regulations as seriously as the altruistic aim it strove for – protecting the public from what they considered to be unsafe midwifery practitioners.

Activity

- In so far as women generally were not well educated at the end of the nineteenth century, did self-regulation give an advantage to elite, articulate and well-educated midwives?
- Would the original CMB have been truly representative of the profession in terms of values, skills and sphere of practice?
- Was self-regulation the best way to proceed?

Self-regulation is important for a profession as it endorses the concept that only the professionals themselves are able to set the standards and tenets by which they should be measured (Shaked and Sutton 1981). Those seeking to practise midwifery are introduced to the profession's values, knowledge and skills during their preparatory education and consequently should enter practice well versed in what is expected and how their peers practise within the defined role. It would seem wholly appropriate therefore that the profession determines what the sphere and domain of its practice are and not take on what others, who are not active practitioners of midwifery, may determine is their function. Indeed, throughout the latter part of the twentieth century the midwifery profession has been fortunate in having a very clear statement about the expectations of a midwife as articulated by the World Health Organisation (2001). This statement adds weight to the direction that the regulatory bodies (e.g. the United Kingdom Central Council and the Nursing and Midwifery Council) pursued over the course of the twentieth century and enables midwives to be clear about what their required and expected behaviours are, as well as what is outside their sphere. Self-regulation therefore has enabled a clear message to be sent to both the professionals and the public as to what is expected of a midwife employed in the UK.

Midwifery education

As the profession was given the responsibility to determine the role and expectations of midwives, it is perhaps not surprising that one of the first actions the CMB addressed was compiling a list of people whom they would register and consequently authorise to practise as midwives in the UK. Initially, midwives were able to register with the CMB either as a 'midwife' who could demonstrate attendance at an approved training course or as a bona fide midwife. The bona fide midwives were those who could provide statements by agreed authorities (e.g. doctors, Midwives Institute) that they were working appropriately, even though they had no training for their role. The CMB therefore allowed these midwives a licence to practise for ten years, within which time they were expected to have attended CMB-approved education to demonstrate their equal standing to midwives who had received some training about childbirth.

Recognising and approving programmes of training and education continues to be a large part of the activities carried out by the current regulatory body for midwives, The Nurses and Midwives Council (NMC). Effectively, midwives have a licence to practise in the UK only because they have been prepared in an institution approved by the NMC, and have demonstrated that they are able to meet the required standards as measured by assessors selected from within the profession. These requirements ensure the 'barriers' preventing anyone practising midwifery are clearly stated whilst simultaneously adding clarity about the quality of care the profession aspires to (NMC 2004a). The midwifery profession was a pioneer in recognising and supporting continuing professional updating and development. Midwives have been required since the establishment of the CMB to undertake statutory refreshment by attending board-approved courses every ten years. This, together with the need to notify their intention to practise with the local supervising authority (see Chapter 19) on an annual basis, enables the midwifery profession to be seen as a leader in establishing continuing professional development and support for its practitioners.

Changes in the midwife–woman relationship

An inevitable and direct consequence of the statutory regulation of a profession is that it creates a monopoly for its practitioners (Johnson 1972; Maks and Philipsen 1999). A professional monopoly will alter the relationship between the professional and the public because the public may now receive care only from practitioners who are registered with the statutory body. This situation, found in a range of service-oriented health care professions, has a potential to create a gulf between the client and professional, not least because the professional must now have a greater knowledge base than the general public. As the knowledge gap inexorably grows between the midwife and woman it can generate communication disparities resulting in the woman having less power and influence over the care she may feel she wants or needs. By the end of the twentieth century a range of interventions were increasingly being used to promote the safety and well-being of the mother and baby. Women's opinions and choices were gradually subjugated with the growth in technology and the science base for childbirth, with the rationale that a woman's compliance with professional advice was the better – safer – way of proceeding.

Implementing the professionals' choice and recommended courses of action to 'save' or prevent problems associated with childbirth from otherwise inevitable mortality or morbidity could not easily be challenged by women looking for a healthy outcome from their pregnancies. Furthermore, this medicalised, scientific approach to childbearing expanded the area of midwifery practice from solely the intrapartum period at the beginning of the twentieth century, to include antenatal and postnatal care. This resulted in pregnancy, childbirth and the puerperium being controlled by the health care practitioners – obstetricians and midwives – and women being expected to comply with the care planned for them for by the professionals for their benefit.

For the childbearing woman, however, the registration of midwives means she is totally reliant on the quality of the skills and abilities of midwives as determined by the NMC's education policies and codes of practice. This situation, although commendable in trying to improve the quality of care women receive, nevertheless does make women reliant on the integrity and commitment of individual midwives to uphold the professional standards. Whilst the legislative action set out to protect the women by providing well-educated midwives, at the same time it created an environment in which midwives could exploit their elite position and coerce women into receiving care that the professionals consider 'best'.

Keenly aware of this situation, midwives have had to consider their fiduciary duty to women. A fiduciary duty is the highest standard of care imposed on a professional. In the case of midwifery it affords the childbearing woman a relationship which has to be established by the midwife, and which should feature loyalty and trust between both partners. Midwives, in accepting the legislatively bound title and role, must not put their own interests before the woman's and should conduct themselves at a level higher than is expected in a non-professional relationship (Allsop and Saks 2002). In order for the midwifery profession to succeed as a self-regulating organisation, midwives have had to establish with the public, and in particular the women in their care, a relationship of trust. The equation which underpins this relationship requires that, in return for the public's trust, the midwifery profession will strive to conduct its duty to care to the highest standard (Klein 1998). The profession achieves this not only by ensuring appropriate education and development of its professionals, but also by providing scrutiny which will bring about the effective exclusion of malpractising midwives who do not meet the standards expected of them.

The nature of a trust relationship for midwives has been shared openly with society and is expressed in the *Code of Professional Conduct* (NMC 2004a). The NMC as the current regulating body has articulated its stance on the values, beliefs, conducts and behaviours expected of its midwifery registrants. The *Code of Professional Conduct* builds upon the statutory instruments, clarifying expectations of midwives in certain spheres of their practice and their duties and responsibilities to the women in their care and the public generally. Over the years the *Code of Professional Conduct* has been expanded and strengthened to acknowledge developments and changes in the expectations of the public. Essentially, however, it can be seen as a form of contract or agreement between the profession and those to whom they owe a duty of care. Failing to address or achieve the standards set in the *Code of Professional Conduct* forms the basis of a breach of care which could be pursued by a dissatisfied woman.

Ensuring standards

The *Code of Professional Conduct* (2004a) and the *Midwives Rules and Standards* (NMC 2004c) can be considered as the NMC's benchmark and informs the public what they may expect to receive and for which each practitioner must be responsible and accountable. A midwife's role continually expands and evolves, but whatever is incorporated, midwives must be able to demonstrate that the care they have delivered is appropriate and relevant (NHS Executive 2000). Measuring this standard is the remit of the Fitness to Practice directorate of the NMC. Ultimately, if a member of the public feels aggrieved by the standard of care they have received, they may take their evidence to the Primary Care Trust for their consideration and response. In these circumstances the midwife is called to give an account of the care given, along with the rationale and basis for her acts of omission or commission.

The hearing held by the NMC will invite appropriate witnesses from within the profession to explore whether the actions taken were those that any midwife would consider reasonable or appropriate in the circumstances. In carrying out this function and using witnesses from within its own professionals the self-regulatory nature of the profession is fully exposed. Peer midwives will determine, based on the best available evidence and practice in use at the time, whether a fellow midwife's standard of care was acceptable, and therefore whether the practitioner should stay within the profession or be dismissed. By creating a self-regulating monopoly the government, and consequently the public, expects a professional body to have procedures and systems available to identify midwives not practising safely and to deal with substandard practitioners appropriately and efficiently.

Activity

Review what the term *duty* means for the profession, the public, the employers of midwives, women themselves. Does each expect the same duty from midwives?

Make a list of what you consider to be the professional duties of a midwife.

Is it only statutory legislation and regulation of a professional group that instils a duty to care, or is this a feature of anyone delivering a service to another person? (Consider bank managers, hoteliers, hairdressers, etc.)

Current challenges to professional self-regulation

A century on from the 1902 Midwives Act the profession is still addressing the public interests and concerns about safe childbirth (Graham and Bell 2001). Both the former regulatory body – the United Kingdom Central Council for Nurses, Midwives and Health Visitors (1983–2002) – and now the Nursing and Midwifery Council have had to embrace the fundamental tenets of these two different professions yet have maintained the specialist and specific interests and concerns relating to midwifery practice through establishing a Midwifery Committee. This professionally appointed, yet statutorily required group leads and affirms the direction and implications of legislation for the midwifery profession, both collaboratively and/or independently to the regulation proposed for nurses. Concurrently, the NMC addresses political debates which challenge the impacts and consequences of being a self-regulating organisation. This appraisal comes especially in light of recent events (Kennedy 2001; Redfern 2001; DH 2004; Smith 2004) which have undermined the public's confidence generally in a range of health professions' ability to police their own practitioners. Furthermore, as many other allied health care workers have also achieved or are pressing for professional regulation and registration with their own self-regulating organisation, the need for so many different health profession regulating bodies is questionable. The commonalities and duplication of approaches associated with the intent to 'protect the public' is exercising the professions to consider being united into one professional health carers' regulating body. These issues will now be explored in order to evaluate the impact that professional self-regulation is having and whether there is evidence that should challenge this practice.

One health regulatory body?

First, we return to the impact that education has had on the profession. We have acknowledged that to have a licence to practise midwives must be educated to professional standards before being registered with the NMC. We have argued that although education can enlighten the evidence base to improve the quality of midwifery care, it can potentially create a power and communication imbalance between the midwives and women. Perhaps even more problematic for the public and profession is the expense that is incurred by improving and increasing the standard of education of midwives. By setting its own standards and determining where the preparation will take place, the midwifery profession, through the NMC, has demanded a continuous striving for greater knowledge, skills and professional conduct.

Currently, preparation programmes are managed by and delivered from universities, with half of the students' programmed time spent in clinical practice. Curriculum designers are challenged with addressing the tension between the higher education demands, ethos and style of education as influenced by the Department for Education and Skills (DfES), whilst also addressing the syllabus and standards for pre-registration midwifery, as required by the NMC (2004b). When successfully integrated it may be anticipated that the student is prepared appropriately for midwifery practice with academic skills underpinning the professional skills, knowledge and behaviours which will keep women safe in their care. The midwife now not only has a licence to practise but a diploma or honours degree associated with it.

Herein lies an increasing problem for both the government and the profession. The NMC stipulates the standards and requirements considered necessary for approved midwifery training inputs and outcomes, with a keen eye being kept to ensure that the standards achieved are appropriate for professional practice, academic award and clinical purpose. The number to be educated annually however is determined by manpower analyses made by the Workforce

Development Directorates of the Strategic Health Authorities. Once registered with the NMC, the majority of midwives are employed by the NHS, with the number required for any particular maternity service being determined through Birthrate Plus (Ball and Washbrook 1996). The government budget-holders therefore determine both how many students it can financially afford to support through the university-based preparatory training *and* the number of midwives it can afford to employ. As the standards of education have increased so too have the associated costs of preparing professionals (Greiner and Knebel 2004). The government is therefore in the powerful position of determining the availability of midwives for the care of women to meet the need for safety – by having midwives educated to the standard recommended by the NMC – with the budget it has available.

This situation exposes the dilemma affecting the public and the profession. This regulatory body sits between two arms of the government – the DfES and the Department of Health. While the NMC's prime focus is the protection of the public by having well-educated midwives, its decisions on the standards it requires influences the costs of education and, as a consequence, the number of midwives available to deliver care for women. Effectively at the start of the twenty-first century, a gulf is opening up between what is desirable – highly skilled and educated midwife practitioners – and what is affordable. This, Allsop and Saks (2002) argue, is an inevitable outcome of professional autonomy over educational standards.

For Greiner and Knebel (2003) this financially driven conundrum typically arises in professions where the education and employment of the professionals is purchased by one and the same body – the government. Whilst some professions (e.g. lawyers and accountants) receive higher education preparatory programmes, their subsequent employers are invariably private individuals or organisations. A tension will always result between what is professionally aspired to and what is affordable. It can therefore be hypothesised that as the number of midwives commissioned declines because of the increasing education costs, so the profession will either have to review the standard of preparatory education it considers adequate, or anticipate that fewer professionals will be trained. The consequence of fewer midwives will be a shortfall in the number of personnel able to deliver care and an environment where other kinds of carers will need to be included in maternity services if women are to enjoy a safe standard of care. Indeed Maks and Philipsen (1999) identify that within this financially tense and driven environment, a range of lay support groups and care assistants can and will enter the arena. Newcomers (Hilton 2005) to the maternity service may have some training in certain skills or aspects of maternity care, delivered locally at maternity units (e.g. breastfeeding support workers) or at further education colleges (e.g. care assistants) and are cheaper to employ than the higher educated midwives. The House of Commons Select Committee on Health – Fourth Report (UK Parliament 2003) encourages further research into how a range of voluntary and support staff could be employed to enhance the maternity services care delivery in a staff-constrained environment which is not conducive to retaining midwives.

Now, after more than 100 years of professional regulation, a familiar yet slightly different regulatory issue will affect the maternity service. Where registration of midwives aimed at protecting the public from poorly educated and substandard practitioners, the maternity service now has to use non-licensed or unregulated carers in order that women can receive *some* attention during their childbirth experience. It could be concluded that, by pursing ever higher standards considered appropriate for the safe practice of its registrants, the regulating body has placed midwives in an exclusive yet unsustainable position.

Activity

Consider the cost of ignorance.

- Having fought for and achieved education for midwives, how can the profession proceed if it has made itself too 'expensive'? To drop standards is neither acceptable nor defensible. How then should midwives continue to protect childbearing women from substandard care?
- Could having a range of care assistants or maternity nurses fragment the care midwives consider should be delivered holistically?
- What models of care delivery do you foresee in future maternity services?
- Will having a range of carers be helpful for women – they at least will have some care – or create sources of more conflicting advice for women?
- Will the partnership and trust built between midwife and woman be undermined by having a range of new carers in the maternity services?
- Is an inevitable outcome of the situation that these new carers will need or want regulation and registration?

Exclusive or inclusive regulatory bodies?

Whilst the implications of these questions are affecting the availability of midwives, there are equally demanding issues to consider – the need for so many regulatory bodies for the different health professions (Johnson 1998; Catto 2003; DH 2005). Currently there are nine bodies that regulate health professionals in the UK, but their statutory powers, decision-making mechanisms and administrative processes vary enormously (NHS Executive 2000).

It is evident that different standards of evidence are required at inquiries, as well as definitions as to what constitutes misconduct or poor performance (Johnson 1998). These regulatory bodies' methods and panel arrangements to investigate professionals differ and as a result their decisions can appear unfair or out of line with the outcomes that other professionals may be given in similar enquiries. For Walshe and Benson (2005) this situation necessitates review. They propose a harmonising approach which, they assert, is more equitable and consistent for both the public and professionals.

Their main assertion is that professions should move away from defining themselves as a group of midwives, doctors and pharmacists and regulate the *actions* that a practitioner can undertake. Such actions, they suggest, are diagnosis, investigation, prescribing, performing restricted interventions. These activities may be considered markers which differentiate between the carers who have specific competencies in these skills which enable them to manage and direct health care and those who can deliver aspects of care but are not bound by a fiduciary duty.

By considering these and similar qualities as the tenets of professionalism and professional status these behaviours can be added to by the various professions by articulating the specific standards and competencies they must have for a named group. This approach, Walshe and Benson suggest, facilitates the inclusion of other health care groups wanting regulation for their sphere of practice as they would be expected to embrace these fundamental activities as part of their care repertoire. Entry to regulatory control, therefore, is based on whether they are required to undertake these 'regulated acts' rather than on the nature or focus of the care provided. Inclusion of these newcomers into the regulating body would therefore be facilitated and monitoring of performance could be more standardised within and among health professions. For Walshe and Benson (2005) it is the activities a health practitioner undertakes which should determine professional status and not the scope or title of the practice which should determine whether a group should be controlled by statutory regulation.

Walshe and Benson (2005) are perhaps the first to acknowledge that these proposals will be challenged and possibly resisted by some of the current regulatory bodies. However, these suggestions do offer an interesting challenge for the midwifery profession to consider as it continues to adjust to the changes in its role and expectations. If, as asserted above, new groups of carers are to be involved in the care of childbearing women, the profession will ultimately have to support their moves for appropriate preparation and, perhaps more importantly, regulation. Not to uphold this development would confront the arguments they pursued for the regulation of midwives over a century ago – that statutory regulation protects women from poor or substandard practitioners and can improve the care women receive. The elite autonomy status of the midwifery profession and others regulated by a regulatory body proposed by Walshe and Benson (2005) would inevitably be moderated, and the professional groups encouraged to function more collaboratively.

Activity

How often have you heard midwives say that 'midwives are independent practitioners, and autonomous in their own right'? Consider what the statement truly means.

- Are we independent?
- Do we have autonomy?
- Is midwifery so different from all other professions that we require our own regulatory body?
- Does retaining our individual regulatory status help support improvements in both care and professional regulatory activity?
- Would one health care regulatory body dumb down the activities traditionally led by the professionally named regulators?

The arguments for change to professional regulation would seem to be timely as moves to reform the regulation of the health professions continue at government level. In the past decade there have been several notorious public inquiries following criticism of the functioning of the health regulatory bodies in dealing with poor practitioners. Although the medical profession has come under particular scrutiny (DH 2004; Smith 2004) the majority of the health professional regulatory bodies have been criticised over many years (Allsop and Saks 2002) for their failure to deal with cases of incompetence, dishonesty and sexual misconduct. As a result, the Council for Healthcare Regulatory Excellence (CHRE) was established, following the NHS Reform Act 2002 and Health Care Professions Act 2002. The CHRE (2006) has a wide range of functions relating to promoting 'best practice and consistency in the regulation of healthcare professionals'. Answerable to Parliament, it ultimately oversees the work of all health professional regulatory bodies by promoting consistency and principles of good regulation. Most importantly, it is able to bring the final decision of a regulating body to the High Court (or equivalent) for the protection of the public and as a last resort, with the endorsement of both Houses of Parliament, to order a regulator to change its rules for the purpose of protecting the public.

This new quality-enhancing organisation therefore has far-reaching powers which will strengthen moves to bring the functioning of the various regulating bodies into line. Similarities rather than differences will be highlighted and promoted, with fitness to practice inquiries more transparent and consistent. It is not difficult to project that with time the CHRE could pave the way for the changes proposed by Walshe and Benson (2005). As the fitness to practise issues are dealt with more reliably, each of the regulating bodies will review its own practice and amend rules to incorporate improved standards of protecting the public. It will then be more of a challenge to sustain all nine of the different regulating bodies when their commonalities are greater than their differences. Furthermore, economies of scale will no doubt be required and the professions more likely to be drawn together to facilitate both their own and the public's interests.

Conclusions

The standards of care a government provides for pregnant women and newborn babies are considered important benchmarks of the overall health care provided by a country (WHO 2006). After a century of regulating midwives and their practice there has been a significant reduction in the maternal and perinatal mortality and morbidity rates and therefore an improvement in the welfare of women and newborn babies. Having well-educated midwives has undoubtedly played an important part in enabling scientific advances to be implemented safely and judiciously and for many high-risk situations to end up with successful outcomes. Furthermore, the academic underpinning skills now developed in midwives at universities – for example, critical appraisal, enhanced judgement and decision-making skills – are enabling midwives to challenge ideas and proposals for care, and negotiate with colleagues and other professionals those approaches which best fulfil safety as well as women-centred and supportive practice.

Government drives for multi-professional education and working are now underpinning a trend to change professional boundaries and attitudes to traditional practices and roles. Whilst midwives are skilled at working with paediatricians, obstetricians and GPs, increasingly their role is requiring that they work alongside a range of social, legal and other health care workers. Furthermore, the public health agenda being promoted by the government means that midwives review their practices and the opportunities they have to influence parents' health and emotional well-being. A current example is the expansion of Children's Centres and the impact that midwives will have in the development of these resources for child-bearing women. Furthermore from the Shribman Report (2007) it is evident the trends for the maternity services will be for more midwifery-led care practice in units within the community. All these initiatives will require the profession to review its preparatory training to ensure that midwives are not only able to carry out the requirements set by the NMC, but also are able to enter employment skilled to work in a dynamically changing maternity service. Challenges to midwifery education are therefore to develop those skills that enable flexible adaptable and innovative midwives, able to lead multi-professional teams in providing quality care for the childbearing women.

Whilst changing the nature and place of midwifery practice has been a regular activity for the profession over the past century, the underpinning ethos of regulating the profession has retained a contemporaneous yet progressive focus on the protection of the public. How this focal point evolves should the NMC merge into a single health regulatory body will be absorbing and no doubt challenging to those tasked with integrating the values and tenets of very different health care groups. If any of Walshe's and Benson (2005) vision does come to fruition it would bring into sharper focus what a united regulatory body would articulate as the standards for health care 'professional practice' and what value-added skills, knowledge and attitudes would then be required to become a midwife. For midwives the influence of the Royal College of Midwives (RCM) may yet again help ensure the concerns of the midwifery profession and childbearing women are articulated and influence policy appropriately. Indeed, any such review of the statutory regulating bodies may instigate a review of the RCM's role and functions in the future, and perhaps to lead future articulations of what the role functions and duties are of UK midwives.

References

Allsop, J. and Saks, M. (2002) *Regulating the Health Professions*. London: Sage.

Ball, J. and Washbrook, M. (1996) *Birthrate Plus – Midwifery Services*. London: Elsevier.

Catto, G. (2003) *Improving Professional Competence – The Way Ahead?* 19th International Conference of the International Society for Quality in Health Care. Paris: International Journal for Quality in Health Care.

Catto, G. (2006) Good doctors, safer patients: a chance to move on. *British Journal of Hospital Medicine* 67: 508–9.

CHRE (2006) http://www.chre.org.uk/Website/about/.

Cowell, B. and Wainwright, D. (1981) *Behind the Blue Door: The History of the Royal College of Midwives 1881–1981*. London: Bailliere Tindall.

Department of Health (2004) *Independent Investigation into How the NHS Handled Allegations about the Conduct of Clifford Ayling*. London: DH.

Department of Health (2005) *Government Widens Review into Healthcare Regulation*. London: DH.

Donnison, J. (1988) *Midwives and Medical Men*. London: Historical Publications.

Fox, E. (1995) Midwifery in England and Wales before 1936. Handywomen and doctors. *International History of Nursing* 1: 17–28.

Galt, J. (1978) *The Howdie. John Galt Selected Short Stories*. Edinburgh: Scottish Academic Press.

Graham, W., Bell, J. et al. (2001) Can skilled attendance at delivery reduce maternal mortality in developing countries? In V. De Brouwere and W. Van Lerberghe, *Safe Motherhood Strategies: A Review of the Evidence*. Antwerp: ITG Press.

Greiner, A. and Knebel, E. (2003) *Health Professions Education: A Bridge to Quality*. Committee on the Health Professions Education Summit, Institute of Medicine US. Washington: National Academies Press.

Hilton, S. (2005) 'Proto-professionalism: how professionalisation occurs across the continuum of medical education. *Medical Education* 39: 58–65.

Hudson, P. (2001) Women's Work. www.bbc.co.uk/history/british/victorians/womens-work.0.

Johnson, J. (1998) Making self-regulation credible through benchmarking, peer review, appraisal and management. *British Medical Journal* 316: 1847–8.

Johnson, T. (1972) *Professions and Power*. London: Macmillan.

Kennedy, I. (2001) *Learning from Bristol: The Report of the Public Enquiry into Children's Heart Surgery at The Bristol Royal Infirmary 1984–1995*. London: HMSO.

Klein, R. (1998) Competence, professional self-regulation and the public interest. *British Medical Journal* 316: 1740–2.

Leap, N. and Hunter, B. (1993) *The Midwife's Tale: An Oral History from Handywoman to Professional Midwife*. London: Scarlet Press.

Lewis, J. (1993) *In the Family Way: Childbearing in the British Aristocracy 1760–1860*. New Jersey: Rutgers University Press.

Llewelyn Davies, M. ([1931] 1977). *Life As We Have Known It. Co-operative Working Women*. London, Virago.

Llewelyn Davies, M. (1978) *Maternity: Letters from Working-Class Women*. London: Virago.

Loudon, I. (1991) On maternal and infant mortality 1900–1960. *Social History of Medicine* 4: 29–73.

Maks, J. A. H. and Philipsen, N. J. (1999) *An Economic Analysis of the Regulation of Professions*. http://www.unimaas.nl/.

NHS Executive (2000) *Modernising Regulation – The New Health Professions Council*. London: DH.

Nursing and Midwifery Council (2004a) *The NMC Code of Professional Conduct: Standards for Conduct, Performance and Ethics*. www.nmc-uk.org.

Nursing and Midwifery Council (2004b) *Standards of Proficiency for Pre-Registration Midwifery Education*. www.nmc-uk.org.

Porter, R. (1997) *The Greatest Benefit to Mankind: A Medical History of Humanity from Antiquity to the Present*. London: HarperCollins.

Redfern, M. (2001) *The Royal Liverpool Children's Inquiry*. London: House of Commons.

Seligman, S. (1980) The Royal Maternity Charter: The first hundred years. *Medical History* 24: 403–18.

Shaked, A. and Sutton, J. (1981) The self-regulating professions. *Review of Economic Studies* XLVIII: 217–34.

Shribman, S. (2007) *Making it Better: For Mother and Baby, Clinical Case for Change*. London: DH.

Smith, J. (2004) *Shipman Inquiry Fifth Report: Safeguarding Patients: Lessons from the Past – Proposals for the Future*. London: HMSO.

Stevens, R. (2002) Themes in the history of medical professionalism. *The Mount Sinai Journal of Medicine* 69(6): 357–62.

UK Parliament (2003) *The Select Committee on Health – Fourth Report*. www.publications.parliament.uk/pa/cm200203/cmselect/cmhealth/464/46402.htm.

Walshe, K. and Benson, L. (2005) Time for radical reform. *British Medical Journal* 330: 1504–6.

World Health Organisation (2001) *Making Pregnancy Safer: The Critical Role of the Skilled Attendant: A Joint Statement by WHO, ICM and FIGO*. Geneva: WHO.

World Health Organisation (2006) *Health Indicators. Reproductive Health and Research. Guidelines for Their Generation, Interpretation and Analysis for Global Monitoring*. Geneva: WHO.

The Impact of Cultural Issues on the Practice of Midwifery

Celia Wildeman

Introduction

The aim of the chapter is to explore contemporary issues that influence midwifery practice in the context of culturally sensitive care so that midwives can address the emerging challenges in the best interest of their clients.

Culture will be defined, and a differentiation between culture, race and ethnicity will be provided. This chapter critically analyses and debates contemporary issues that arise in the context of culturally sensitive midwifery care. Finally, you are asked to evaluate personal/professional practice and think about how to construct a workable philosophy of client care that will make a difference to provision and the delivery of high-class, culturally sensitive care.

The importance of the role and function of an inter-professional team approach to midwifery care and how this can create a climate of tolerance and change will be outlined. You are prompted to reflect on and critically examine the impact of power dynamics on the inter-professional team and clients.

Culture

Literature and research have consistently highlighted the extent of the motivation or lack of motivation of midwives to engage with the concept of culture and even to embrace people from the diverse cultural mix who entrust their lives to them (Rowe and Garcia 2005).

The essential nature of midwives working in a culturally sensitive manner has long gained a steady footing in midwifery circles (Bowler 1993; English National Board 2001). Midwives live and work in a complex multiracial and multicultural society, one in which she is perceived as a role model, friend, confident and advocate (Hunt 2001). It is therefore vital that she is able to think, feel and act inside and outside the societal box to enhance midwifery care to clients who are considered already to be at a disadvantage. It could be suggested that some midwives may shy away from political issues that have a direct impact on care. Two such issues are poverty and health inequalities. Thinking outside the box requires the midwife to move away from what is considered safe territory (Wickham 2007). She would need to network with agencies and personnel not normally considered part of the health care team. Agencies such as the Citizen's Advice Bureau have the resources and expertise so potentially useful to the very clients to whom this chapter intends to give a voice.

Case Notes

Amy is sixteen years old, single and has limited social support. She is at the antenatal clinic for a routine check-up at 28 weeks' gestation. Your practice mentor has asked you to do the antenatal examination. This includes questioning Amy about her wellbeing. On enquiring about her nutritional status, she tells you she is not eating regularly or sufficiently. She is worried about money and identifies this as the main reason why she is neglecting to eat adequately.

How would you go about finding a solution to this problem?

When responding, it is important that Amy is treated with respect and concern. This includes not falling into a parent–child mode of conversation (Walsh 2005). The student is in a powerful position because Amy, like most women, wants the best for her baby and is therefore receptive to advice, even when it is not given sensitively. It would be helpful to show genuine curiosity about the reasons why she felt that she could not afford nutritious food. Once you have gathered the relevant information, it is important to consult your practice mentor so that a possible solution can be found. This might be to:

- Arrange for the community or teenage pregnancy midwife to visit Amy at home. This might enable her to feel supported and the midwife to assess her social situation and needs

- Refer her to a dietician so that her nutritional needs can be determined and she can increase her motivation to meet the dietary requirements necessary to sustain a healthy pregnancy
- Provide her with information about the Citizen's Advice Bureau so that she can enquire about her eligibility for social benefits
- Think further outside the box and make an appointment to see her MP to discuss pregnancy-related issues in the context of poverty and inequalities

Having considered this scenario, the student midwife should be in a position to construct a definition of culture. This may facilitate a mindset that supports a personal and professional position where she treats her clients as individuals irrespective of their cultural or other differences.

Activity

What is your definition of culture?

There is no one definition of culture and it is important not to be constrained by any one definition; however, it is useful to have ideas around the concept of culture. This may offer the student guidelines that can enhance her understanding of the diverse needs and expectations of people who may be similar to or different from herself. It may also facilitate a mindset in which she is receptive to change in the way she perceives clients who do not apparently conform to the norms of society. These norms are not usually transparent, particularly to people who have limited language skills and also low or infrequent exposure to people and or experiences from the dominant culture.

There is no one way to construct a definition of culture (Hoffman 1990). This is because the midwife is often unconsciously aware of her thinking, feelings and actions that may be influencing her decision-making and attitude to a particular client. Burr (2001) warns against the tendency to believe that knowledge and assumptions that guide us in our dealings with other people are 'truths'. She is of the opinion that *'our current accepted ways of understanding the world, is a product not of objective observation of the world, but of the social processes and interactions in which people are constantly engaged with each other'*. This view is supported by Reynolds and Manfusa (2005), who argue that a significant number of midwives do not believe that cultural issues are relevant or significantly important. Their lack of awareness and familiarity with interacting with people from diverse cultural backgrounds militate against them gaining deeper understanding of the cultural aspects of midwifery care. They therefore suggest that midwives give greater priority to getting to know about their clients' cultural beliefs and expectations so as to meet their individual needs and preferences.

For the purpose of this chapter various definitions will be suggested to facilitate the student's autonomy in determining a personal working definition of culture. This free choice is in keeping with the philosophy that underpins the contents and tone of the text. The expectation is that midwives and student midwives will feel committed to working culturally sensitively with their clients rather than believe it is a professional obligation.

Schott and Henley (2001) express the view that culture is a set of norms, values, assumptions, perceptions (both explicit and implicit) and social conventions which enable members of a group, community or nation to function cohesively. Schott and Henley (2001) are of the opinion that *culture vitally affects every aspect of our daily life, how we live, think, behave and how we view and analyse the world*'. Burnham and Harris (1996) argue for the usefulness of understanding the difference between three interrelated concepts: race, ethnicity and culture. They define race as '*a personal biological inheritance*'. Clearly, a person's race is immediately apparent and assumptions, stereotypes and equally dangerous judgements can be readily made which are believed to be truths (Burr 2001). Culture is defined by Burnham and Harris (1996) as '*the social network within which conversations about race and ethnicity evolve*'; and ethnicity is the '*way a person thinks about the biological inheritance*'. Burnham and Harris imply that the meaning of ethnicity and culture is constantly emerging and changing. They are not static concepts but dynamic. This suggests that as the practitioner familiarises herself with the client's cultural norms and expectations she will be more willing to become transparent about prejudices, ideas and practices so that the ideas and biases may become more open and available for refreshment and reconstruction (Burnham and Harris, 1996).

Helman (2001) defines culture as a '*set of guidelines that individuals inherit as members of a particular society, and that tell them how to view the world, how to experience it emotionally and how to behave in it in relation to other people, to supernatural forces or gods and to the natural environment*'. Norms and rules are usually opaque and only come to light when they are broken. Midwives are in a privileged position in which they have the education and training to be able to be tolerant of difference in their clients' knowledge and behaviour without judging them too harshly.

There are many similarities in the authors' definitions of culture in that they have personal, familiar and societal connotations. However, Helman (2001) highlights the significance of an individual's belief system around the kind of person she is or can become, personal responsibility or even duty to transmit these beliefs across generations by the *'use of symbols, language, art and ritual'* (Helman 2001). It is apparent that the client's cultural lens through which she perceives and understands the world is extremely important to her and will be fiercely protected from threat or perceived threat by anyone, including the midwife, who may seem likely to do harm.

The morality of working in a cultural context

Hart et al. (2001) discuss the positive ways in which health professionals carry out their work. They often do this in stressful and under-resourced contexts in order to achieve health benefits to disadvantaged groups. Indeed, though they acknowledge this positive approach, they are cognisant of the fact that this is not universal. Hart et al. highlight the consistent nature of evidence of how interactions between health professionals, health care institutions and service users result in clients feeling oppressed and humiliated rather than cared for, particularly in the case of disadvantaged service users. It is important that practitioners feel good about the way they work with their clients. However, it is also necessary for midwives to be willing to reflect on and face the challenges and criticisms about any shortfall in care provision and/or delivery that negatively impact on client's who already suffer social disadvantages.

Carter (2001) asserts that by having a *'greater understanding of ourselves through developed self-awareness we are more likely to have increased self-respect, which in turn leads to a greater respect of others'*. It appears that the practitioner's sense of self, who she is, how she arrived at this awareness and the social and professional context in which she operates, provides a rich source of information that will inform her moral and ethical position.

The NMC (2004) supports an ethico-legal position of equity for all the midwife's clients/patients. It states that, *'all registered nurses, midwives and specialist community public health nurses are personally accountable for their practice and that they should in the exercise of their duty'* (NMC, 2004a):

- Respect the patient/client as an individual
- Obtain consent before you give any treatment and care
- Protect confidential information

- Co-operate with others in the team
- Maintain your professional knowledge and competence
- Be trustworthy
- Act to identify and minimise risk to patients and clients

Case Notes

Jane has arrived on the delivery suite and is in established labour. She is a single white woman with no supportive birth partner. She is extremely scared and appears not to be coping with the pain.

You have been allocated as the student midwife to care for Jane. After the initial history taking and measuring of vital signs, you inform your practice mentor of your findings and discuss the plan of care. Jane did not complete her birth plan. She has, however, stated that she does not want any male professionals involved in her care.

What are the ethical issues here?

The student midwife may be aware that she has a duty to care for Jane in as non-judgemental a way, as is appropriate. Ethically, she needs to take the time to interact with Jane and find out what her needs and expectations are. In this case there are no visible clues about how or what Jane's decision not to accept care from male health care professionals is based on. She had a usually considered British name and speaks English fluently.

An exploratory approach based on Jane's right to choose would have discovered that she is a Muslim, something that she did not disclose at her booking assessment as she felt that this information would be perceived negatively. It is also useful to be aware that Jane in the past may have experienced violence, sexual abuse or inappropriate treatment which would cause her to be distrustful of men. She was extremely afraid of being judged by health professionals and did not want to jeopardise her care and that of her baby.

In this case it would be good practice for the midwife/student midwife to keep an open mind, listen actively, be supportive and show empathy. The midwife/student midwife would also be acting as an advocate by informing the multi-professional team on a need-to-know basis and documenting Jane's wishes to ensure that quality care can be continued and a record is maintained.

In the *Code of Professional Conduct* the NMC (2004a) states that registrants must *'recognise and respect the role of patients and clients as partners in their care and the contribution they can make to it'*. It continues that the practitioner should identify the client's preferences regarding care and respect these within the limits of professional practice, existing legislation, resources and goals of the therapeutic relationship. These ethical ideals are well supported by the Equality Act 2007, which is discussed later in the chapter.

You are personally accountable for ensuring that you promote and protect the interests and dignity of patients and clients, irrespective of gender, age, race, ability, sexuality, economic status, lifestyle, culture and religion or political beliefs. In Jane's case the support of a non-judgemental, culturally sensitive midwife who could see beyond her decision not to have male health care professionals involved in her care was required. The potential for upholding difference and therefore inducing conflict would then be avoided and a more positive alliance ensured. Jane's right to 'autonomous' (NMC 2004a) decision-making in this instance would get the NMC's approval and that of the Equality Act 2007 which '*aims to ensure that people are treated fairly and equally*' and '*enjoy the privileges of fairness and respect irrespective of who or where ever they are*' (Commission for Equality and Human Rights 2006).

Similar ethical/moral positions are expressed by various authors. For example, Quinn and Harding (2001) endorse the government's view that '*NHS care has to be shaped around the convenience and concerns of patients*'. To achieve this, '*patients must have more say in their own treatment and more influence over the way the NHS works*' (DH 2000).

Clearly, the morality of midwifery care is complex. In professional practice the practitioner's ethical position can conflict with her beliefs about how she would like to conduct herself as a midwife and the image she portrays. Ethical decisions are not straightforward.

Case Notes

Chloe has stated in her birth plan that she wishes to have a natural birth. This means that she does not want technology as a means to monitor progress of the baby.

She is admitted to the antenatal ward as her blood pressure is elevated, there is protein in her urine and oedema of her face and sacral area. It is normal professional practice as part of the assessment of her care to carry out a cardiotocograph. However, Chloe has refused to give her consent to have fetal monitoring.

How would you deal with this situation?

In response to this scenario there are several approaches that could be considered. You could try to persuade Chloe to think about her options, after showing her that you are receptive and sensitive to her decision by acknowledging positively that she made this decision in the best interest of herself and her baby. However, her circumstances have changed and she and her baby are at increased risk of obstetric complications that could affect their wellbeing. Her blood pressure is elevated; there is proteinuria and non-dependent oedema. All three signs are suggestive of pre-eclampsia, an obstetric complication of pregnancy that increases the chances of a poor outcome for the client and her baby. It is important to document Chloe's wishes and concerns and refer the case to a midwife or your mentor for further action.

The ethical dilemma in this case is enormous. The right of Chloe to be autonomous and make her own decisions created tensions with the professional duty of the midwife to *act to identify and minimise risk to patients and clients'* (NMC 2004). Indeed, to exercise her accountability and responsibility the midwife must provide safe and competent care (NMC 2004a).

Midwifery practice in a culturally sensitive climate of care

Today, midwives work in a climate of change, one in which collaboration and partnerships need to be forged to ensure delivery of good standards of care. Fletcher (2001) expresses the view that the midwife should build on existing partnerships (e.g. with obstetricians, paediatricians) and develop new ones (e.g. with the private and voluntary sectors) that will enable them to respond positively to the challenges of 'the new NHS'. One of the biggest challenges for the midwife of the twenty-first century is her ability to understand and act on the diverse needs and expectations of a multicultural clientele. Helman (2001) observes that the tendency to generalise is ever-present. For example, blanket policies and procedures are put in place to meet the needs of clients of all cultures irrespective of the relevance to them as individuals. Breastfeeding policies, for example, sometimes create immense stress and unhappiness for many clients and their families, who are expected to accept rules and customs that are alien to them.

The potential for conflict is ever-present, one of the reasons being that people, including health care professionals, make assumptions that they believe to be truth. Helman (2001) asserts that one should differentiate between *'the rules of a culture, which govern how one should think and behave, and how people actually behave in real life'*. This guideline is worthy of note in particular because generalisations can be dangerous, for they often lead to stereotypes and then to cultural misunderstandings, prejudices and discrimination (Helman 2001). The midwife's professional practice must therefore be grounded in best available evidence and guided by her employer's policies and procedures.

Activity

Find and read the equal opportunities policy associated with your current placement. This should be available in whichever setting or context you work. It might be useful to organise a study group and share the content and your ideas.

Following this invite your mentor(s) to a discussion group and reflect on what is required from you by your employer.

What are the possible implications for your developing midwifery practice?

Some of the following may emerge:

- The employer's expectations of the practitioner's interactions with clients
- The legal framework that governs the practice of midwives in the context of equal opportunities, fairness and justice
- The sanctions that are in place to monitor, control and discipline practitioners who do not achieve the legal and or professional standard
- Your and others' theoretical and personal codes of ethics for delivery of client care

The values you hold personally and professionally will influence you when you treat clients, irrespective of the culture. Fry (2002) is of the opinion that '*a value is a worthwhile standard or quality of a person or social group*'. She reminds practitioners that '*cultural values are the accepted and dominant standards of a particular cultural group*'. Indeed, these values function in conjunction with belief systems and serve to give '*meaning and worth to the existence and experiences of the group*'. The midwife in daily practice needs to be cognisant that '*every culture has values and beliefs about health and illness and about what is morally acceptable behaviour in the provision of health promoting care to people*' (Fry 2002). The British, for example, '*place a high premium on the sovereignty of the individual and the rights of the individual to make choices about their lives*' (Fry 2002). Others, for example, Greeks, Italians and many groups found in South Asia, place a high value on the family, collective and communal decision-making and the '*overriding obligation of individual family members to place the interest of their family above their own*'.

Clearly, these descriptions of some cultural ways of being are not absolute. There are bound to be subcultures within these that may not necessarily comply with the majority of their cultural group. This highlights the need for clarity by the midwife in her dealings with cultural group members. It is important for her to be aware that sameness is not synonymous with those who appear to be from the same or similar cultural groups. Racial (and indeed cultural) stereotyping in midwifery has been shown to influence care of Asian women, for example, negatively (Kirkham et al. 2002; Rowe and Garcia 2005). Informed choice and decision-making by clients can be influenced significantly by the predisposition to place clients in the straitjacket of stereotyping.

The Confidential Enquiry into Maternal and Child Health (Royal College of Gynaecology 2004), *Why Mothers Die*, in providing its findings and recommendations for midwifery practice, highlights the following risk factors for maternal deaths:

- Social disadvantage
- Poor communities
- Minority ethnic groups
- Late booking and poor attendance
- Domestic violence

All these are of key relevance to the culturally diverse groups that midwives interact with on a daily basis. This heightened awareness, with compounding evidence to support it, has the potential to persuade midwives to take the lead in pushing for change. This is necessary to improve the lives of their clients by facilitating acceptance rather than exclusion.

Skinner (2001) warns of the difficulties that midwives face if they are unable to cultivate a culture of change. The significant factors according to Skinner (2001) are empowerment, autonomy and increasing confidence that the care they give their clients is relevant to their needs and preferences. The issue of self-belief needs to be added. Midwives are the lead professionals in over 70 per cent of maternity cases, and the challenge of change is believed to be an exciting venture by some (Skinner 2001). The opposing view is that traditional beliefs and attitudes to care inevitably will be affected and lead to dissonance and possibly fear. However, midwives need to be prepared to lead the campaign for change in the best interest of their disadvantaged clients.

Royal College of Gynaecology (2004) emphasises the important role of midwives in ensuring that local maternity services reach and maintain contact with all pregnant women. This, it suggests, could be achieved through various basic yet essential processes – for example, advocating for professional interpreters for women who do not speak English and the *'strengthening or development of a robust and effective communication system'* (Royal College of Gynaecology 2004). The important value of the mechanism of statutory midwifery supervision (Royal College of Gynaecology 2004) in providing impetus for change in the form of the midwife developing and utilising skills of advocacy, anti-discriminatory and anti-oppressive practices is relevant to midwifery care in the twenty-first century and beyond. Midwifery practice must embrace the high principles and values that put clients at the centre of all that is done by the midwife. As Royal College of Gynaecology (2004) points out, the midwife carries out her work in the context of deprivation, poverty and with women having difficulty accessing services. At the same time, *'the midwife may often be the only professional who is able to build an element of trust with the woman'* (Royal College of Gynaecology 2004). How the midwife organises and delivers her practice will influence the quality of the maternity experience that the client receives as well as the midwife's satisfaction in her work. The midwife must be aware that *'where the services are not meeting the medical or cultural needs of women, midwives act as advocates to ensure that appropriate services are delivered, interpreting services are available and cross-organisational communication are of the highest standard'* (Royal College of Gynaecology 2004). That is the stuff that midwifery practice should be made of and maybe the power dynamics will change to one of equity rather than midwife domination as appears presently to be the case.

The power dynamics of midwifery practice

The *Code of Professional Conduct* expects registered practitioners, including the midwife, to *'recognise and respect the role of patients and clients as partners in their care and the contribution they can make to it'* (NMC 2004a). Indeed, the practitioner is accountable for ensuring that she *'promotes and protects the interests and dignity of patients and clients, irrespective of gender, age, race, ability, sexuality, economic status, lifestyle, culture and religion or political beliefs'*. Thus the midwife is accountable to her clients to ensure that they receive as good a quality of care, however they define it, as anyone from the dominant culture. Kitzinger (2000) asserts that *'birth is women's business, takes place in women's space and is choreographed by women'*. Though Kitzinger (2000) made her comments in the birth context, they are also relevant to any situation in which midwives interact with their clients.

Burr (2001) believes that power can be thought of as the *'extent of a person's access to sort-after resources, such as money, leisure time, rewarding jobs and the extent to which they have the capacity to have some effect on their world'*. The ability to influence your environment can only become a reality through empowerment brought about as a result of being treated equally. The White Paper *Fairness for All* (DH 2004) states that *'unjust treatment can make a person feel isolated, scared and misunderstood'*. This is a situation that midwives can through pro-activity and insightfulness prevent.

Midwives possess resources (knowledge and skills) that put them in a powerful position. Clients want and need these resources, particularly those who are disadvantaged because of cultural differences. They are positioned within the minority groups rather than the dominant cultural groups, which means that they constantly jostle for scarce resources, both human and material. Midwives should not be complacent but humble and appreciative of their powerful position. They can use it to influence policy and change and to empower rather than exclude clients who already suffer the effects of substandard care (Royal College of Gynaecology 2004). Burr (2001) supports the notion that knowledge increases a person's power. She reiterates Foucault's (1976) idea that *'knowledge is power over others, the power to define others'*.

To change the dynamics of unequal power between the midwife and her culturally disadvantaged clients, midwives need to be committed to instigating and delivering care that is anti-discriminatory and anti-oppressive, to meet the individual needs of clients and their families and to comply with the legal requirements. *'Individuals have no control over the cultural background in which they are born'* (Millen, 2002). The midwife, though, can voluntarily sanction her behaviour by showing sensitivity and respect. Thompson (2002) asserts that professionals should *'value diversity'* and that *'developing anti-discriminatory practice is an essential part of good practice'*. However, he acknowledges that issues to do with this aspect of care are a 'minefield of difficulties at both a theoretical and practical level' (Thompson 2002).

Giving and receiving information is time-consuming. In the current climate where clients and midwives alike perceive her as extremely busy, the midwife needs always to be aware that the power of communicating at all levels and contexts is essential to her very survival.

Activity

The student midwife may find the following cultural awareness quiz useful and interesting. It will enable her to develop curiosity about her clients. Interest in clients (Henderson 2005) enhances familiarity and this in turn breaks down cultural barriers (Reynolds and Manfusa 2005).

Cultural awareness quiz

Please complete the quiz. It can be completed individually or as a group. It might be useful to arrange a study room at your university's Learning and Resources Centre or invite your mentor(s) on your practice site to complete the quiz with you.

The answers to the quiz can be found at the back of the book.

Cultural Awareness Quiz
Questions

1. When is Ramadan and what must Muslims <u>not</u> do during this period?
2. Why do Spanish people have two surnames?
3. Why does the Christian festival of Easter move dates each year?
4. What group is defined by the 5 Ks and what are they?
5. What is Halal meat?
6. What is the origin of Halloween?
7. What religion is practised by most Indians?
8. What religion is practised by most Pakistanis?
9. What is the official language of India?
10. What are the main religions of Afro-Caribbeans?
11. What is the official language of Pakistan?
12. From which West Indian island do most Afro-Caribbean people in the UK come?
13. Who is/was St Christopher?
14. What is a Bar Mitzvah?
15. What is Rastafarianism?
16. What information about Rastafarianism would enhance medical and midwifery care?
17. How many times each day do Muslims have to pray and what do they have to do beforehand?
18. What is Nirvana?
19. Where do most Buddhist international students come from?
20. What food is acceptable to most religions?
21. What is the ethnic origin of a person with a white British father and a black Trinidadian mother?

The activity in itself is useful. However, it is the focusing on individual difference, familiarity around cultural groups and the willingness to orient to the needs and expectations of these client groups that will put the student midwife in good stead. Axten (2003) is of the opinion that *'feeling secure means being in control and that placing ourselves in positions where we can control others increases our sense of security'*. Midwives need to disown any false sense of security and instead embrace the challenge of really getting to know and understand the diverse client groups that entrust their care to them. Indeed, facing cultural issues provides her with the opportunity to reduce the 'widening gap' that exists between the dominant and minority cultures (DH 2005). This is indeed a position of humility and privilege.

Conclusion

Royal College of Gynaecology (2004) notes that the '*midwife may often be the only professional who is able to build an element of trust with the woman*'. This puts her in a privileged and powerful position.

Midwives have an opportunity to make a difference to the lives of clients who may already experience disadvantage from all quarters. It is consistently stated and noted that '*midwives are perfectly placed as advocates for the safe delivery of maternity care*' (Royal College of Gynaecology 2004). The challenge is and always will be: are midwives prepared to stand up and be counted to ensure that her clients are central to her work?

There are professional directives and guidance, for example the *Midwives Rules and Standards* (2004c), *Code of Professional Conduct* (2004a) and, most recently, the Equality Act 2006. This Act provides for the establishment of the Commission for Equality and Human Rights (CEHR). This new framework is a part of the government's wider programme of reform to challenge discrimination and inequality and to promote equality and diversity. The CEHR must also take on responsibility for the promotion of human rights. Midwives essentially must keep themselves up to date with these changes in order to work in a culturally intelligent and sensitive manner. This should enable them to truly advocate for and empower their clients.

References

Axten, S. (2003) Power: how it is used and sometimes abused. *British Medical Journal* 11(11): 681–4.

Bowler, I. (1993) They're not the same as us: midwives' stereotypes of South Asian descent maternity patients. *Sociology, Health and Illness* 15(2): 157–78.

Burnham, J. and Harris, Q. (1996) Emerging ethnicity: a tale of three cultures. In K. Dwivedi and V. Varma (eds), *Meeting the Needs of Ethnic Minority Children: A Handbook for Professionals*. London: Jessica Kingsley.

Burr, V. (2001) *An Introduction to Social Constructionism*. London: Routledge.

Carter, D. (2001) Developing self-awareness. *Midwives in Action* 1(2): 10–18.

Commission for Equality and Human Rights (2006) *Fairness for All: A New Commission for Equality and Human Rights*. London: CEHR.

Department of Health (2000) *The NHS Plan: A Plan for Investment, a Plan for Reform*. London: DH.

Department of Health (2004) *Fairness for All: A New Commission for Equality and Human Rights*. London: DH.

Department of Health (2005) *Tackling Health Inequalities: Status Report on the Programme for Action*. London: DH.

English National Board (2001) *Midwives in Action*. London: ENB.

Fletcher, S. (2001) Partnership working. *Midwives in Action* 2(3): 28–33.

Foucault, M. (1976) *The Will to Knowledge*. Paris: Gallimard.

Fry, F. T. (2002) *Ethics in Nursing Practice: A Guide to Ethical Decision-Making*, 2nd edition. London: Blackwell.

Hart, A., Lockley, R., Henwood, F. et al. (2001) *Researching Professional Education, Addressing Inequalities in Health: New Directions in Midwifery Education and Price*. London: NMC.

Helman, C. (2001) *Culture, Health and Illness*, 4th edition. London: Arnold.

Henderson, C. (2005) Midwives can help reduce inequalities. *British Journal of Midwifery* 11(11): 681–4.

Hoffman, L. (1990) Constructing realities: an art of lens. *Family Processes* 29(1): 1–12.

Hunt, S. (2001) Tackling disadvantage in maternity care. *Midwives in Action: A Resource*. London: NMC.

Kirkham, M., Stapleton, H., Curtis, P. and Thomas, G. (2002) Stereotyping as a professional defence mechanism. *British Journal of Midwifery* 10(9): 549–52.

Kitzinger, S. (2000) Some cultural perspectives of birth. *British Journal of Midwifery* 8(12): 746–50.

Millen, R. (2002) *Anti-Discriminatory Practice: A Guide for Workers in Child Care and Education*, 2nd edition. London: Continuum.

Nursing and Midwifery Council (2004a) *Code of Professional Conduct*. London: NMC.

Nursing and Midwifery Council (2004b) *Guidelines for Records and Record-keeping*. London: NMC.

Nursing and Midwifery Council (2004c) *Midwives Rules and Standards*. London: NMC.

Quinn, P. and Harding, C. (2001) Involving clients and responding to women's needs. *Midwives in Action: A Resource*: 2(4): 34–48.

Reynolds, F. and Manfusa, S. (2005) Views on cultural barriers to caring for South Asian women. *British Journal of Midwifery* 13(4): 236–42.

Rowe, R. and Garcia, J. (2005) Ethnic minorities' access to antenatal screening. *British Journal of Midwifery* 13(2): 101–4.

Royal College of Gynaecology (2004) *Confidential Enquiry into Maternal and Child Health: Why Mothers Die*. London: RCOG.

Schott, J. and Henley, A. (2001) *Culture, Religion and Childbearing in a Multi-racial Society*. Oxford: Butterworth-Heinemann.

Skinner, G. (2001) Developing the culture. *Midwives in Action: A Resource*: 41–8.

Thompson, N. (2002) *People Skills*, 2nd edition. Basingstoke: Palgrave Macmillan.

Thompson, N. (2003) *Communication and Language: A Handbook of Theory and Practice*. Basingstoke: Palgrave Macmillan.

Walsh, D. (2005) Professional power and maternity care: The many faces of paternalism. *British Journal of Midwifery* 13(11): 708.

Wickham, S. (2007) A decade of polarity. *The Practicing Midwife* 10(3): 44–5.

Legislation and the Midwife

Cathy Hamilton and Lisa Nash

Introduction

This chapter considers the practice of midwifery within a contemporary legal framework. The importance of the midwife understanding key legal terms and ethical principles in order to carry out her practice within the law is highlighted. It is beyond the scope of this chapter to discuss in depth all aspects of legislation in relation to midwifery, and the reader is referred to other key texts to obtain the relevant detail. However, information relating to legislation of particular relevance to midwifery is included, such as referral to current health and social care legislation.

What is the law?

Law can be defined as a rule of conduct or procedure established by custom, agreement or authority. It is the mechanism by which society regulates the order and control of people who live in it. The legal system itself is enforced by a political body (Jones and Jenkins 2004). The law produces rules by which all members of society are expected to abide. There are rules to deal with conflict, punish unacceptable behaviour and protect society's members from harm (Jones and Jenkins 2004). If someone is accused of 'breaking the law', the accuser should be able to cite the source of the law to which reference is being made (Dimond 2006). If the statement is accurate, then the appropriate Act of Parliament or a previous decided case can be cited. Without the law, there would be anarchy, fear and confusion (Jones and Jenkins 2004).

They law is classified as criminal or civil. A criminal offence is said to have been committed when the accused takes part in a forbidden activity. As a result he or she will face criminal proceedings in a court of law (Dimond 2004). In this case, the prosecution must prove 'beyond reasonable doubt' the guilt of the accused. In the Crown Court if the accused pleads 'not guilty', the case is put before a jury of twelve randomly selected members of the public, who will determine among themselves the defendant's guilt or innocence.

Civil law relates to the rights of private citizens or institutions. Civil proceedings take place between individuals with a view to obtaining compensation or a remedy, such as an injunction preventing contact between two individuals (Dimond 2004). The standard of proof in civil courts is based on the 'balance of probabilities'. This means that it must be demonstrated that it is 'more probable than not' that the accused is guilty of misconduct.

There are three main sources of English law: statutory law, common law and European law.

Statutory law

A statute is a formal written rule of a country or state. Statutes are Acts of Parliament and as such are the most important source of law. An Act creates a new law or changes an existing one. An Act is a Bill approved by both the House of Commons and the House of Lords and formally approved by the reigning monarch (given royal assent). Once implemented, an Act becomes law and applies to the whole of the United Kingdom (UK) or to specifically defined countries within the UK. In contrast to an Act, a Bill is a proposal to produce a new law or amend an existing one that is presented for debate before Parliament.

In order to be passed, an Act of Parliament needs to proceed through a number of stages for consideration and debate. When the government is considering introducing new legislation it has various ways to proceed. It can bring the issue straight to Parliament or it can consult the public first. A Green Paper is a government consultative document, which is circulated in order to obtain the views of the general public, civil servants and ministers – in fact, any interested parties who may add to the debate. Following this, a White Paper is issued, which sets out in everyday language the government's intentions in relation to implementation of the proposed law.

Examples of Green and White Papers relevant to midwives are *Our Healthier Nation* (DH 1998), a Green Paper which formed a background to the White Paper *Saving Lives: Our Healthier Nation* (DH 1999), which was presented to Parliament the following year.

Activity

Visit the Department of Health website (www.dh.gov.uk) to access these Green and White Papers. Search the website to see what other consultations of relevance to midwifery are currently being undertaken. Consider contributing to these.

Statutory Instruments (SIs) are a form of legislation which allows the provisions of an Act of Parliament to be brought into force or altered without Parliament having to pass a new Act. They are also known as secondary, delegated or subordinate legislation (House of Commons 2007).

An example of how this system works is the Nursing and Midwifery Order 2001 (SI 2002 No. 253). In 2002 the Nursing and Midwifery Council (NMC) replaced the United Kingdom Central Council for Nursing, Midwifery and Health Visiting (UKCC) following this Order. The SI is complicated but comes from section 60 of the Health Act 1999, which allows secondary legislation to amend primary legislation in the regulation of health care professions. The Order repealed the Nurses, Midwives and Health Visitors Act 1997 and placed all the relevant regulations in the Order. The NMC was then enabled to produce a new *Code of Professional Conduct* (NMC 2002) (Jones and Jenkins 2004).

Secondary legislation has the same legal power as primary legislation provided the content remains within the authority of the original Act (Jones and Jenkins 2004).

Common law or case law

This type of law is determined by the decisions of judges in relation to particular cases. The decisions of the courts create precedents which can not be overridden by a court lower down in the hierarchy. For example, a judge in a County Court may not go against a decision made in a similar case in a High Court; the Court of Appeal may not go against decisions made in the House of Lords. However, a judge may decide that the case being heard is different from

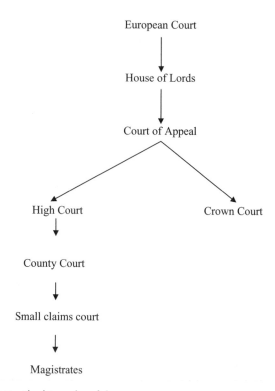

Figure 13.1 The hierarchy of the court system

previous ones which allows the judge to reach a different decision as long as the different feature is clearly highlighted in the judge's summing up. See Figure 13.1 for an overview of the hierarchy of the court system.

Decisions are recorded in All England Law Reports (All ER) or Weekly Law Reports (WLR) so that everyone associated with the law can have easy access to them.

An example of a case which has great relevance in health care is *Bolam v Friern Hospital Management* [1957] 1 WLR 582. The reference lets you know that it was reported in 1957 in the first volume of Weekly Law Reports on page 582. This case is also reported in All England Law Reports as *Bolam v Friern Hospital Management* [1957] 2 All ER 118.

This case concerned a man who had been given electroconvulsive therapy without a muscle relaxant or anaesthetic and suffered a fractured jaw as a result. He claimed that his doctor had been negligent in his care. However, the judge, Mr Justice McNair, ruled that a doctor is not guilty of negligence if a responsible body of medical opinion considers that he has acted properly even if not all members of the medical profession share this view. This landmark case put peer judgement at the centre of assessing clinical care and led to the instigation of the so-called Bolam test.

European law

Since Britain joined the European Community (EC) in 1973 and following the signing of the Maastricht Treaty in 1992, which led to the formation of the European Union (EU), it is obliged as a member state to ensure that EU directives and regulations are enforced in the UK. All UK law must also fit within the framework of EU legislation and appeals can be made to the European Court of Justice.

A regulation is binding on all member states from the time it is developed without the need for the states to pass any enabling laws. A directive, however, is binding only in terms of the outcomes which must be achieved and not how they are brought about. In these cases the member states themselves may decide what laws are required in order to fulfil the directive.

An example of a directive relevant to midwifery is the inclusion in the *Midwives Rules and Standards* of the Midwives Directive 80/155/EEC, indicating the minimum activities that midwives should undertake. The *Midwives Rules and Standards* (NMC 2004b) also indicate that this directive must be met in educational programmes leading to registration as a midwife.

The law and the issue of consent

Consent is defined as a client's agreement for a health care professional to provide care. Consent may be given verbally, non-verbally (such as a woman holding out her arm to have blood taken) or in writing (DH 2001).

The NMC's (2004) *Code of Professional Conduct* clearly states the health care professionals' responsibilities in relation to obtaining consent before any treatment or intervention is undertaken. This is a general legal and ethical principle and reflects the fundamental right of all individuals to decide for themselves what is to happen to their bodies (DH 2001).

All adults are presumed to have the mental capacity to give consent or refuse treatment unless they are unable to take in information about the treatment, are unable to understand the information given and are unable to consider the information given as part of the decision-making process (NMC 2006). Issues relating to minors are discussed later in this chapter.

There are two areas of the law relating to consent:

1. The actual giving of consent by the client
2. The duty of the midwife to give appropriate information before the client gives consent

If consent is not given but treatment is undertaken, the client may have grounds to sue the practitioner for trespass to the person. An assault is when a person perceives that there is a threat that she may be touched without her consent. On the other hand, if she is actually touched without giving consent, this is battery. Threatening verbal behaviour, for example, without any physical contact is assault, while a vaginal examination undertaken without a woman's consent is battery (Dimond 2004).

The person who has suffered the trespass can sue for compensation in the civil courts. In these cases the individual does not have to prove that harm has occurred as a result of the interaction, just that touching occurred without her consent. However, it is worth remembering that the touching behaviour must refer to care or treatment being undertaken by the practitioner. An arm around the shoulder of a distressed person would not count as trespass to the person in these cases.

A health care professional also has a duty to give the client all information relating to the treatment, including risks, benefits and alternative treatments. If this is not undertaken, then a woman could sue if she suffers harm as a result of accepting a treatment but then claims that the health care professional did not alert her to the possibility that harm could occur. A charge of negligence could then be brought against the health care professional.

Consent is valid only if it is given voluntarily by an individual who is fully informed and has the mental capacity to consent to the treatment or care (DH 2001). A midwife attempting to gain consent from a woman for any particular procedure should consider whether the woman has the capacity to give consent, whether she has been given enough information, with time to consider her options and discuss them with a health care professional. It is suggested that 'seeking consent' should be considered as a joint decision-making process between the client and the health care professional (DH 2001). Once consent has been given, the midwife should consider whether consent was given voluntarily or whether the woman was under pressure from her partner, family or others to make a particular decision (Jones and Jenkins 2004).

Usually the health care professional who is proposing to undertake the procedure will obtain consent (NMC 2004). However, in certain circumstances this may be delegated to another health care professional who has been appropriately trained for that specific area of practice (NMC 2004a). The midwife, according to the NMC (2006), has three main professional responsibilities with regard to obtaining consent:

1. Always act in the best interests of the client
2. Ensure that the process of establishing consent is rigorous and transparent
3. Documentation is accurate and clearly records all discussions and decisions relating to obtaining consent

There is further guidance concerning consent issued by the Department of Health, which includes twelve key points for health care professionals to consider in relation to this issue (DH 2001).

Activity

Access the DH website for further guidance about the complex issues relating to consent: www.dh.gov.uk

Emergency situations

Case Notes

A woman, who has given birth at home unaided and unattended arrives at the maternity unit in a paramedic ambulance in a state of severe collapse. She is bleeding very heavily from her vagina and it would appear that she is suffering from a massive primary postpartum haemorrhage. No medical notes are available and she is unaccompanied. She is unconscious on arrival. She has lost approximately 1 litre of blood and it is clear that she will need a blood transfusion and possibly an operation to save her life.

An adult who is unable to give consent because she is unconscious may receive whatever treatment is required in order to save her life, provided it is in the best interests of the client (NMC 2006). In such cases the health care professionals would not be committing a trespass to the person (Dimond 2004). Exceptions are when the client has already issued an advanced direction (often referred to as a living will) indicating that any further treatment is refused (NMC 2006). Another exception would be if a woman had made a decision while she was still mentally competent and alert. A Jehovah's Witness, for example, may refuse a blood transfusion or the use of any blood products and it would be unlawful for midwives or doctors to administer these even if she loses consciousness and her condition becomes critical.

It is not possible for anyone to give consent for treatment for another adult. In this case the practice of midwives asking a partner or other next of kin for consent is unlawful (Jones and Jenkins 2004).

The rights of the fetus?

Case Notes

Gina is 38 weeks' pregnant and expecting her first baby. She has high blood pressure and has been diagnosed as suffering from pre-eclampsia. The doctor advises urgent admission to hospital with a view to inducing her labour. The concern is that as her condition worsens, her life and the life of her baby will be at risk. Gina fully understands all the risks involved and after careful consideration decides that she does not want to be induced. She would prefer to wait for labour and delivery to occur naturally.

Despite the fact that the law states that a mentally competent person has the absolute right to consent to or refuse medical treatment for any reason (or even no reason at all) it is suggested that in the past this has not been fully understood by health care professionals in relation to maternity care. There seems to have been an assumption that pregnant women are obliged to give consent to various procedures and interventions for the sake of her unborn baby (Jones and Jenkins 2004).

A case illustrating this is *Re F (in utero)* [1988]. A woman with a history of drug abuse and mental illness went missing late in her pregnancy. The local authority was concerned for the welfare of the unborn baby and sought to make the fetus a ward of court, which would mean that the woman would be found, housed and required to attend for hospital appointments.

The judges in this case, although sympathetic to the concerns of the local authority, rejected the application. They stated that the fetus had no legal rights and that a court order of this kind would override the rights of the woman.

Another controversial case, *St George's Health Care Trust v S* [1998], highlights similar issues. In this instance, a woman refusing a caesarean section was detained under section 2 of the Mental Health Act 1983 and a caesarean section was carried out without her consent. The woman later sought a judicial review of her case and the Court of Appeal ruled that she had been unlawfully detained under the Mental Health Act. Although her thinking processes were unusual and contrary to the views of most other people, she was not suffering from a mental disorder which warranted her detention in hospital. Furthermore, a woman detained under the Act for mental disorder could not be forced into a procedure (in this case, a caesarean section) unconnected with her mental condition. S was not held to be mentally incompetent and so the compulsory caesarean section was a trespass to her person.

The cases above illustrate the position of the law in relation to the fetus: the fetus as an unborn child is not a separate person from its mother. The need of the fetus for medical assistance to save its life does not override the rights of the mother.

Consent of minors

Case Notes

Renuka, a community midwife, visits a young mother at her home. Katrina is 14 years old and has a seven-day-old baby. Renuka wants to undertake the Guthrie test on the baby but Katrina is on her own as her parents are out.

Can Katrina give consent for Renuka to undertake the Guthrie test on her baby?

In England, Wales and Northern Ireland adulthood is deemed to start from 18 years of age (in Scotland this legal capacity is reached at 16 years of age). However, young people between 16 and 18 years have been given the absolute right to consent to or refuse treatment in relation to diagnostic investigations, care and treatment in the same way as a competent adult (Family Law Reform Act 1969). This does not apply to certain areas though, such as the donation of blood or organs which are not being used in the treatment of the young person him/herself. Parents or those with parental responsibility may override the refusal of a young person up to the age of 18 years.

Until 1986, consent by parents or those with parental responsibility was always needed for children and young people under 16 years. Following the court ruling in the case of *Gillick v West Norfolk and Wisbech Area Health Authority* [1986] the law was changed. Victoria Gillick was concerned that the government was going to allow doctors to give family planning advice and treatment to girls under 16 years without parental consent if it was considered to be in the best interest of the girl. Mrs Gillick claimed that to do so was unlawful. The House of Lords eventually ruled that it was lawful in those cases where the girl possessed sufficient understanding and intelligence to understand fully the proposed treatment. This level of understanding was termed Gillick competence, but is now more likely to be referred to as following the Fraser Guidelines. The principles apply to all areas of health care, not only contraceptive advice, and were incorporated into the Children Act 1989.

The test for Gillick competence involves the health care professional considering three key questions:

1. Does the client understand the situation she is in?
2. Have the options available to her been explained and does she understand them?
3. Does she understand the possible consequences of these options?

Although midwives' clients will have reached physical maturity, there is a great deal of variation between the emotional and mental maturity of young people aged 12–16. A 13-year-old may pass the test while a 15-year-old may not. In either case, it is just as lawful to act on the wishes of the 13-year-old as it is to seek parental consent for the 15-year-old (Jones and Jenkins 2004). Accurate record keeping (NMC 2005) is extremely important in these cases, so that the midwife can clearly demonstrate that the young person has passed the test and that all aspects of care have been discussed. The competence principle described here also applies to decisions which a young mother may need to make regarding treatment for her baby.

Parental consent for babies

There may be times when the parents will not give consent for their baby to undergo a medical procedure which doctors believe is essential to the wellbeing of the child. In these cases, health care practitioners may need to apply for a judicial ruling in the best interests of the baby (Jones and Jenkins 2004). This scenario is illustrated in the practice dilemma described below.

Case Notes

Sextuplets were born to a Canadian couple who were Jehovah's Witnesses. The six babies were born nearly three months prematurely. Two died within a week and the doctors told the parents that the remaining four babies needed urgent blood transfusions if they were to stand any chance of survival. The parents refused to give their consent as their religion strictly forbids the use of blood products. The hospital in Vancouver applied to the British Columbia government to take the surviving babies into protective custody so that the transfusions could be given. The authorities complied and the babies were transferred to the care of the state. Two of the babies received blood transfusions. The parents were devastated and accused the doctors of violating their children (Philp 2007).

Legislation used by the midwife

There are many Acts which are used by the midwife in everyday practice, which this chapter will now consider. It will address the following:

- The Human Rights Act 1998
- Equal Opportunities legislation (e.g. Sex Discrimination Act 1975)
- Access to Patient Records (Data Protection Act 1998, Access to Health Records Act 1990)
- Abortion Act 1967
- Registration of births and stillbirths
- Human Fertilisation and Embryology Acts 1990, 1991, 1992
- Criminal law and attendances at birth (Nurses, Midwives and Health Visitors Act 1997)
- Children Act 1989
- Congenital Disabilities (Civil Liability) Act 1976

The Human Rights Act 1998

Under the Human Rights Act, the following articles are pertinent in midwifery:

- Article 2: the right to life
- Article 3: the right not to be tortured or subjected to inhumane or degrading treatment or punishment
- Article 5: the right to liberty and security

- Article 6: the right to a fair trial
- Article 8: the right to respect privacy and family life

There is some debate surrounding prisoners being handcuffed to a bed whilst giving birth in relation to Article 3: being subjected to inhumane or degrading treatment. There was also some initial anxiety surrounding Article 8: the right to respect privacy and family life. The concern was that there would be a conflict with the protection of children. However the intervention of a public authority to protect the child does not contravene that right.

Equal opportunities legislation

For the purposes of midwifery the equal opportunities legislation (European Communities Act 1972; Sex Discrimination Act 1975; Employment Rights Act 1996; Employment Act 2002) gives the pregnant woman certain rights which protect her against discrimination. It is against the law for employers to treat pregnant women unfairly, dismiss them or select them for redundancy for any reason connected with pregnancy, childbirth or maternity leave. A pregnant woman:

- Does not have to tell a potential employer if she is pregnant when going for an interview
- Does not have to tell her employer that she is pregnant until the 15th week before her baby is due
- Is entitled to take time off for antenatal appointments and other appointments without loss of pay

In addition, if a pregnant woman is:

- Made redundant whilst on maternity leave her employer must offer her any suitable alternative that is available. If there is none, they must give the woman notice and redundancy pay
- Dismissed when she tells her employer of her pregnancy she has three months to go to an employment tribunal

The pregnant woman must inform her employer that she is pregnant in writing. Regarding returning to work:

- She should give her employer 28 days' notice before returning to work
- Her employer can write from 15 weeks into the woman's maternity leave asking if she is coming back to work and her expected date of return. A reply must be given within 21 days, although the date of return can be changed

Access to patient records

Patients have a right to access health information about themselves (DH 2004) as governed by the Data Protection Act 1998. The data controller (e.g. a GP).is responsible for giving the patient access to their records

The following principles apply:

- A request has to be made in writing
- The access request should be verified
- Ensure that enough data are present to check the identification matches with the record
- If a previous request has been made, a second request can be refused unless a significant change has occurred in the condition of the patient
- A patient can be charged to gain access to their records
- The request must be logged appropriately
- The health professional responsible for the clinical care must be consulted

There are two reasons why the information does not have to be disclosed:

1. Where the information could cause significant harm to the mental or physical well-being of the patient or another party
2. Where the information has been disclosed by a third party who does not give consent for the information to be made available

Abortion Act 1967

This Act requires two medical practitioners to agree to a termination of pregnancy, the following stipulations apply with regards to the procedure:

- The pregnancy is less than 24 weeks' gestation, and that to continue it would involve a greater risk than a termination to the woman's physical or mental health, or that of her existing children; or

- The termination is necessary to stop permanent damage to the physical or mental health of the woman; or
- If the pregnancy were continued it would involve a greater risk to the life of the pregnant woman than if it were terminated; or
- If the child were born there would be a substantial risk of it being seriously handicapped, mentally or physically

However, in an emergency situation the necessity to have the agreement of two medical practitioners can be waived, provided that the medical practitioner holds the opinion that a termination is immediately necessary to save the life of the pregnant woman or prevent her from being permanently mentally or physically injured.

Registration of births and stillbirths

By law every birth is required to be registered (Births and Deaths Registration Act 1953). This is applies to births and stillbirths taking place after 24 weeks' gestation (as amended by the Stillbirth Definition Act, 1992). Where the neonate is born alive (whatever the gestation) and then dies the birth and death must both be registered. Where a miscarriage occurs before 24 weeks' gestation there is no requirement to register it. However, the wishes of the parents must be taken into consideration along with public decency when disposing of the body.

Activity

Find out if there is a stillbirth folder available on the unit where you work. Familiarise yourself with the associated paperwork.

Human Fertilisation and Embryology Acts 1990, 1991 and 1992

Following the 1990 Act, the Human Fertilisation and Embryology Authority (HFEA) was set up to issue licences, oversee the clinics and monitor them. The 1991 Act influenced the Abortion Act, changing the gestation for a legally induced abortion to the end of the 24th week. The law allows for a selected reduction of fetuses if one or more of the fetuses is seriously abnormal or if to continue with that number of fetuses would cause the woman ill health or threaten her life. The 1990 and 1992 Acts influence where fertility treatment can take place.

Criminal law and attendances at birth

Under the Nurses, Midwives and Health Visitor Act 1997, section 16 it is a criminal offence for someone other than a midwife or registered medical practitioner (or their students) to attend a woman in childbirth. The exception to this is in an emergency. This legislation is reiterated in the Nursing and Midwifery Order 2001, Article 45. People have been prosecuted for breaching this order. If a midwife struggles with an aggressive partner, she should call the police to provide assistance in dealing with the matter.

Children Act 1989

The midwife must be familiar with child protection, taking immediate action to inform the appropriate person if they suspect that a child or minor in the care of one of their clients is being physically, emotionally or sexually abused. The nature of child protection dictates that different professionals will be working in these instances so good relations need to be fostered. It is imperative that the midwife has contact details of local agencies. Inter-agency communication is of the utmost importance. In the case of Victoria Climbié (Laming 2003) inter-agency working broke down. Victoria had come into contact with various aspects of health care provision and other professionals but no one had taken the lead to deal with the problems that subsequently led to her death. In cases of child protection it is everybody's responsibility and where there is any doubt about whether neglect or abuse is taking place health care professionals must not assume that another professional has raised any concerns. We must remember that the main priority is the safety of the child. (See Chapter 14 for more information on inter-professional working.)

Many health care professionals worry about the consequences if they suspect that a case of child abuse or neglect is taking place but their concerns are unfounded. In cases such as these the name of the professional who raised the concerns will not be divulged.

The underlying principles of the Children Act 1989 are as follows:

- The welfare of the child is the main consideration in court proceedings
- Children should be brought up by and cared for in their own families wherever possible

- Courts should make an order only where it is better than making no order at all and should ensure that any delay is avoided
- Children should be kept informed of the proceedings and should be involved with the decision-making processes about their future
- When the children no longer live with their parents the parents continue to have parental responsibility. They should therefore be included in the decision-making process in relation to their children's future (it is only if children are adopted that the birth parents lose parental responsibility which then becomes the responsibility of the adopted parents)
- Parents with children in need should be facilitated to bring up their children themselves
- The help that the parents receive to enable them to do this should:
  - Be provided in partnership with them
  - Meet the identified needs of each child
  - Appropriately address the child's race, culture, religion and language
  - Be open to 'effective independent representation and complaints procedures'
  - Use effective partnerships between the local authority and other agencies, including voluntary organisations

Activity

Familiarise yourself with your local policy in relation to child abuse cases. Find out where information on cause for concern cases is kept in your unit. Try to attend a case conference where possible (you will need to agree this with the chair prior to attending)

Congenital Disabilities (Civil Liability) Act 1976

This Act enables children who are born with a disability due to a negligent act before birth to claim compensation from the person who was negligent. In the case of a road traffic collision where the mother has been negligent, it is her insurance company which pays any compensation. This is the only scenario in which a child can sue its mother. Recently provisions have been made in relation to children who have been disabled during IVF treatment.

Conclusion

This chapter has considered the practice of midwifery within a contemporary legal framework. It has introduced the reader to the law and its principles, exploring what the law is, and the differences between criminal and civil law, and statutory, case and European law. It has raised key areas for discussion such as consent and the rights of the fetus and highlighted the legislative requirements in which the midwife is expected to practise regarding consent. The chapter then looked in more detail at specific legislation which midwives use to enable them to be put into context.

References

Department of Health (1998) *Our Healthier Nation: A Contract for Health.* London: HMSO.

Department of Health (1999) *Our Healthier Nation: Saving Lives.* London: HMSO.

Department of Health (2001) *Good Practice in Consent Implementation Guide: Consent to Examination and Treatment.* London: HMSO.

Department of Health (2004) *The Confidentiality and Disclosure of Information: General Medical Services, Personal Medical Services and Alternative Provider Medical Services Code of Practice 2004.* London HMSO

Dimond, B. (2004) Law and the midwife. In C. Henderson and S. Macdonald (eds), *Mayes Midwifery: A Textbook for Midwives.* London: Baillière Tindall.

Dimond, B. (2006) *Legal Aspects of Midwifery*, 3rd edition. Edinburgh: Books for Midwives.

Henderson, C. and Macdonald, S. (eds) (2004) *Mayes' Midwifery A Textbook for Midwives*, 13th edition. Edinburgh: Baillière Tindall.

House of Commons (2007) *Statutory Instruments.* Information sheet L7. London: House of Commons.

Jones, S. and Jenkins, R. (2004) *The Law and the Midwife*, 2nd edition. Oxford: Blackwell.

Laming, W. H. (2003) *The Victoria Climbié Inquiry. Report of an Inquiry by Lord Laming.* London: TSO.

Nursing and Midwifery Council (2002) *Code of Professional Conduct.* London: NMC.

Nursing and Midwifery Council (2004a) *Code of Professional Conduct: Standards for Conduct, Performance and Ethics.* London: NMC.

Nursing and Midwifery Council (2004b) *Midwives Rules and Standards.* London: NMC.

Nursing and Midwifery Council (2005) *Guidelines for Records and Record Keeping*. London: NMC.

Nursing and Midwifery Council (2006) *A–Z Advice Sheet: Consent*. London: NMC.

Philp, C. (2007) Babies seized after Jehovah's Witness mother refuses blood for sextuplets. *The Times* (23 February): 3.

Legislation

The Children Act 1989. London: HMSO.

The Family Law Reform Act 1969. London: HMSO.

The Mental Health Act 1983. London: HMSO.

Cases

Bolam v Friern Hospital Management [1957] 2 All ER 118.

Gillick v West Norfolk and Wisbech Area Health Authority [1986] CLR 113 (HL)

Re F (in utero) [1988] 2 All ER 193, [1988] Fam 122 (CA)

St George's Health Care Trust v S [1998] 3 All ER 673 (CA)

14 Confidentiality

Celia Wildeman

Introduction

Patient information is generally held under legal and ethical obligations of confidentiality (DH 2003b). From a professional, legal and ethical perspective, information provided to the midwife by her clients in confidence should not be used or disclosed indiscriminately. This particularly applies to disclosure in a form that might reveal the identity of the client who may not have consented to this revelation about her.

It is prudent to be aware from the first day as a student midwife that the patient is entitled to confidentiality with respect to information about her (Dimond 2006). Historically, midwives enjoy an enviable position in their relationship with women and their families. In whatever setting she works, mutual trust and respect for the individual are key requirements for the job. And the midwife's sensitivity and openness are axiomatic to her feelings of worth and enhancement of job satisfaction.

In no other aspect of the role of the midwife are these principles more relevant to than confidentiality. The midwife's personal and professional philosophy about right and wrong and her stance on advocacy and other ethical issues that influence interaction between client and professional will hold her in good stead. On the other hand, her ethical principles may cause tensions that inhibit harmonious dealings with clients, their families and the wider community.

The student midwife will come with personal belief systems. These can be modified and may change as she engages in education and training activities and as the highs and lows of professional life are experienced. Deeply entrenched personal beliefs and values are extremely difficult to change as they form the core of the person. The individual can feel threatened and challenged by the constraints of professional life as this might require her to think, act and even conform in ways that are unfamiliar. Indeed, it is important for practitioners, including midwives, to be aware that their perceptions, ideas and beliefs determine how they act towards others. However, the midwife has a duty of care to the woman, the unborn child, the neonate and, for some clients, their partners. In order to achieve the professional, ethical, legal and contractual requirements involved in confidentiality the midwife must be receptive to change. She must be ever aware of the depth of responsibility to clients, her employer, the Nursing and Midwifery Council (NMC) and the community to uphold confidentiality. However, there are exceptions to absolute confidentiality – for example, breach of confidentiality in the public interest – and these will be discussed later in the chapter.

This chapter explores, analyses and discusses the concept of confidentiality. It includes guidance and direction from the NMC for practitioners and in particular how midwives should conduct themselves in the day-to-day care of clients and their families. The legislative framework is also outlined.

The overall aim is to highlight the role and responsibilities of the midwife in order to work in a confidential manner when providing care for clients and their families to promote their dignity and trust. The chapter can help the reader to define confidentiality and explore why it is essential to professional midwifery practice. The reader will be able to analyse the different approaches to confidentiality, evaluate the meaning of the concept and discuss the implications that may arise when confidentiality is breached. The NMC's position regarding confidentiality is outlined allowing the reader to evaluate the ethical issues and to develop a personal/professional philosophy that will ensure continuing learning and change.

Confidentiality

The professional stance

The NMC (2004b) holds a very firm position on confidentiality. It asserts that *'registrants have a responsibility to deliver safe and effective care based on current evidence, best practice, and where applicable, validated research'*. This must be based on the concept of confidentiality to ensure that the midwife–client relationship is strengthened through transparency, trust and mutual respect.

Activity

How would you define confidentiality?

In your response your definition of confidentiality may include the following: confidentiality covers information (private or sensitive) revealed to a chosen other but which is protected from being shared with others (McKeown and Weed 2002).

It is essential that clients feel able to trust midwives with personal and confidential information and the client has every right to expect that such information will be kept in the strictest confidence. This means not sharing it with a third party unless it was made explicit to the client that it was likely to be shared. An explanation of why information may be shared should be given.

Confidentiality means keeping records which contain information given by or about an individual in the course of a professional relationship secure from others (Dimond 2006). It means that a professional must not disclose anything learned from a person who has consulted her, or whom she has examined or treated, without that person's agreement.

The essential nature of confidentiality for professional practice

It requires a huge amount of trust for a client to disclose personal information to the midwife. Some women will not have previously shared such details with anyone outside their family, and in some cases with no one, including their partner, until they divulge the information to the midwife. The midwife is therefore in a very privileged position and should understand the sensitive nature of her interaction with the client.

The NMC (2006, Clause 5) sets strict guidelines on the midwife's role and responsibilities regarding confidentiality. It states:

- You must treat information about patients and clients as confidential and use it only for the purposes for which it was given. As it is impractical to obtain consent every time you need to share information with others, you should ensure that patients and clients understand that some information may be made available to other members of the team involved in the delivery of care (for example, if an obstetrician has prescribed a particular treatment and the client refused to consent to the treatment then this information must be divulged to the obstetrician so that appropriate action can be taken). You must guard against breaches of confidentiality by protecting information from improper disclosure at all times. In the example given above, the midwifery practitioner would have complied with the employer's policy and professional guidelines to facilitate proper disclosure of client information

- You should seek patients' and clients' wishes regarding the sharing of information with their family and others. When a patient or client is considered incapable of giving permission you should consult relevant colleagues for example, a midwifery manager or senior midwife
- If you are required to disclose information outside the team that will have personal consequences for patients or clients, you must obtain their consent. If a patient or client withholds their consent, or if consent cannot be obtained for whatever reason, disclosures may be made only where:
  - They can be justified in the public interest (usually where disclosure is essential to protect the patient or client or someone else from the risk of significant harm)
  - They are required by law or by order of a court
- Where there is an issue of child protection, you must act at all times in accordance with national and local standards. These are based on legislative principles which give powers and duties to those involved in protecting children, the central standard being that the children's welfare should be 'paramount' in making decisions about their life and property (Kay 2003)

The NMC is therefore clear about the reasons why the midwife should uphold confidentiality and the way she must act to ensure this is achieved.

Activity

What does improper disclosure of information mean to you?

You might have begun your response by asking yourself the following questions:

- Who owns the records?
- What is the employer's (work-context) policy about disclosure?
- What does my professional body have to say about the issue?
- What is my personal/professional ethical position?

Answers to these questions will help you arrive at an understanding of the complex issue of disclosure of sensitive, private information. It is important that the midwife understands that the duty of confidentiality exists to protect the client.

Case Notes

You are a student midwife on duty on the postnatal ward. While at the midwifery station, a telephone call comes from a man claiming to be Jane's partner. He is enquiring about her and the baby's wellbeing.
How would you deal with this enquiry?

There are several possible responses. One is to seek answers to the following questions:

- What do I need to ask the enquirer to clarify who he is?
- Who do I need to consult before responding to this request?
- How much information do I need to give?

Additional information is required from the caller, for example his name and how much information he already has. It is important that Jane is consulted prior to divulging any information in order to confirm her relationship to the caller and in particular what, if any, information she consents to be divulged about her and the baby. This is important because Jane should be the main decision-maker in this instance. The student should document the communication between herself, the caller, Jane and any other personnel involved, then date and sign the entry.

Whatever decision you have made about what may be considered as improper disclosure of information should be taken in the knowledge that the practitioner should not make a unilateral decision (NMC 2004a). She should take into account, for example, that the records belong to the organisation where you work (if you work in the NHS, this is the Secretary of State), and not the professional staff who write them. The legal right to access information is not automatic. Clients have the right to request access to their records, whether manual or electronic. This right to access is based on the following:

- Data Protection Act 1998
- Access Modification (Health) Order 1987
- Access to Health Records Act 1990
- Access to Health Records (North Ireland) Order 1993
- Data Protection and the Freedom of Information (Scotland) Act 2000

Procedures for access must be in accordance with the Freedom of Information Act 2000, the Freedom of Information (Scotland) Act, 2002, the Data Protection and Freedom of Information (Scotland) Act 2002 as well all other relevant legal frameworks. These are in place to ensure that the practitioner carries out their duties with regard to client confidentiality in a knowledgeable and confident manner. The midwife's responsibility not to disclose confidential information applies not only to clients who are alive but also to patients and clients who are deceased. The midwife is personally accountable for any disclosure.

The midwife is obliged to keep information which she obtains from or about her clients confidential, and she should be aware that her contract of employment endorses this. Either the NMC or the client could bring an action for negligence if harm was caused as a result of the breach of duty to maintain confidentiality or an action for an allegation of breach of trust.

To facilitate the midwife's accountability and responsibility, the NMC (2006) supports the view that they should 'respect people's confidentiality'. The client's right to be informed about how and why information will be shared with the multidisciplinary team is mandatory. Should it become apparent that the midwife needs to divulge private and sensitive information to a third party, it must be made clear to the client and a rationale given. In all instances it is necessary if possible to gain the client's consent; such an approach can facilitate and enhance the client–midwife relationship. Awareness of the complex nature of working collaboratively with members of the multidisciplinary team is worthy of note. The dual professional message of respect for client's confidentiality and keeping colleagues/the team informed requires the practitioner to have a good working knowledge of her responsibilities and accountability.

Alternative approaches to confidentiality

Confidentiality is key to the midwife–woman relationship. Women traditionally have had a close relationship with their midwife, one that facilitates trust. Any doubt that the midwife will respect the confidence may make the woman reluctant to give vital information that could influence the outcome of her care.

The ethical stance

Haegert (2000) is of the opinion that *'care together with compassion, forms the foundation of morality'*. What does this mean in the context of midwifery? This is the essence of 'being with woman' and is a reminder to students of midwifery and midwives that their prime purpose is to 'care' for clients in a sensitive, compassionate manner, unconditionally and non-judgementally. This philosophy should be extended to private information and secrets revealed to them.

Information equates to power (Burr 2000). The midwife should be mindful that she occupies a powerful position in the client–midwife relationship. How she acknowledges and executes this power depends, among other things, on her ethical perspective. There are various things she might decide to do depending on the personal belief system, professional and legal directives, and guidance.

Utilitarian theory suggests that human nature is such that it seeks pleasure and avoids pain (Fletcher et al. 1995). If one adopts this view, it is feasible to assume that one's awareness of one's own pleasure and pain preferences ensures awareness of others'. From a professional midwifery perspective, a practitioner who considers the disclosure or non-disclosure of sensitive information to be harmful to the client may make an ethical decision that ensures the greater good is achieved.

Gillon (1986) asserts that *'the commonest justification for the duty of medical confidentiality was undoubtedly consequentialist'. 'People's better health, welfare, happiness are more likely to be attained if doctors and other professionals are fully informed by their patients/clients'*, and this is more likely if they undertake not to disclose their patients'/clients' secrets.

The deontological view is based on the theory of the absolute and the principle of individual rights to autonomy and privacy. *Deon* is Greek for duty and deontology considers duty to be central. Deontologists believe that good emanates from people doing their duty Hendrick (2004). This principle prevails irrespective of the consequences. From a midwifery professional perspective the concept of 'duty' fits well, and the duty of confidentiality may necessitate disclosing or not disclosing information in the interest of the client.

Ethically it could be argued that the professional's decision to disclose information that could be helpful to a third party should be based on the principle of the greatest good for the greatest number Hendrick (2004). The opposing view supports the position that disclosure leads to erosion and even breakdown of the woman–midwife relationship. The utilitarian view is not without problems, with conscience and tension around value systems. It could be argued though that midwives, working in a climate of scarce resources, are faced with difficult decisions every day. This often necessitates a bias towards the majority rather than the minority and adoption of the utilitarian approach. So what determines the position that the professional will take? This depends on the ethical belief system to which she subscribes and the balance she achieves through exposure to other ethical views, for example, the deontological perspective.

The ethics of professional practice are not easy. However, professionals make difficult, far-reaching decisions every day. These choices may affect their clients positively or negatively. Guidance should be sought from the NMC (2004b), among other sources of help, including the policy of the employer for whom you work and the Local Supervising Authority (LSA 2003). The key awareness should be the practitioner's commitment to her clients and her willingness to be their advocate. By the very nature of their situation, they are vulnerable to possible breaches of confidentiality. Continuously updating knowledge and understanding of the professional guidance currently available is essential to the midwife's practice in this and other areas of care.

The NMC's (2007) draft *Code of Professional Conduct* states that *'people must be able to trust you with their lives and health'*. It continues that the professional should *'respect people's confidentiality'*. Indeed, it asserts that professionals should *'make the care of people their first concern'*. Clearly, from a midwifery professional perspective the rights of the client enjoy prime position. This, however, can generate tension between professional, legal and ethical positions.

Case Notes

Tanya informs you that she is having difficulty bonding with her baby. You have been delegated their care for the shift by the midwifery mentor.

How would you deal with this situation?

A student midwife may be faced with this scenario. Clients frequently confide in them as they feel that they have more time to listen to their concerns. It is important to be aware of the limits to the student midwife's practice. It is helpful to Tanya to be reassuring by showing empathy and offering to consult your mentor and/or the midwife in charge.

The confidential nature of the situation is evident and documentation is crucial. The entry should include the following details:

- The person who was consulted
- The response of the consultant (if appropriate)
- The information the client received about the action that would be taken to support her
- Who will be involved in finding a solution that will satisfy the client

All this should be documented along with a plan of care, designed in partnership with the client and appropriate health care professionals (e.g. community public health nurse and/or obstetrician). The date, time, who was involved and the student's signature countersigned by the mentor should be included in the documentation.

The legal framework of confidentiality

The psycho-social context of midwifery practice supports the view that the midwife compared to other caring professionals is at particularly high risk of becoming involved in litigation (Rae 1990). This occurs because she has potentially three persons for each case in her care, the woman, the unborn child and the partner (Schott and Henley 2001). The woman's priority will be her own personal health and safety, that of her child (born or unborn) and that of her partner if this is relevant. Women appear to be far more informed today, possibly as a result of increased reading, access to the Internet and consulting the NMC's various documents that are available to the public. They are therefore more empowered and alert to any actions or omissions that her midwife makes. Rae (1990) also highlights the fact that midwifery clients *'by being comparatively alert and well, will be more willing to seek legal treatments against any health care practitioner who may be considered to be the cause of harm to the family unit'*.

Indeed, Rae (1990) reminds us of the legal maxim that states *'the higher the risk, the greater the duty of care'*. The midwife makes professional decisions that increase her risk both in *'professional malpractice and in legal liability'* (Rae 1990). With the greater risk and indeed the higher duty of care, the midwife must ensure that she weighs up carefully the consequence of the risk in relation to the benefit of undertaking it. The law makes it clear that the practitioner must balance the importance of the object to be achieved against the consequences of taking the risk (Rae 1990). The midwife is reminded that she should be guided at all times by the statutory instruments including the *Midwives Rules and Standards* (NMC 2004a), *Records and Record-keeping* (NMC 2004), *Code of Professional Conduct* (NMC 2004b) and any other legal and/or professional guidance (e.g. the LSA Standards 2003). Midwives traditionally have cultivated a sound relationship with women. Informed consent, therefore, has become the usual way for midwives to go about their work. Indeed, litigation is seldom directed at midwives and other safeguards, such as midwifery supervision, facilitate midwives to enhance their practice and at the same time protect the public (LSA 2003). Midwifery supervision is a statutory provision which ensures quality of client care based on best available evidence and research. (Chapter 19 discusses the issue of statutory supervision in more detail.)

In your response it may be useful to consider the impact on you and your feelings and the actions you might consider to seek remedies to rectify the situation. This should enable you to think about how a similar situation could affect someone in your care. The exploration of your own thoughts, feeling and potential actions should enable the student midwife to empathise, think about and support women in a sensitive way so that the women will not have cause to take legal action. Women are more likely to consider legal action when communication does not meet the accepted quality standard.

The crux of the matter is that the concept of confidentiality should not be ignored but be uppermost in the thoughts and deeds of the midwifery practitioner.

Exceptions to the rule of non-disclosure of client information

A duty of confidence arises when one person discloses information to another in circumstances where it is reasonable to expect that the information will be held in confidence (DH 2003b). This situation includes the divulging of private information from the client to the midwife.

This legal obligation derives from case law, is a requirement established in the *Code of Professional Conduct* (NMC 2004b) and must be included in NHS and private employment contracts as a specific requirement associated with disciplinary procedures. Midwives who work independently also have these professional responsibilities.

Women in the care of the midwife entrust the NHS, private and independent sector to elicit sensitive information relating to their health and other matters. They do so in confidence and have high expectations that midwives and the multidisciplinary team will respect this trust. Even if the woman is unconscious, the duty to uphold confidentiality is not exempt. '*It is essential, if the legal*

*requirements are to be met and the trust of the women is to be retained,
that the NHS provides, and is seen to provide a confidential service'* (DH
2003b).

Activity

Go back the previous activity. Did you include sanctions you would take
in your pursuit of your legitimate expectation to confidentiality?

It could be suggested that women generally trust midwives. The
relationship between the woman and midwife is extremely intimate
physically, socially and psychologically. Good self-awareness
enhances the practitioner's ability to be aware of the needs of their
clients and their expectations. The realisation that you expected
confidentiality to be respected in your situation should enable you
to extend that right to the women in your care.

Civil law (statutory and case) enables citizens to claim remedies
against other citizens or organisations as a result of a civil wrong
(Dimond 2006). A large group of civil wrongs are known as torts, of
which negligence is the main one, but the group also includes action
for breach of statutory duty, nuisance and defamation (Dimond
2006).

Communication is central to the client–midwife relationship and
all clients have a right to quality information communicated in a
form they can understand regardless of race, age, culture or any
marker of disadvantage (Schott and Henley 2001). The duty of care
in the law of negligence may include the duty to give information.
Failure to communicate important information relating to treatment
and care is considered in relation to the laws on trespass to the
person and negligence (Dimond 2006).

There are various Acts, professional guidance and ethical ways of
doing and thinking that ensure women come to no harm. The following Acts are central to confidentiality and the student of midwifery needs to be aware of them in order to understand and execute
her role effectively.

The Data Protection Act 1998

The European Directive on Data Protection, European Commission,
Schedules 1and 2 was implemented in the UK by the Data Protection
Act 1998. This Act requires that patients be told how their information will be used, who will have access to it and the organisations
to which data will be disclosed.

Human Rights Act 1998

Article 8 of the European Convention on Human Rights, which is given effect in the UK by the Human Rights Act 1998, establishes a right to respect for private and family life. It emphasises the requirement to protect the privacy of individuals and preserve the confidentiality of their health records.

Understanding the concept of confidentiality and the stance of the midwife must take cognisance of the Data Protection Act 1998 and Human Rights Act 1998.

Public interest

The law does, however, provide for exceptions to the duty of confidentiality. Statute requires or permits the disclosure of confidential patient information in certain circumstances, and the courts may exercise its right to disclosure (DH 2003a).

Under common law, staff are permitted to disclose personal information in order to prevent and support detection, investigation and punishment of serious crime and/or to prevent abuse or serious harm to others (DH 2003b), where they judge that the public good that would be achieved by the disclosure overrides the obligation of confidentiality to the individual patient and the broader public interest.

Serious crime and national security

Disclosures to prevent serious harm or abuse also justify breach of confidentiality. Serious crime is difficult to define, but includes murder, manslaughter, rape, treason, kidnapping, child abuse or other cases where individuals have suffered serious harm (DH 2003b). The student of midwifery may encounter some of these issues – for example, child abuse, particularly in the community midwifery setting. This would be a situation for child protection.

In the interest of improving quality care

It is absolutely essential that patients are told that information may be disclosed in order to improve the quality of care that they receive (Currie et al. 2004). Instances when disclosure may be necessary include clinical governance and clinical audits (Currie et al. 2004). These are legitimate reasons for disclosure, particularly in a climate of accountability, financial and professional constraints. Disclosure may be requested for research purposes, but the client's written consent and the approval of an ethics committee must be sought.

From the student midwife's and midwife's perspective, in the interest of protecting the client and infant, information may sometimes be disclosed either directly or through the midwife mentor, to the Supervisor of Midwives or the LSA Responsible Officer. This would be for health improvement, quality advancement and to safeguard the interest of the client (LSA 2003). The consent of the client is still a prerequisite.

Protecting client information

Guidelines on the protection and use of patient information require that when the use of patient information is justified, only the minimum necessary information should be used. It is also states that this information should be anonymised wherever possible.

To ensure that this ruling is followed, the Caldicott Committee (DH 2003a) was established. As the committee found there was little standardisation in the way patient information was handled, it set guidelines and the establishment of a network or organisational guardians. Their role is to ensure that information that identifies patients is protected from abuse. Guardians are also responsible for agreeing and reviewing protocols governing the disclosure of patient information across organisational boundaries.

Activity

Find out where the Caldicott principles are kept in your maternity unit.

* Read and make a written summary.
* What does it expect from the midwife practitioner?

In whatever sector you are employed, you are required to follow the Caldicott principles as laid down by the NHS Executive. The principles explain why, how, when, who and the legal framework for professional practice. The Department of Health has provided guidance in the form of a confidential model (DH 2003b) (see Figure 14.1). This should enable practitioners to meet the legal, ethical and professional standards of practice.

Confidentiality model

The model outlines the requirements that must be met in order to achieve a confidential service. The four main requirements are:

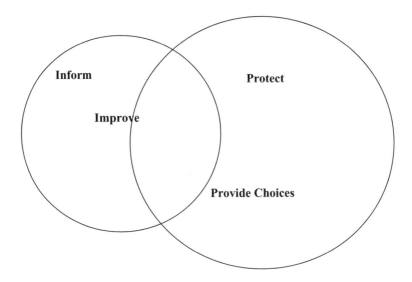

Figure 14.1 Confidentiality model (Source: adapted from DH 2003b)

1. Protect
2. Inform
3. Provide choice
4. Improve

All the four aspects are interrelated and mutually dependent.

Protect
Practitioners and student midwives must act to protect the client's confidential information. This includes manual, electronic and, for some groups of clients (especially teenagers), text messages, emails and telephone calls. The Caldicott ruling also includes storage, handling, communication between NHS and non-NHS staff, and the methods for recording information.

Inform
Clients must be aware of how the information held about them will be used. This includes actually and potentially, who will have access, under what circumstances, what is likely to be divulged and how the sharing of information will influence their care (DH 2003b).

Provide choice
The informed choice of clients must be part of best professional practice. Women should be empowered to decide whether their information can be disclosed or used in particular ways. Each client is an

individual and therefore what is considered confidential will vary from woman to woman. The DH (2003b) advises health care practitioners to ask patients for their consent before using their personal information, to respect patient's decisions to restrict the disclosure or use of information, except where exceptional circumstances apply, and to ensure that clients understand what the implications may be if they choose to agree to or restrict the disclosure of information. The key message is that even if, in the practitioner's judgement, the patient's/client's decision will be detrimental to their health and well-being, the patient's/client's decision must be respected.

Improve

The DH (2003b) advises that it is the role of the practitioner to *'always look for better ways to protect, inform and provide choice'*. The importance of keeping up to date with legal, ethical and professional changes that affect client confidentiality is essential to professional practice. There is also the expectation that breaches or possible breaches of confidentiality will be reported. This is and has always been a difficult and complex issue for health care students, including student midwives, particularly when senior practitioners are involved. They may experience a conflict between their education and training needs and the disclosure and possible breach of confidentiality.

The complex nature of whether the practitioner is bound to disclose information may generate immense stress for some students as they grapple with the demands of professional practice. The guidance of the practice mentor, education tutor and the Supervisor of Midwives should be sought. They are facilitators, guides and confidantes in professional matters. They act in the best interest of clients and this facilitates a mutual alliance with their students.

Conclusion

Midwives are expected to maintain high standards of ethical conduct in a professional context. This must be evidence-based, which necessitates them being motivated to continue to learn and be receptive to change.

The guiding principles for professional midwifery practice are:

- Respect for persons
- Respect for autonomy
- Justice
- Beneficence
- Non-maleficence

(Fletcher et al. 1995)

In addition to the midwife's duty of care to the client is the issue of the multidisciplinary team. It is important for the midwife to understand how and when sharing confidential client information will be in the best interest of all concerned. In all situations the overriding factor is whether or not client consent has been sought and received.

There are two exceptions to this: compulsion of law and the public interest. The NMC states that midwives have a responsibility to protect confidential information about clients (NMC 2007). The reciprocal nature of confidentiality is important to bring to awareness (Johnson 2006) in order to ensure that the best interest of the client is served by the multi-professional team. Information-sharing between practitioner and client is necessary to facilitate the assessment, planning, delivery and evaluation of care. Therefore, understanding the value of reciprocity and how it benefits clients and practitioners is vital.

References

British Medical Association (1999) *Confidentiality and Disclosure of Health Information*. London: BMA.

Burr, V. (2000) *An Introduction to Social Constructionism*. East Essex: Routledge.

Currie, L., Morrell, C. and Scrivener, R. (2004) Clinical governance: quality at centre of services. *British Journal of Midwifery* 12(5): 330–4.

Department of Health (2003a) *Patient Confidentiality*, London: DH.

Department of Health (2003b) *Confidentiality: NHS Code of Practice*. London: DH.

Dimond, B. (2006) *Legal Aspects of Midwifery*, 3rd edition. Edinburgh: Books for Midwives.

Fletcher, N. et al. (1995) *Ethics, Law and Nursing*. Manchester: Manchester University Press.

Gillon, R. (1986) *Philosophical Medical Ethics*. Chichester: John Wiley.

Haegert. S. (2000) An African ethic for nursing. *Nursing Ethic* 7(6): 492–502.

Hendrick, J. (2004) *Law and Ethics*. Nelson Thornes: Cheltenham.

Johnson, G. (2006) Confidentiality and standards of care. *Midwives* 9(12): 486–7.

Kay, J. (2003) *Protecting Children*, 2nd edition. London: Continuum.

Local Supervising Authority for England (2003) *Statutory Supervision of Midwives. National Standards for England*. LSA National Forum.

McKeown, R. E. and Weed, D. L. (2002) Ethics in epidemiology and community health. Applied terms. *Journal Epidemiology Community Health* 56: 739–41.

Nursing and Midwifery Council (2004a) *Midwives Rules and Standards*. London: NMC.

Nursing and Midwifery Council (2004b) *Code of Professional Conduct: Standards for Conduct, Performance and Ethics*. London: NMC.

Nursing and Midwifery Council (2006) *Confidentiality*. Advice Sheet C. London: NMC.

Rae, K. (1990) *Legal Aspects of Midwifery*. Midwives' Information and Resource Service (MIDIRS). Information Pack 14: 18–19. Bristol: MIDIRS.

Schott, J. and Henley, A. (2001) *Culture, Religion and Childbearing*. Gateshead: Butterworth-Heinemann.

Clinical Decision-Making

Marianne Mead

Introduction

Chapter 17 on evidence-based midwifery reminds midwives of the importance of understanding research principles and methods in order to appraise the quality of reported studies and therefore to judge whether or not the conclusions of such studies should or should not be taken into consideration in practice.

Decision-making is closely linked to the appreciation of evidence, but needs to be seen in the context in which women, midwives and other health care professionals, as well as economists, politicians and ethicists to name but a few, live, practise and relate to each other. However, the concept of decision-making is extremely complex and brings to bear a multitude of aspects that can only be partly considered in this chapter.

The management and prioritising of competing demands through all aspects of midwifery practice will be given consideration. This includes decisions relating to the referral of care to appropriate health care professionals when interventions to maintain the safety of the woman and her baby are required.

This chapter considers fundamental principles of decision-making as they complement or challenge evidence, experience or accepted practice. Two main areas are examined: diagnostic decision-making and treatment decision-making. Proposals for principles are then put forward that can be followed by midwives to improve their judgement and decision-making skills.

Decisions

We make a multitude of decisions every day and they are wide-ranging: the time we get up in the morning, whether or not we believe our boyfriend or girlfriend to be a good partner, whether we should back horse X or Y running in the 2 pm at Cheltenham, whether we should move out onto a main road or wait for more space, whether unprotected sex is OK. The examples are endless, but essentially there are two main types of decision that health professionals make: diagnostic and treatment. Examples of diagnostic choices in midwifery may be that a mother is or is not in labour, or that a baby suffers or does not suffer from neonatal jaundice. Examples of treatment choices include the recommendation to use or not to use syntometrine for the management of the third stage of labour, or to use or not use an epidural for a mother diagnosed with pregnancy-induced hypertension.

The fact is that the choices we make are not necessarily always correct: the majority of people who gamble do not win, otherwise running a casino would not be such a lucrative business; some people miscalculate the space they have to get onto the road and that explains the existence of insurance companies and the legal requirement to be insured to drive; and not all boyfriends or girlfriends are long-term relationship material as demonstrated by the break-up rate of marriages or relationships, and the existence of divorce lawyers. The same goes for unplanned and at times unwanted pregnancies, together with the rate of termination of pregnancies. Bearing in mind that marriage and pregnancy are major decisions, and that people do not generally wilfully enter into marriage or sexual activity with the express wish of making a mistake, it is worrying to see that the divorce rate was 53 per cent in the UK in 1998 (European Foundation for the Improvement of Living and Working Conditions 2007) and there were about 279 terminations of pregnancy (TOPs) for 1000 deliveries in the UK, but 841/1000 deliveries for women under the age of 20 (WHO 2007). The same database reveals that in some countries, often shown as an example to the UK, the figures are somewhat controversial, e.g. Sweden has an higher overall abortion rate (341 TOPs for 1000 deliveries), but a rate that is about five times the UK rate for women under 20 – 4175 TOPs for 1000 deliveries, with the consequence that only 1.6 per cent of all births are to women under 20 in Sweden, compared to 7 per cent in the UK (WHO 2007).

These types of error are relatively well documented, but people tend to think that this situation may be different in health care. This is probably nothing more than wishful thinking, although the rate of errors is thankfully not on the same scale! The majority of health care professionals aim to do the best they can for the people they look after, yet errors occur with alarming frequency. We know that this is the case because of the publication of enquiries into maternal mortality (Confidential Enquiry into Maternal and Child Health 2004b) and perinatal mortality (Confidential Enquiry into Maternal and Child Health 2004a). Indeed, the confidential enquiry into maternal death refers to 'substandard' care that could be classified as either 'major' or 'minor'.

In this context major substandard care is defined as care that '*contributed significantly to the death of the mother, i.e. different management would reasonably have been expected to alter the outcome*'. Minor substandard care is defined as a relevant contributory factor, but with the mention that different management might have made a difference although the mother's survival was unlikely (Confidential Enquiry into Maternal and Child Health 2004b).

The midwives and doctors caring for these women were probably doing their best, yet failures led to the death of some women. This demonstrates that even in the best of intentions, errors can and do occur. Often, they do not lead to major problems, but occasionally they do. That goes some way to explaining 'There but for the grace of God, go I'.

Errors

Maternal death is the most negative outcome of pregnancy in midwifery and obstetrics. There are cases that are inevitable because of severe pathology – for example, women with severe congenital heart malformation complicating pregnancy or cancer during pregnancy – but these events are rare. The majority of maternal deaths in the West are not associated with inevitable causes, but mostly with human error. The errors can be broadly classified as:

- Under-diagnosis, if they originate from a failure to recognise risk factors, or a failure to appreciate the significance of the presenting signs and symptoms, and therefore failure to recognise the real pathology and therefore act swiftly and correctly
- Over-diagnosis, if a condition that does not exist is diagnosed, usually instead of the correct diagnosis, leading to inappropriate treatment

Clinical expertise is closely related to clinical experience, and as severe maternal pathology is by definition unusual since pregnancy is usually a physiological state, it is likely that many midwives and obstetricians will never come across a maternal death, or if they do, their experience will be very limited because this untoward event is rare. It is therefore easy to underestimate the severity of symptoms in a condition that most practitioners will not have encountered. This may go some way to explain the poor interpretation of some of the presenting symptoms and therefore the delay in action leading to a catastrophic outcome. Indeed, there is evidence that although more experienced practitioners, and practitioners who are more certain of their diagnosis, are more likely to be right, some diagnoses are more likely to be under-diagnosed, and the misdiagnoses can at times be associated with ineffective or even harmful treatments (Cameron et al. 1980; Pounder et al. 1983; Stevanovic et al. 1986; McKelvie 1993; Sarode et al. 1993; Ermenc 1999).

Pulmonary embolism, a rare event, but one of the main causes of maternal death in the UK, is also one of the most likely diagnoses to be missed in a general population of people who have died and on whom an autopsy has been carried out. In their study, Stevanovic et al. (1986) identified an 84 per cent missed diagnosis rate; whereas a Scottish study identified 189 cases of pulmonary embolism, with 45 cases confirmed at autopsy, 35 cases not confirmed (i.e. over-diagnosed) and 110 cases where the condition was identified at autopsy, but not identified as a cause of death. On the other hand, the more common diagnosis of myocardial infarction was much more likely to be correctly diagnosed (98 cases) than under-diagnosed (51 cases) or over-diagnosed (58 cases) (Cameron and McGoogan 1981).

Perception as a source of errors

There are two main areas of medical error: what you believe is wrong with a particular individual, i.e. the diagnosis; or the choice of treatment. Clearly the wrong diagnosis may lead to the wrong choice of treatment because one is trying to cure a disease that does not exist. If the treatment is the same for the wrong diagnosis as it would be for the correct one, then the patient is lucky and the error does not matter that much. However, in some cases, an incorrect diagnosis may be associated with the choice of treatment that may do more harm than good. For example, administering an anticoagulant to a person diagnosed with a myocardial infarction, but who is in fact suffering from a gastric ulcer, may lead to severe haemorrhage and subsequent death. It is easy to think that this is farfetched and would not happen, but the literature demonstrates that such errors are not uncommon (Cameron and McGoogan 1981).

Sometimes an incorrect diagnosis is arrived at because practitioners rely too much on intuition and gut-feeling than factual analysis of hard data. Sometimes an incorrect interpretation of the statistics leads to error. This has been very well demonstrated in the case of Professor Sir Roy Meadows. He acted as an expert witness for the prosecution in a number of child abuse cases, and on the basis of his evidence, parents were convicted of the murder of their children. Later their convictions were overturned when it was demonstrated that his statistical interpretation of the likelihood of a second and subsequent infant death from natural causes occurring in one family had been flawed.

So, there is evidence that a poor understanding of some very basic statistical principles may lie at the root of many errors. An understanding of some statistical terminology may help midwives question and interpret diagnostic tests more accurately, or at least be more aware of their potential limitations. In a very recent article on a new technique aimed at diagnosis of Down syndrome without the need of invasive procedures (Dhallan et al. 2007), the authors report:

> *'Amniocentesis or newborn reports from the clinical sites confirmed that the copy number of fetal chromosomes 13 and 21 was determined correctly for 58 out of the 60 samples analysed; our method correctly identified 56 of the 57 normal samples, and two of the three trisomy 21 samples (samples 4 and 31). Sample 18 was a false positive (p = 0·05) on the basis of a negative amniocentesis report for the sample. Sample 55, which was identified as trisomy 21 by amniocentesis, was falsely identified as a normal sample by our methods ... The sensitivity of our test was 66·7% (95% CI 12·5–98·2), specificity was 98·2% (89·4–99·9), positive predictive value was 66·7% (12·5–98·2), and the negative predictive value was 98·2% (89·4–99·9)' (p. 478).*

At first reading, this may appear daunting, but if we break down the text, we can make sense of it. A little background information may be helpful.

Down syndrome is one of the most common congenital malformations, occurring in about 1 in every 800 pregnancies, but with a risk known to rise with an increase maternal age (Cuckle et al. 1987). Individuals with Down syndrome have learning disabilities, and the diagnosis is also associated with a high level of congenital heart disease and other long-term health problems, as well as some behavioural problems. Tools aimed at screening for or diagnosing Down syndrome (also known as trisomy 21) have been developed for at least 30 years. However, for the moment, the only positive way to diagnose a fetus with Down syndrome is amniocentesis. In this procedure a needle is inserted in the uterus and some amniotic fluid is withdrawn and analysed to identify an extra chromosome 21. Amniocentesis has been associated with a spontaneous abortion rate of 0.5–2 per cent depending on the skill and experience of the operator. The risk of carrying a baby with Down syndrome in women under the age of 20 is about 1 in 1500, so the risk of an amniocentesis of between 1 in 50 and 1 in 200 is substantially higher than the risk of the fetus having Down syndrome. This level of risk is generally unacceptable and this is the reason why so much effort has been expended in the development of more sophisticated screening tools that can identify women who have an increased risk. Only these women would then be offered an amniocentesis to reduce the number of fetuses spontaneously aborted because of the invasive amniocentesis.

A screening tool is not as accurate as a diagnostic tool. It only provides an indication that a higher risk may exist. It can be compared to the alcohol breath test that a police officer can request from a driver stopped for a motoring offence. This test provides an indication that the driver may be over the legal alcohol limit, but it is only the later blood test that will determine the actual alcohol blood level.

The study undertaken by Dhallan et al. (2007) aimed at testing the presence of fetal cells in the maternal blood and to see whether the analysis of these cells could reliably be used to diagnose Down syndrome in the fetus. An excellent test would always be positive when a condition is present and always negative when the condition is absent. But there are very few perfect tests. In reality, the majority of tests miss some cases and identify others as present when they are in fact absent. That sounds impossible, but it is true. Statisticians have devised some analyses that enable the calculation of some of these concepts, and in particular sensitivity, specificity and predictive value of a test. The sensitivity of a test (its true positive rate) is the ability of a test to produce a positive result when the condition is present, whereas the specificity of a test (its true negative rate) is its ability to produce a negative result when the condition is absent. By contrast, the false positive rate is the proportion of positive test results obtained when the condition is absent, and the false negative rate is the proportion of negative tests obtained when the condition is present. The positive predictive value of a test calculates the proportion of true positive tests for all positive tests, whereas the negative predictive value calculates the proportion of true negative tests for all negative tests.

The sensitivity, specificity and predictive values can be represented in a 2×2 table, considering the presence or absence of a

Table 15.1 Sensitivity, specificity and predictive value

	Condition			
Diagnostic test	Present	Absent		
Positive	True + **a**	False + **b**	Total Test + **a + b**	PV+ **a/a + b**
Negative	False − **c**	True − **d**	Total Test − **c + d**	PV− **d/c + d**
	Total Condition + **a + c**	Total Condition − **b + d**	**a + b + c + d**	
	Sensitivity **a/a + c**	Specificity **d/b + d**		

particular condition, and the predictive values of the test used for its diagnosis (see Table 15.1).

$$\text{Sensitivity} = a \:/\: a + c$$

'a + c' are the people who have the condition, but 'a' obtained a positive test and 'b' a negative test. So the sensitivity of the test, or the ability of the test to be positive when the condition truly exists, is the proportion of positive tests for the people who have the condition.

$$\text{Specificity} = d \:/\: b + d$$

'b + d' are the people who do not have the condition; 'd' was correctly identified as not having the condition with a negative test. So the specificity of the test, or the ability of the test to be negative when the condition does not exist, is the proportion of the negative tests for the people who do not have the condition.

$$\text{Predictive value of a positive test} = a \:/\: a + b$$

'a + b' are the people who have a positive test, even though only 'a' has the condition. The predictive value of a positive test refers to the proportion of positive tests that are accurate.

$$\text{Predictive value of a negative test} = d \:/\: c + d$$

'c + d' are the people who have a negative test, even though only 'd' actually does not have the condition. The predictive value of a negative test refers to the proportion of negative tests that are accurate.

Dhallan et al. (2007) were able to analyse the fetal cells and identify the presence of Down syndrome in 58 of the 60 cases they examined; they were also able to say that the results were normal for 56 of 57 normal cases, but they identified one case as having Down syndrome when in fact this fetus did not have this condition.

If the sensitivity of the test is the rate of correct diagnoses made by the test for all actual diagnoses, $58/60 = 96.7$ per cent, yet the authors report that the sensitivity was 66.7 per cent (95% CI 12.5–98.2). The difference between the simple calculation of 96.7 per cent and the reported 66.7 per cent is explained by the fact that this diagnostic tool was tested on a relatively small number of cases. The authors identify that they are 95 per cent confident (CI = confidence interval) that if this study was repeated on many more cases, the sensitivity would not be lower than 12.5 per cent or higher than 98.2 per cent. Of course, if the sensitivity was 12.5 per cent or thereabouts, it would not be a very good test, but if it was 98.2 per cent, it would be very good test, but still not as sensitive as an amniocentesis. On the other hand, a negative test is very specific – 98.2 per cent (89.4–99.9). However, this test does not carry any danger for the fetus and that has major advantages since the very fact of conducting an amniocentesis is itself associated with the loss of between 1 in 200 and 1 in 50 fetuses, depending on the skill of the doctor performing the test. This demonstrates the difficulties that parents face when deciding to go for a non-invasive test that might not be totally accurate, or an invasive one that is accurate but associated with an risk of miscarriage of a healthy fetus. Nothing is simple!

Midwives are regularly confronted with such questions when deciding whether observations are diagnostic of a particular condition or not, but it is likely that the presentation of the information and its analysis are not always clearly identified, so that a positive test is usually seen as being indicative of a condition, and the analysis of the likelihood of a false positive test is not examined. Indeed, the rise in caesarean section is causing concern because this increase in maternal morbidity has not recently been associated with a corresponding fall in neonatal problems. It is likely that when a baby delivered by emergency caesarean section cries loudly, that baby was just fine and therefore the diagnosis of fetal distress was incorrect, or that this baby is so relieved that he cries for joy – but this is highly unlikely! Midwives and obstetricians must do better if unnecessary interventions, including caesarean sections, are to be avoided.

The art of medicine – and by extension midwifery – is the skilled application of medical science (Schwartz and Griffin 1986), the processing of information (Lilford 1990) or the choice of decisions

(Thornton 1990). However, as seen when examining the quality of judgements or diagnoses, common decisions can also appear quite complex when they are translated into a statistical model or framework.

The choice between active and physiological management of the third stage of labour provides a relatively simple example. If one considers only the lower risk of a postpartum haemorrhage (PPH), there is little doubt that the active management of labour should be favoured, but this is not without side-effects, in particular nausea, vomiting and hypertension. This information renders the choice more complex, particularly if the midwife or obstetrician is confronted with a situation of increased risk of PPH, but in a mother who has a phobia of vomiting or injections.

Judgement often involves the manipulation of large amounts of information yet there is evidence that the brain can only manipulate small amounts at any one time. So we often use rules of thumb or cognitive shortcuts, otherwise known as heuristics, to explain phenomena, come to decisions or solve problems (Bursztajn et al. 1990). By definition, rules of thumb cannot be accurate, and heuristics fail systematically to process some information that is necessary to make sense of the whole issue under consideration. It follows that any heuristic decision has a higher chance of being the result of only partial consideration of all the dimensions of any problem. Human beings are extremely prone to these shortcomings, but computers are not. This is why, wherever possible, computers have replaced human judgement.

This is particularly true in many modes of transport. It is more accurate to use radar readings than the naked eye of even the best control tower technician, or satellite navigation than map reading when driving, or on-board instruments measuring the altitude of an aircraft than the pilot's estimation. Similarly, it is more accurate to use electronic blood pressure machines than the old-fashioned mercury measurement tools or the naked eye of the doctor looking at the patient to see whether their blood pressure is normal or not. Similarly, it is better to use a calculator to make even simple, never mind complex, calculations. Electronic tools make far fewer errors than humans, and more importantly, when they do make errors, the errors are systematic and can therefore be rectified more easily; whereas human beings make random errors that have no real patterns to them and are therefore much more difficult to correct.

But medicine – and midwifery – relies heavily on human judgement and there are therefore inevitably many errors. The under-diagnosis of conditions such as thrombosis and/or thromboembolism in pregnancy or the postnatal period is an example of the application of heuristics in maternity care where the severity of symptoms is not recognised or the symptoms are attributed to other causes (Confidential Enquiry into Maternal and Child Health 2004b). The rarer an event, the more likely it is not to be recognised because of lack of experience in putting all the pieces of the puzzle together.

Some approaches aimed at reducing errors

The previous section has looked at the errors that professionals make. The decision about what treatment is best for an individual often follows a diagnosis. As we have seen, diagnoses or clinical judgements can be the subject of a multitude of errors, often developed because of a poor understanding of statistical principles. The same can be said of clinical choices or decision-making, and often for the same reasons: inadequate or inaccurate weighing of options and their consequences. In the same way that computerised calculations help diagnosis or judgement, they can also support decisions about the most judicious choice of options for treatment. When a systematic approach is used to come to a choice, it is said to be subjected to decision analysis. Decision analysis originates mostly from psychology because psychologists have for some time been preoccupied with how and why people make errors. One such psychologist is Arthur Elstein and he defined decision analysis as:

> 'a formal analytic framework that is increasingly being applied to the problem of selecting an action in clinical situations in which the optimal choice is not intuitively clear or the judgments of competent physicians differ. These situations often involve complex combinations of uncertainty, values, risks, and benefits, precisely where human judgment may encounter difficulty in reaching an optimal solution and where a decision aid may be useful' (Elstein et al., 1986).

Some decisions are relatively easy to make. If I need to cross the road, it is best that I wait for a gap in the traffic. As I have not yet been run over when crossing a road, I have either correctly calculated the distance and the speed at which cars are travelling, or drivers have been driving carefully and within the speed limit, or they have had extremely good reflexes and applied an emergency braking procedure very effectively instead of colliding with me. That is true for the majority of us most of the time, but as some people are run over, it is obvious that human beings make errors in their decisions of when or how to perform an action. The same is true for health practitioners – we make mistakes; in fact, we make a lot of mistakes. Most of these lead to no significant consequences for the patients, but some do.

In an effort to avoid errors, formal analytical models have been developed to guide good decisions. One of the best known is Bayes' Theorem. Bayes' Theorem is based on the fact that people hold basic beliefs about various phenomena, but these can be altered in the presence of new probabilistic information (Thompson 1999). Decision analysis combines probabilities of the potential outcomes:

1. The prior probability of this outcome based on experience (Rayburn and Zhang 2002), or on epidemiological studies (Haynes de Regt et al. 1986; Spiegelhalter et al. 1999)
2. The conditional probability of a positive test, a concept that is similar to the true positive rate or sensitivity of a test
3. The posterior probability that combines the prior probability and the condition probability

Bayes expresses that theorem as:

$$P(\text{disease} \mid \text{findings}) = \frac{P(\text{findings} \mid \text{disease}) \times P(\text{disease})}{P(\text{findings})}$$

if:

$P(\text{disease} \mid \text{findings})$ = probability of a disease given a positive test, i.e. the posterior probability or odds

$P(\text{findings} \mid \text{disease})$ = probability of a positive test given the presence of the disease

$P(\text{disease})$ = probability of the disease, i.e. the prior probability or odds

$P(\text{findings})$ = probability of the findings

Bayes' Theorem provides an answer to the question: 'What is the probability of a particular outcome given a particular action?' For example, what are the chances of someone having a car accident given that they are over the alcohol limit?

$$P(\text{car accident} \mid \text{over the alcohol limit})$$
$$= \frac{P(\text{over the alcohol limit} \mid \text{car accident}) \times P(\text{car accident})}{P(\text{over the alcohol limit})}$$

The chances of having a car accident given that the driver is over the alcohol limit is not the same as the chance of being over the limit given that the driver has had a car accident. In other words, the majority of people who are over the limit do not – fortunately for the innocent others – have car accidents, but a sizeable proportion of people who have a car accident are over the alcohol limit. This justifies the police breathalysing all drivers involved in the accident or those who are driving erratically, but not all drivers who are driving apparently normally.

An example that is more relevant to midwifery is: 'What are the chances of a woman becoming pregnant given that she has had sexual intercourse?' Clearly the majority of women who are pregnant have had sexual intercourse, but the majority of women who have intercourse do not get pregnant every time!

$$P(\text{pregnancy} \mid \text{intercourse})$$
$$= \frac{P(\text{intercourse} \mid \text{pregnancy}) \times P(\text{pregnancy})}{P(\text{intercourse})}$$

These examples explain why we can only say that there is an increased chance or risk that one action will lead to a consequence, e.g. people who are over the alcohol limit are more likely to be involved in accidents; women who have sexual intercourse are more likely to get pregnant. But statistically, one does not *cause* the other, because if it did, that same action would *always* be followed by the same consequence. That is clearly not the case – increased risk, but not cause and effect.

Because of the elements that the Bayesian model takes on board, this process of decision-making can be said to be prescriptive, that is, if the Bayesian model is applied, the results should be accepted because the equation will have taken into consideration all the potential aspects of the problem. As the equation is only used in the presence of uncertainty, and the model provides clarity, it would not make sense to dismiss the results because they do not quite match our *feelings*. It is presumed that the outcome that combines the best chances and the best values for the outcomes will be the decision of choice.

This model of decision-making would be ideal if the level of information that is required in such a process was readily available to midwives and obstetricians, but that is not necessarily the case. There is now evidence that using the Internet search engine Google may help some physicians identify diagnoses in difficult cases (Tang and Ng 2006). However, following some basic principles may help clinicians come to a better quality of decision-making. These principles have been identified:

1. The problem must be correctly defined
2. Values, preferences and trade-offs must be clearly articulated
3. A wide range of creative solutions to the problem must be explored
4. Credible relevant data must be used for evaluating these alternatives

5. Logically correct reasoning must be used to evaluated alternatives
6. All the proper stakeholders need to be involved to ensure a commitment to acting on the results of the analysis

(Bordley 2001).

Most of the steps are relatively self-explanatory and are common sense. It is essential that a problem or a question should be framed correctly if it is to answered efficiently, and to find the most suitable answer, it is essential that all the potential answers ought to be stipulated so that they can be explored in turn. As seen when referring to Bayes' Theorem, it is essential that accurate data should be available not only on the likelihood of a condition, but on the likelihood of treatment success or failure for each of the considered alternatives. All stakeholders must be involved in the decision-making process, and this includes clinicians, health economists, policy managers and above all service users. The inclusion of service users and the exploration of their views will enable the identification of values, preferences and trade-offs and their inclusions in the decision-making process. The inclusion of values in the equation is called the maximising of utilities (O'Leary et al. 1995; Schackman et al. 2002).

The example of the active management of labour has already been identified as a potential clinical decision-making situation. To be able to come to a decision about how best to manage this clinical situation for a specific woman, information must be available: the incidence of postpartum haemorrhage generally, the specific risk assessment for this mother, bearing in mind her own specific risks, the alternatives available and the likelihood of outcomes given each alternative. Maximising utilities by adding the values that this mother would attach to each outcome would ultimately make the decision pertinent to this specific situation. The adoption of clinical guidelines rather than more rigid protocols enable midwives to include the values of the woman they are caring for in the equation. In the example of the management of the third stage of labour, the incidence of postpartum haemorrhage can be gathered from epidemiological data and calculated according to the various decision options. The risk can then be more specifically calculated bearing in mind the specific risk factors of this mother. Finally, given that any choice involves both potentially positive and negative outcomes, e.g. a reduced blood loss, but an increased chance of nausea and vomiting (Prendeville et al. 2000), the midwife can present the likelihood of the outcomes given the various choices and then ask the mother to provide her own values on the outcomes. It is important to identify that the likelihood of the outcome does not affect a change in the values that the mother would attach to it, so that the chance of normality, or postpartum haemorrhage or nausea and vomiting does not affect the values that the mother would attach to these outcomes. Including the values in the equation that would be used to arrive at the final decision then leads to a decision that is tailored to the calculation of risk and values for individual mothers. Examples of this approach have been given elsewhere (Mead and Sullivan 2005).

Conclusion

This short introduction to clinical judgement and decision-making might lure the reader into the false sense of security that these principles are simple and easy to follow. Nothing could be further from the truth. These disciplines are complex and have developed from the work of a few visionaries like Paul Meehl, Amos Tversky, Daniel Kahneman, Arthur Elstein, Harold Burztajn and Robert Hamm, to name but a few. However, even the briefest of introduction to the subject should be enough to whet the appetite of any midwife because the ultimate aim of the care they provide is maximising normality and reducing unnecessary risk. At a time when the caesarean section rate is at its highest, with no obvious benefit for either neonates or mothers, it is time that midwives, with their medical colleagues, adopt a more systematic approach to maternity care. A better understanding of the scale of the level of clinical errors and of the cognition processes that lead to the development of such errors ought to help clinicians bring about processes that will challenge poor judgement and, in conjunction with the elicitation of the values of women, lead to more personalised but safer care.

References

Bordley, R. (2001) Naturalistic decision-making and prescriptive decision theory. *Journal of Behavioral Decision-making* 14(5): 355–7.

Bursztajn, H., Feinbloom, R., Hamm, R. and Brodsky, A. (1990) *Medical Choices, Medical Chances: How Patients, Families and Physicians Can Cope with Uncertainty.* London: Routledge.

Cameron, H. M. and McGoogan, E. (1981) A prospective study of 1152 hospital autopsies: II. Analysis of inaccuracies in clinical diagnoses and their significance, *J Pathol* 133(4): 285–300.

Cameron, H. M., McGoogan, E. and Watson, H. (1980) Necropsy: a yardstick for clinical diagnoses. *British Medical Journal* 281(6246): 985–8.

Confidential Enquiry into Maternal and Child Health (2004a) *Stillbirth, Neonatal and Post-neonatal Mortality 2000–2003, England, Wales and Northern Ireland.* London: RCOG Press.

Confidential Enquiry into Maternal and Child Health (2004b) *Why Mothers Die 2000–2002. Report on Confidential Enquiries into Maternal Deaths in the United Kingdom.* London: RCOG Press.

Cuckle, H. S., Wald, N. J. and Thompson, S. G. (1987) Estimating a woman's risk of having a pregnancy associated with Down's syndrome using her age and serum alpha-fetoprotein level. *British Journal of Obstetrics and Gynaecology* 94(5): 387–402.

Dhallan, R., Guo, X., Emche, S. et al. (2007) A non-invasive test for prenatal diagnosis based on fetal DNA present in maternal blood: a preliminary study. *The Lancet* 369(9560): 474–81.

Elstein, A. S., Holzman, G. B., Ravitch, M. M. et al. (1986) Comparisons of physicians' decisions regarding estrogen replacement therapy for menopausal women and decisions derived from a decision analytic model. *American Journal of Medicine* 80(2): 246–58.

Ermenc, B. (1999) Minimizing mistakes in clinical diagnosis. *Journal of Forensic Science* 44(4): 810–13.

European Foundation for the Improvement of Living and Working Conditions (2007) *Quality of Life Survey.* Dublin: EFILWC.

Haynes de Regt, R., Minkoff, H., Feldman, J. and Schwartz, R. (1986) Relation of private or clinic care to the caesarean birth rate. *The New England Journal of Medicine* 315(10): 619–24.

Lilford, R. (1990) Limitations of expert systems: intuition versus analysis. In R. Lilford (ed.), *Bailliere's Clinical Obvstetrics and Gynaecology.* London: Bailliere Tindall.

McKelvie, P. A. (1993) Medical certification of causes of death in an Australian metropolitan hospital. Comparison with autopsy findings and a critical review. *Med J Aust* 158(12): 816–18, 820–1.

Mead, M. and Sullivan, A. (2005) Processes and challenges in clinical decision-making. In M. Raynor, J. Marshall and A. Sullivan (eds). *Decision-making in Midwifery Practice.* Oxford: Elsevier Science.

O'Leary, J. F., Fairclough, D. L., Jankowski, M. K. and Weeks, J. C. (1995) Comparison of time–tradeoff utilities and rating scale values of cancer patients and their relatives: evidence for a possible plateau relationship. *Medical Decision-Making* 15(2): 132–7.

Pounder, D. J., Horowitz, M., Rowland, R. and Reid, D. P. (1983) The value of the autopsy in medical audit – a combined clinical and pathological assessment of 100 cases. *Australian and New Zealand Journal of Medicine* 13(5): 478–82.

Prendeville, W. J., Elbourne, D. and McDonald, S. (2000) Active versus expectant management in the third stage of labour. *Cochrane Database Systematic Review* (3), CD000007.

Rayburn, W. and Zhang, J. (2002) Rising rates of labor induction: present concerns and future strategies. *Obstetrics & Gynecology* 100(1): 164–7.

Sarode, V. R., Datta, B. N., Banerjee, A. K. et al. (1993) Autopsy findings and clinical diagnoses: a review of 1,000 cases. *Human Pathology* 24(2): 194–8.

Schackman, B. R., Goldie, S. J., Freedberg, K. A. et al. (2002) Comparison of health state utilities using community and patient preference weights derived from a survey of patients with HIV/AIDS. *Medical Decision-Making* 22(1): 27–38.

Schwartz, S. and Griffin, T. (1986) *Medical Thinking – The Psychology of Medical Judgment and Decision-making*. New York: Springer-Verlag.

Spiegelhalter, D., Myles, J., Jones, D. and Abrams, K. (1999) An introduction to Bayesian methods in health technology assessment. *British Medical Journal* 319(21 August): 508–12.

Stevanovic, G., Tucakovic, G., Dotlic, R. and Kanjuh, V. (1986) Correlation of clinical diagnoses with autopsy findings: a retrospective study of 2,145 consecutive autopsies. *Human Pathology* 17(12): 1225–30.

Tang, H. and Ng, J. H. K. (2006) Googling for a diagnosis – use of Google as a diagnostic aid: Internet-based study. *British Medical Journal* 333(7579): 1143–5.

Thompson, C. (1999) A conceptual treadmill: the need for 'middle ground' in clinical decision-making theory in nursing. *Journal of Advanced Nursing* 30(5): 1222–9.

Thornton, J. (1990) Decision analysis in obstetrics and gynaecology. In R. Lilford (ed.), *Baillière's Clinical Obstetrics and Gynaecology*. London: Baillière Tindall.

World Health Organisation (2007) European health for all database http://www.euro.who.int/hfadb (accessed February 2007).

Health, Safety and Environmental Issues

Lisa Nash

Introduction

This chapter considers issues around health and safety, and the environment. It is important that the midwife understands the effect of these issues and has the knowledge and understanding to deal with them appropriately. Key legislation is examined, including the Health and Safety at Work Act 1974, the Workplace (Health, Safety and Welfare) Regulations 1992 and the Management of Health and Safety at Work Regulations 1999. The chapter begins by dealing with the following health, safety and environmental issues, although it is by no means exhaustive:

- Assessing risk
- Slips, trips and falls
- Mental health and stress
- Looking after your back
- Infection control
- Dealing with sharps
- Working in isolation
- Violence and aggression
- Working with computers
- Reporting of Injuries, Diseases and Dangerous Occurrences Regulations
- Control of Substances Hazardous to Health

Assessing risk

It is a legal requirement for employers to assess all potential risks in the workplace. It is important to do so to prevent injuries, accidents and ill health. Carrying out a risk assessment is largely common sense and has been condensed into five steps (HSE 2006):

1. Look for any hazards
2. Decide who might be harmed and how
3. Evaluate the risks and decide whether the existing precautions are adequate or whether more should be done
4. Record your findings
5. Review your assessment, revising it if necessary

Within the maternity unit there are potential risks everywhere as there are in any workplace – for example, a blocked emergency exit. Those at risk include midwives, health care assistants, domestic or portering staff, new and expectant mothers, visitors, including partners and family, any contractors that may be working there, doctors and other allied health care professionals. In the event of a fire or any other reason to evacuate the ward an obstructed exit will impede the safe evacuation of those present and could be life-threatening. This is a high risk and will need to be remedied by unblocking the emergency exit.

You need to reduce the possible of any risk occurring, therefore you may wish to think of measures to prevent the same event recurring by educating staff, finding suitable storage for the object(s) blocking the area and putting up notices. You may be able to think of other ways to achieve this.

To control risks the following principles should be applied:

- Try an alternative option which will be less risky
- Prevent access to the hazard, for example by guarding
- Reduce exposure to the hazard by organising work accordingly
- Issue personal protective equipment
- Provide facilities to aid welfare in the event of an occurrence, for example first aid and washing facilities to enable the removal of substances on the skin

You need to record what you found and what you did about it. You must tell the employees about your findings. Although it is recognised that risk cannot be completely removed, every possible means should be taken to reduce any risk.

Activity

Find out who conducts the risk assessment in your clinical area. You may find it helpful to discuss with them how they conduct the risk assessment and look at any paperwork that they use.

Activity

Following steps 1 and 2 above, look for areas where hazards could exist and therefore what you need to check. It is not anticipated that you will identify risks, but the exercise should enhance your observations of potential risks. An example of avoiding a potential risk would be the electrical testing of all electrical devices and plug sockets.

Slips, trips and falls

Slips and trips account for a third of all accidents in the workplace (HSE 2002). Avoiding them is largely common sense and it is every-one's responsibility to ensure that their working environment is as safe as it can be. Often where serious accidents or falls occur, someone else has first slipped or tripped at floor level prior to this occurring.

As a member of staff you are responsible for:

- Attending any training sessions that are offered
- Following health and safety procedures and policies within your working environment
- Tidying up as you go
- Being aware of potential hazards at all time

This means that you should:

- Look at what is going on around you and be aware of where you are going and what you are doing
- Look where you are going and do not run or rush
- Use any safety equipment provided
- Be especially careful on uneven ground and steps, using hand-rails where provided
- Follow safety guidelines in your area
- Use lighting in dark areas (it is surprising how many people fumble around in dark or dimly lit storage areas)
- Not attempt to carry out any activity beyond your capability. You may need some assistance

- Conduct yourself in an appropriate fashion. Playing practical jokes on colleagues may seem like fun, but can be a serious risk to you and your colleagues if it results in an accident

Preventing slips:

- Deal with any spillage (e.g. blood, liquor or vomit) immediately; do not wait for someone else to clear it up
- Take care on slippery surfaces, including those which have recently been waxed or washed
- Non-skid mats should be used around washing areas, such as showers and baths
- Ensure that mats and carpets are secured to the floor surface, maintain any areas which are frayed, worn or curled up
- Flooring may have uneven surfaces or be damaged in some way; take extra care when walking on these surfaces. Similar hazards exist on pavements and walkways around your workplace, so take care here too
- Be aware of your footing as the level may change unexpectedly, for example when you go round a corner
- Proceed with caution when walking on icy surfaces and alert your employer to enable precautions to be implemented
- Wear shoes that are fit for your job. They should offer support, have enough grip on them and should not be open-toed

Activity

Find out how you would deal with a blood spillage in your area, including where you would go to find cleaning equipment.

Preventing trips:

- Get into a daily routine of ensuring that your working environment is kept tidy, with items returned to where they belong
- Keep floors free from rubbish and any other debris such as swabs, incontinence pads, wrappers, and so on
- Do not leave anything on the stairs
- Keep drawers and cupboard doors closed
- Store equipment such as cardiotocograph machines, stools and ventouse apparatus out of the way safely
- Make sure that electrical leads and cables attached to resuscitaires, cardiotocograph machines and ventouse apparatus, etc. are not across walkways or where anyone can trip over them
- Have a place for everything and keep it there. Do not store anything in corridors

- Be mindful of where any furniture is placed, allowing easy access for anyone needing to come into the area
- Move obstacles out of the way; do not attempt to step over them

Preventing falls:

- When going upstairs do not carry anything that obscures your vision and use the handrail
- Ensure that adequate lighting is available. Stair lighting especially should be bright
- Ask for help when carrying heavy loads
- Do not stand on chairs. If you need a stepladder use one
- Make sure that chairs are fit for the purpose and use them appropriately, for example not standing on them or rocking
- Use a ladder to get down from a height, such as when getting out of a store room or closing a high window
- If you are using a ladder, for example to get to equipment out of your reach, know how to use it properly

Remember, it is your responsibility to:

- Dress appropriately. You should not wear jewellery, long hair should be tied back and you should ensure that your footwear is sturdy with closed toes
- Only carry out the work that you are trained to do
- Take time to organise and plan how you are going to do your work. For example, if you need equipment which is out of reach, ensure that you can reach it safely using the appropriate equipment

Activity

Reflect on your work in the last week. Can you recall any incidences when you have taken unnecessary risks? If so, think about how you could reduce the risk in future. If not, think of a risk activity that you have undertaken in the past and how you would prevent yourself being in that situation in the future. An example is using a chair to get something that is out of your reach.

Mental health and stress

Under the Disability Discrimination Act 1995, employers may not discriminate against people with a mental health disorder (including depression or schizophrenia). This means that they cannot deny someone a job or career progression on the grounds of mental ill health. It also means that the employer is legally obliged to make 'reasonable adjustments' to prevent the employee being disadvantaged by their illness.

It is recognised that stress affects the smooth running of any business, including an increase in staff turnover, and is therefore costly. Thus, it makes good business sense to reduce stress in the workplace. The employer has a legal obligation to protect employees against ill health, including the effects of stress. A risk assessment should be conducted and precautions taken (Amicus 2006). Stressors in the workplace include:

- Boring or repetitive work
- Too little to do
- Too much to do or too little time to do it
- Inadequate or excessive work-based training
- Uncertainty about roles within the team
- Having responsibility for others
- Lack of flexible work schedules
- The threat of violence
- Poor working conditions
- Lack of control over work activities
- Lack of communication and consultation between managers and staff
- Negative culture, for example a blame culture
- Lack of developmental support

When dealing with stress it is important for the employer to listen to staff. The following measures can be taken to prevent stress from becoming a problem (Amicus 2006):

- Take stress seriously
- Show an understanding attitude to those affected
- Make sure that staff have the appropriate skills, training and resources to enable them to carry out their job confidently and competently
- Allow staff to have a say in how they do their work
- Where possible, vary working conditions
- Treat all staff fairly and consistently
- Deal effectively with bullying and harassment
- Ensure good communication in the workplace between managers and staff, paying particular attention in times of change
- Design and implement an effective mental health policy, taking into account the view of all sectors of staff

Within the maternity unit many pressures are put on staff which may cause stress. In current practice the massive changes that maternity units are undergoing, such as hospital mergers, are a good example. Mergers cause anxiety due to the uncertainty that they cause and changes within the team, such as a change of management; shift times; working environment; and working with different staff who may have different working practices.

Activity

Reflect on a recent change which has affected you. This could be relatively small, such as a change in hospital policy, or major, such as a change in job role.

- How did you feel about the change and how did you adapt to it?
- Did you find anything particularly difficult?
- Did you adapt quickly or was it a slow process?

Stress at work can lead to mental and physical ill health, including depression. Stress is caused when you are under excessive pressure for some time. You may notice the following signs in someone suffering from stress (HSE 1998b):

- Increased sick leave
- More unexplained absences
- Poor time-keeping
- Poor performance
- Increased intake of alcohol, drugs, tobacco or caffeine
- Social withdrawal
- Frequent headaches or backaches
- Indecisiveness
- Poor decision-making
- Fatigue or low energy levels
- Mood changes (irritability, tearfulness)

Activity

Reflect on a time when you experienced a stressful situation – a new job, a house move, bereavement or a busy day at work when you felt pulled in many directions. Think through the following points:

- How did you deal with the situation?
- Did you deal with it adequately?
- How did you feel about it?
- Who supported you?
- Were you able to take time out for yourself?
- Did the situation change your perceptions in any way?

Looking after your back

In practice we use and abuse our backs in all manner of ways. All staff are required to attend mandatory moving and handling sessions on an annual basis. As midwives and allied health care professionals we unnecessarily put strain on our backs in many different scenarios, including the following:

- Conducting deliveries
- Moving beds around bays or to the operating theatre
- Conducting a postnatal examination on the mother and neonate
- Conducting an antenatal examination on the women in our care
- Attaching a cardiotocograph machine
- Collecting equipment from store rooms
- Facilitating infant feeding

We should all be mindful of our posture when completing the tasks necessary to carry out our work.

Activity

Reflect on the following:

- How your colleagues care for their backs.
- In which situations do you rush without thinking of the damage that you are potentially doing to your back?
- Do you need to alter your behaviour in order to care for your back?

Infection control

Infection control is important to prevent cross-infection and thereby maintain our clients' as well as our own well-being. Midwives can be contaminated with human immunodeficiency virus (HIV) or hepatitis C, etc., or women and their babies can be contaminated with methicillin-resistant staphylococcus aureus (MRSA) or group B streptococcus (GBS).

Infection control has been the focus of publicity recently with a various campaigns running to highlight this basic but essential aspect of health care. Cases of MRSA are frequently reported, along with other organisms. The Royal College of Nursing is currently campaigning for minimum infection control standards, including: mandatory basic training for all new staff, 24-hour cleaning teams and a module on infection control to be introduced into all training programmes, among other things.

We all play a vital role in maintaining standards for the prevention of infection and should follow the standard precautions (RCN 2005), ensuring that we:

- Maintain the highest standards in hand hygiene
- Use personal protective equipment
- Handle and dispose of sharps safely
- Handle and dispose of clinical waste safely
- Manage blood and bodily fluids appropriately
- Decontaminate equipment
- Keep the clinical environment clean and well maintained
- Use indwelling devices appropriately
- Manage accidents effectively
- Communicate well with our colleagues, patients and visitors
- Attend training and educate those around us

Activity

Examine your own actions when dealing with these areas of clinical practice. For example:

- Do you wash your hands before and after *every* client contact?
- Do you educate parents about maintaining hand hygiene before and after changing their baby's nappy?

Activity

Find out:

- Who your infection control nurses/midwives are for your unit.
- Where the infection control policy is in your workplace.
- What equipment is available for you to carry out your duties safely.

Dealing with sharps

Midwives deal with sharps on a regular basis, including amniocentesis hooks, needles, fetal scalp electrodes and drug vials. It is vital that you use and dispose of sharps appropriately to prevent infection of hepatitis B, hepatitis C and HIV. After back injuries, sharps injuries are the second most common injury in the NHS. The RCN (2005) reports that over the five-year period 1997–2002 there were

1550 incidences of exposures of blood-borne viruses to health care workers, 42 per cent of whom were nurses or midwives.

To ensure that the risks of sharps injuries are kept to the minimum you should maintain the following practice (RCN 2005):

- Never pass sharps from hand to hand. Always use a receiver
- Keep the handling of sharps to a minimum. There should be no unnecessary handling
- Check that needles are not damaged before use or disposal
- Never dismantle syringes and needles but dispose of them as a single unit
- Never re-sheath needles
- Take responsibility for the disposal of your own sharps. Always dispose of them appropriately when you have finished with them, do not ask someone else to do it
- Sharps containers must comply with British Standard 7320 and UN standard 3291
- Never fill a sharps box more than two-thirds to ensure that injuries are not caused by sharps sticking out
- Sharps boxes must be stored away from the public to prevent them being tampered with or injury
- Sharps trays should have integral sharps bins
- Sharps should be disposed of immediately after they are used
- Be aware of your local sharps policy

In the event of a sharps injury you must (RCN 2005):

- Encourage the wound to bleed (but do not suck)
- Wash well with running water
- Cover with a plaster
- Report the injury to occupational health (A & E if out of hours) and to your manager
- Complete an accident report form
- If the injury is from a used needle you should seek advice from a microbiologist, infection control doctor or consultant for communicable disease control

In the event of contamination with body fluids you should:

- Wash mouth out with water if fluids enter the mouth
- Irrigate the eyes if fluids enter them

Activity

Read through your local policy on sharps injuries, ensuring that you know what to do in the event of an injury.

Working in isolation

We will all be working alone at some point in our career. For some it will mean being in a delivery room on our own, for others it will be mean being in someone's home on our own. Although many of us will only need to call for help to a colleague, those of us working in the community are very isolated and therefore the potential risks are greater as generally your location will be unknown, no one will know that you are in trouble and when help is summoned it will not be immediately available.

Under the Health and Safety at Work Act 1974 (HSE 1998a) employers are required to assess risks to those working in isolation and minimise them. Of course, as an employee it is our responsibility to take precautions too. As with any area covered by the Act employers must discuss this aspect with the employees that it affects and put in place controlling measures. These can include instruction, training, supervision and protective equipment.

Considerations for lone workers:

- Emergency situations, such as maternal collapse in the home
- Physical activities/situations. For example, you may have to consider how you would transfer a labouring woman down five flights of stairs
- Mental stressors. For example, you might walk into a stressful situation, such as a couple having a row, or find that you have too much work to do
- Adequate training to ensure that the lone worker can practise safely. For example, being able to deal with emergency situations such as a postpartum haemorrhage

Activity

Take time to consider any vulnerable situations that you may find yourself in when working alone, for example, attending a born before arrival to find that the woman is having a postpartum haemorrhage and you are the only person there, or conducting a delivery where the partner becomes aggressive (in the home or in hospital).

- What would be your immediate actions?
- How would you raise an alarm for help?
- What other considerations may you have to take into account?

Precautions to increase your safety (HSE 1998a):

- Identify exits when entering a building
- Ensure that you can handle all your equipment safely
- Do not work alone if you have a medical condition that would make it dangerous or impractical to do so
- Consider which tasks can be carried out on your own and which require assistance. For example, in case of an emergency during a home delivery it is standard practice to have a second midwife in attendance
- Undertake any training offered, including any that helps you handle an aggressive situation
- Seek advice from a manager as and when necessary
- Maintain regular contact with colleagues
- Ensure that someone (e.g. a colleague) knows where you are due to go each day
- Use your judgement. Walk away if you feel threatened, you can return later with the police or a colleague
- Consider whether you need to take a colleague with you, for example, if there has been an aggressive incident on the premises in the past
- Consider whether you are the most suitable person. If you have already had some degree of misunderstanding/altercation with the client or their partner, it may be wise for another colleague to attend who may be able to handle the situation differently (for example, they may be perceived differently by the client and/or their partner) and therefore better suited
- Ensure that you have the equipment necessary to deal with emergency situations
- Check in with colleagues when you return to your base site or home
- An alarm system should be used which will send an alert out when you have had periods of inactivity

Violence and aggression

People working in a health care setting are up to four times more likely to experience violence in the course of their work than anyone else. Periodic inspections are carried out by the HSE to check what arrangements are in place to deal with workplace violence (HSE 2004).

The HSE (2004) reports that the following factors increase the risks of violent or aggressive situations:

- Impatience
- Frustration

- Anxiety
- Resentment
- Alcohol, drugs or mental instability

Activity

Reflect on how these factors could manifest themselves in your clinical environment. It may help to talk to colleagues about their experiences of dealing with violent or aggressive clients, partners or visitors.

As with any other health and safety issue the employer has to assess the risk and put appropriate measures in place. These measures may include:

- Providing training and information
- Reviewing and improving the environment in which you work
- Altering staff roles

Working with computers

However infrequently we work on a computer, using one incorrectly can result in health risks. These need to be addressed. Some users report getting upper limb disorders, including aches and pains in the hands, arms and neck. Under the Health and Safety (Display Screen Equipment) Regulations 1992, the employer has an obligation to ensure that these risks are minimised by the effective design of the workplace and jobs.

Good practice when working with a computer includes (HSE 2008b):

- Take frequent breaks or change your activity
- Ensure that there is adequate lighting
- Sit in a comfortable position with knees at right angles (adjusting the height of your chair accordingly)
- Your eyes should be positioned level with the top of the screen
- If you straighten your arm out the screen should sit an arm's length away
- The keyboard should be at the correct height, ensure that your arms are bent at 90 degrees
- Make sure that you have adequate space for documents that you are working on
- Your mouse should be relatively near you, so that your wrist is straight and your forearm is supported whilst using it

- You should maintain an upright posture and sit near the desk
- Make sure that the screen is free from glare and bright reflections
- You should have plenty of room to move your legs under the desk
- Ensure that your knees and back of your legs are not experiencing excessive pressure
- Consider where your keyboard is placed. It should be relatively near you, although some room in front of it may be useful for resting your hands when not typing
- Good keyboard technique is essential, your fingers should not be overstretched and you should touch the keys softly
- Make sure the screen is clean
- Ensure that the text is large enough to read and that the characters do not flicker
- Be mindful of the colours that you are working with on the screen, ensuring that they are easy on the eye
- Avoid using a laptop where possible
- When using a laptop you must take extra precautions to ensure that the keypad is at the correct height
- Employers should have a designated person who assesses workstations. Ensure that you have yours assessed as various equipment can be provided to improve your comfort
- Have your eyes tested regularly. Employees regularly using computers are entitled to get their employers to pay for their eye examinations

Reporting of Injuries, Diseases and Dangerous Occurrences Regulations 1995

Under RIDDOR some work-related accidents, dangerous occurrences and diseases must be reported (HSE 2008a):

- The reported incident will be investigated by the Health and Safety Executive (HSE), along with local authorities to ascertain the causes of serious incidents
- They will identify where and how risks arise
- They will give advice on the reduction of injury, ill health and accidental loss

The following need to be reported (HSE 2008a):

- Death or major injury
- An injury which is not serious but causes you to be absent from work for three days or more

- Disease
- Any dangerous occurrence

The midwife may suffer from a major injury due to equipment failure, equipment falling over or splashes, etc. A major injury includes the following (HSE 2008a):

- Fractures (excluding to fingers, thumbs or toes)
- Amputation
- Dislocation of the shoulder, hip, knee or spine
- Loss of sight (temporary or permanent)
- Chemical or hot metal burn to the eye or any penetrating injury to the eye
- Injury resulting from an electric shock or electrical burn leading to unconsciousness; or requiring resuscitation; or admittance to hospital for more than 24 hours
- Any injury that leads to hypothermia, heat-induced illness or unconsciousness; or requiring resuscitation; or requiring admittance to hospital for more than 24 hours
- Unconsciousness caused by asphyxia or exposure to a harmful substance or biological agent
- Acute illness requiring medical treatment, or loss of consciousness arising from absorption of any substance by inhalation, ingestion or through the skin
- Acute illness requiring medical treatment where there is reason to believe that this resulted from exposure to a biological agent or its toxins or infected material

The HSE (2008a) describe dangerous occurrences as:

- Collapse, overturning or failure of load-bearing parts of lifts and lifting equipment
- Explosion, collapse or bursting of any closed vessel or associated pipe work
- Electrical short-circuit or overload, causing fire or explosion
- Dangerous occurrence at a well (other than a water well)
- Failure of any load-bearing fairground equipment, or derailment or unintended collision of cars or trains
- A dangerous substance conveyed by road involved in a fire or released
- Unintended collapse of any building or structure under construction, alteration or demolition where over 5 tonnes of material falls; a wall or floor in a place of work; any false work
- Explosion or fire causing suspension of normal work for over 24 hours
- Sudden, uncontrolled release in a building of:

- 100 kg or more of a flammable liquid; or
- 10 kg or more of a flammable liquid above its boiling point; or
- 10 kg or more of a flammable gas; or
- 500 kg of these substances if the release is in the open air
- Accidental release of any substance which may damage health

Diseases which are reportable:

- Some poisonings
- Some skin diseases, including occupational dermatitis
- Infections, including leptospirosis, hepatitis, tuberculosis, anthrax, legionellosis and tetanus
- Other conditions, for example occupational cancer and some musculoskeletal disorders

What to do when an incident occurs:

- Notify the HSE area office immediately by telephone in the event of a death, major injury or dangerous occurrence
- Complete an accident report form whenever there is an accident
- A record of any occurrence must be kept for three years and should include:
  - The date and method of reporting
  - The date, time and place of the event
  - Personal details of those involved
  - A brief description of the nature of the event or disease

Activity

Although uncomfortable to discuss, find out the procedures needed to be carried out following a maternal death.

Control of Substances Hazardous to Health Regulations 2002

Under the COSHH the employer has certain obligations requiring substances. The following constitute hazardous substances:

- Those used directly in work activities (such as cleaning agents)
- Biological agents (such as bacteria and other microorganisms)

Substances which are hazardous to health (e.g. bleach, drugs and chemicals) carry a warning label (see Figure 16.1), and as such they should be treated appropriately as according to COSHH.

Figure 16.1   An example of a warning label

Effects of hazardous substances:

- Skin irritation/dermatitis
- Asthma
- Unconsciousness
- Cancer
- Infections

Activity

Identify hazardous substances in your workplace which could cause an adverse effect. For example, latex gloves cause an allergic reaction in some people leading to dermatitis.

COSHH requires you to undertake the following eight steps in relation to substances which can be hazardous to health (HSE, 04/05):

1. Assess the risks – who is likely to be at risk and how likely a risk does the substance pose?
2. Decide what precautions are needed
3. Prevent or adequately control exposure
4. Ensure that control measures are used and maintained
5. Monitor the exposure
6. Carry out appropriate health surveillance
7. Prepare plans and procedures to deal with accidents, incidents and emergencies
8. Ensure that employees are properly informed, trained and supervised

Conclusion

This chapter has examined some of the common issues surrounding health and safety and environmental issues in the workplace.

Legislation which has been put in place to protect employees has been brought to the attention of the reader to expand their knowledge and understanding. Together with the activities, this should have increased awareness of the issues. Throughout the chapter some common principles have become apparent which the midwife should follow. These include: using common sense when dealing with anything; not rushing unnecessarily; planning your work before you carry it out; attending any training that is offered; taking responsibility for your actions; looking out for hazards; seeking advice from your Supervisor of Midwives, manager or colleagues; and documenting everything.

References

Amicus (2006) *Stress*. Bromley: Amicus.

Health and Safety Executive (1998a) *Working Alone in Safety*. Sudbury: HSE Books.

Health and Safety Executive (2002) *Preventing Slips, Trips and Falls at Work*. Sudbury: HSE Books.

Health and Safety Executive (2004) *Work-Related Violence*. Sudbury: HSE Books.

Health and Safety Executive (2006) *Five Steps to Risk Assessment*. Sudbury: HSE Books.

Health and Safety Executive (2008a) *RIDDOR in Detail*. Sudbury: HSE Books. http://www.hse.gov.uk/riddor/guidance. Accessed 10 January 2008.

Health and Safety Executive (2008b) *Working with VDUs*. Sudbury: HSE Books. http://www.hse.gov.uk/pubns/indg36.pdf. Accessed 10 January 2008.

Royal College of Nursing (2005) *Good Practice in Infection Control*. London: RCN.

Evidence-Based Practice

Marianne Mead

Introduction

The midwife's role in contributing to the development and evaluation of guidelines and policies to ensure the best care for women
and children is the basis of this chapter. This includes discussion on
research and best available evidence concerning midwives, women
and children. The importance of critical appraisal of knowledge and
research evidence is emphasised as well as keeping up to date with
evidence, applying evidence to practice and the dissemination of
new evidence to others.

Background

Midwives are asked to be 'effective' and this is demonstrated by the
wording of several chapters in this book: 'Effective postnatal care',
'Effective emergency care', 'Effective documentation'. This fits in the
context of major changes that have emerged in the last 30 years or
so, namely the development of the number of peer-reviewed journals and therefore published information and research, and in paral-
lel, the development of electronic information and more recently
access to the World Wide Web, resulting in information becoming
readily available not only to professionals, but also to women and
their partners.

These changes have engendered a transformation in the quality
of the information on what constitutes good care and therefore of
the way care is delivered. Today health care professionals must

develop sound library skills, including searching skills and the organisation of references in a system such as EndNote (http://www.adeptscience.co.uk/), the understanding of fundamental research principles so that they can read the published literature effectively and select the most appropriate care for individual women and their families based on best evidence. The availability of electronic facilities has also meant that care can be audited, evaluated and compared to other centres of excellence, thereby raising the overall quality of the care available to patients, who can themselves explore a large amount of information to ensure that what is proposed best suits their needs.

The movement for evidence-based practice began with medicine as early as in post-revolutionary France and was later developed more formally at McMasters University, Canada, by a group led by Gordon Guyatt (Sackett et al. 2000). It reached world-wide recognition with the first edition of *Evidence-based Medicine* (Sackett et al. 1997). Does this mean that practice was not based on evidence before then? Certainly not, but health care practitioners were less likely to be asked to justify their practice on scientific grounds. Indeed, in the mid-1970s nursing and midwifery school libraries were small and just two textbooks were used: one for anatomy and physiology and the other for midwifery. At that time, the ninth edition of *Myles' Midwifery* was used and not a single statement in the book was referenced, except for those relating to the *Midwives Rules* of the then statutory body for midwives, the Central Midwives Board. Needless to say, student midwives were not asked to reference any statement they made in their handwritten course work either. Times have certainly changed!

In nursing and midwifery, the changes began with the publication of the Briggs Report (Committee on Nursing 1972) which recommended that the nursing profession, and therefore midwifery, should become more research-oriented. It also recommended that the nine professional bodies that regulated nursing, midwifery and health visiting at the time should merge into one institution. This eventually became the United Kingdom Central Council for Nursing, Midwifery and Health Visiting (UKCC), later replaced by the Nursing and Midwifery Council (NMC).

In May 1986, the UKCC published a revised version of the *Midwives Rules* and for the first time, student midwives were required to demonstrate *'an awareness of the importance of research-based practice'*. This was later updated and required midwives to *'be able to use relevant literature and research to inform their practice'* (UKCC 1991). The latest version is the *Midwives Rules and Standards* (NMC 2004) and this uses the term 'evidence' rather than research. It clearly states: *'Your practice should be based on the best available current evidence'*. These changes beg the question of what is the difference between research and evidence, and in turn the difference between research-based or evidenced-based practice.

Research- or evidence-based practice?

Sackett et al. (2000) provide a number of definitions that are useful in distinguishing the various concepts:

- Evidence-based medicine is *'the integration of best research evidence with clinical expertise and patient values'*
- Research-based evidence is clinically relevant research, often from the basic sciences of medicine, but especially from patient-centred clinical research into the accuracy and precision of diagnostic tests (including the clinical examination), the power of prognostic markers, and the efficacy and safety of therapeutic, rehabilitative and preventive regimens
- Clinical expertise is the ability to use clinical skills and past experience to rapidly identify each patient's health state and diagnosis, their individual risks and benefits of potential interventions, and their personal values and expectations
- Patients' values are the unique preferences, concerns and expectations each patient brings to a clinical encounter and which must be integrated into clinical decision if they are to serve the patient

These aspects together are the integral parts of evidence-based practice. The definitions provided by Sackett et al. (2000) identify a number of issues that are relevant to medicine, but also to midwifery. Diagnostic tests can, for example, include abdominal palpation, vaginal examination, postnatal examination including the detection of postnatal depression, to give but a few examples, because the purpose of these examinations is to identify that the pregnancy or postnatal period is progressing normally. Midwives are slightly different from most of the other health care practitioners because they seek to diagnose normality rather than abnormality, which is more the province of medical practitioners, since the majority of patients visit a doctor because they have a problem whereas the majority of women visit a midwife because they are embarking on the generally normal physiological process of pregnancy and childbirth. In their assessment of any mother or infant they are looking after, midwives use prognostic markers, i.e. specific observations that enable them to identify that the pregnancy is progressing normally, and only if they fail to identify these will they suggest that a deviation from the norm may be present.

Personal experience, tradition, authority, common sense and trial-and-error are no longer accepted as valid bases for midwifery practice. To be able to adopt an evidence-based approach to practice, midwives must ensure that they understand basic scientific principles, and in particular research methods and epidemiology (the study of the distribution of diseases in the population). There are many textbooks on research methods. Some have been written specifically for professional groups, e.g. nurses, doctors or psychologists, but the principles are the same whatever the discipline. It is important that midwives understand the principles of the main research approaches that they are likely to encounter in the scientific literature relevant to maternity services so that they can appraise the quality of published work and therefore decide if research findings should or should not be implemented. The following section provides a very short introduction or reminder of the main research methods that midwives may encounter when examining research that is relevant to their practice.

Research methods

The purpose of research is to increase the body of knowledge available to practitioners, consumers, managers, economists and educationalists. It is a systematic scientific approach characterised by order and control, empiricism and generalisation (Polit and Hungler 1991). The scope of research methods is as large as befits the scope of knowledge that is to be gained. Indeed a 'continuum of evidence' has been described from the purely qualitative perspective at one end to the purely quantitative at the other end (see Figure 17.1).

The methods used depend on the questions that are to be addressed. Several classifications of research methods are available, e.g. quantitative or qualitative, prospective or retrospective, descriptive, exploratory or explanatory, phenomenological or positivist, holistic or reductionist, to name but a few. Methods are sometimes

Qualitative perspective

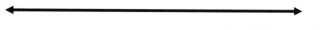

Quantitative perspective

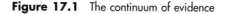

Figure 17.1 The continuum of evidence

but not always mutually exclusive, although some characteristics can be, e.g. an experiment cannot be retrospective, descriptive studies cannot be experimental.

Research methods situated at the more qualitative or phenomenological end of the research continuum are more likely to be associated with the social sciences because the questions they answer are based on an assumption that the world in which events occur is socially constructed. This type of research does not aim to test a hypothesis, but to generate one, based on the understanding of the values and meanings of observed phenomena, from the perspective of participants. Qualitative research approaches typically include in-depth interviews, focus groups, case studies, non-participant observations and ethnography.

At the other end of the spectrum, quantitative or positivist research methods are based in the natural sciences and aim to test a stated hypothesis. This area of research is reductionist rather than holistic (e.g. the level of cortisol in the presence of stress), but not how the individual experiences/feels about stress, which would be addressed via a more holistic qualitative approach. Hypothesis testing is based on empirical, objective and measured observations. Measurements are statistically tested so that the initial hypothesis can be either supported or rejected. This type of research is concerned with testing cause-and-effect relationships, or at least correlations.

The method previously referred to as the gold standard of positivist research is the randomised controlled trial, but other methods are also included, e.g. case-controlled studies, cohort studies, some surveys, systematic reviews and meta-analyses.

Each research method has its own specific aims, characteristics, strengths and limitations. For further in-depth knowledge, it is important that readers consult research methods textbooks. Only a very small example of research methods are presented here – experiments and surveys, together with a very brief introduction to qualitative studies, because they are some of the most common research methods that midwives will encounter when searching and exploring the literature.

Experiment

Quantitative methods include the experimental methods and some aspects of surveys. Experimental research includes studies such as randomised controlled trials, experimental trials and quasi-experimental trials. In experimental research, control is the most important aspect. The purpose of control is to ensure that the results of any experiment cannot be biased by extraneous variables (a variable other than the experimental variable that could explain the outcome of the experiment). Aspects of this control include randomisation or random *allocation* (not to be confused with the random *selection* of surveys) of subjects to either the experimental or the control trial groups, blind or double blind trials where the subjects, or the subjects and the researchers, do not know whether the subjects have been allocated to the experimental or the control group.

The quality of the randomisation should always be checked by readers of research publications to ensure that both the experimental and the control groups are similar at the point of entry to the study. If the group characteristics are similar, and the results of the experiment show differences between the two groups, these can be attributed to the experiment, but if the groups are not similar in the first instance, it will be impossible to attribute ultimate differences to either the differences in group characteristics or the experimental variable itself. Blinding and double blinding will ensure that the participants, or the participants and the research staff, are not able to introduce bias in the experiment or the interpretation of the results.

Although control is a very strong feature of experimental studies, representation is less important. It is though important for the generalisation of findings. However, experiments are more likely to be involved in a reductionist research (e.g. uterine activity) and representation is less important in such studies because it is easy to see that, for example, one nulliparous uterus is very much like another nulliparous uterus. This explains why the results of drug trials on the prevention or treatment of postpartum haemorrhage could be undertaken on one side of the world and be applicable to the rest of the world population.

Where experiments deal with factors that are not universal, the generalisation of the findings is less likely to populations that do not share these characteristics, e.g. the findings of experimental studies on the introduction of a particular system of midwifery care might not generalised to countries where the culture and the health system are different from the place where the study took place. In such instances, replication of studies in different countries will add to the weight of the initial study if the findings are replicated.

Survey

A survey is a means of gathering information on particular populations by questionnaires or interviews. These include opinion polls, telephone interviews and focus groups. A survey can be a research design by itself, whereby people are asked to provide information on their attitudes, perceptions, opinions, behaviours or views. Alternatively, it can be a research tool used in the context of a study – for example, an experimental study comparing obstetric and midwifery antenatal care, whereby women are randomly allocated to an obstetrician or a midwife at the onset of pregnancy. It might ask women for their opinion via a questionnaire, an interview or a focus group. In this case, the study would be experimental, using a survey as one of the data collection tools.

In the context of surveys, a population is defined as a group of people who share the same characteristics, e.g. student midwives in the UK; male midwives in the Scottish Highlands; nulliparous women. In studies where the relevant population is small, e.g. male midwives in the Scottish Highlands, any study aimed at gathering their perspective on a given topic may involve the whole population. Such a study is defined as a census: the whole population is investigated. Censuses are uncommon because relevant populations are usually rather large and it is therefore unnecessary to include the whole population if a representative sample can be investigated 'on behalf' of the whole population. In this case, researchers speak of a survey.

The most important aspect of surveys is therefore representation. The researchers must ensure that the sample selected to represent the population is truly representative of that population. Several means can be used to ensure this. The most common is random *selection* (not to be confused with random *allocation* of experimental studies) because each subject in the population has an equal chance of being selected. This is quite useful where the characteristics of individuals are relatively well distributed in the population, but not so useful if some sub-groups are more likely to be more represented than others, e.g. a survey of midwives may need to have a greater proportion of independent midwives in the sample to ensure that enough are surveyed to achieve valid and reliable findings. Where random selection is neither appropriate nor feasible, other sampling procedures can be used (e.g. stratified, purposeful, snowball, convenience), but it is important for readers of surveys to understand that different types of sampling procedures may threaten the representation of the population and therefore the external validity or generalisation of the findings.

Qualitative studies

Whereas experimental studies tend to be reductionist and base their analysis mostly on statistical methods, qualitative approaches are more suitable for the exploration of social or cultural phenomena or lived experiences. An experimental study will work out that the administration of maternal corticosteroids will benefit premature babies, but it will not be able to capture the experience of the mother who is given these drugs. Qualitative approaches are needed to explore such an experience. There are a number of qualitative research designs, each specifically targeting specific types of question, from the single case study to the participant or non-participant observational studies. Main approaches have been defined and described, e.g. ethnography, case studies, phenomenology, action research, heuristic inquiry or grounded theory. The scope of this chapter does not permit an exploration of any of these in any detail, but it is useful to note that these methodologies have only relatively recently become accepted by the medical establishment (Mays and Pope 1995; Greenhalgh and Hurwitz 1999; Donovan et al. 2002).

The analysis of qualitative data requires skills that are very different from either experimental studies or quantitative surveys. Whereas statistical packages are available for statistical analyses, e.g. SPSS (www.spss.com), Minitab (www.minitab.com), qualitative data analysis packages have also emerged, e.g. NVivo, formerly NUD.IST (www.qsrinternational.com) and Atlas/ti (www.atlasti.com). Most novice researchers are advised to use the simpler paper analysis approach to learn how to develop their themes and their thematic or content analysis.

Systematic reviews and meta-analysis

Randomised controlled studies used to be seen as the gold standard of positivist research, but this status has been taken over by the systematic review that locates, appraises and synthesises evidence from scientific studies in order to provide informative, empirical answers to research questions (NHS Centre for Reviews and Dissemination 2001). As can be seen, a systematic review is not a literature review, although it does include a thorough and systematic exploration of the available literature, both published and unpublished, and subsequent critical analysis of that literature. Generally speaking, the purpose of systematic reviews is to provide the best evidence of effectiveness, i.e. clinical but also economic evaluation.

The principles underpinning systematic reviews have been developed because of the vast amount of literature that has been published in the last 25–35 years. Some of the research findings can be confusing if not contradictory, and the very quantity of the information available makes exploring and making sense of the research a very complex and time-consuming task. Good reviews are therefore the end-result of a very systematic research process that includes the formulation of a precise research question, the systematic and as exhaustive as possible retrieval of relevant research studies, the selection of entry and exclusion criteria to ensure that only relevant studies are included in the final analysis, a very sound analysis of the strengths and limitation of each study included in the final selection of studies, the extraction of the data from each study, the statistical analysis of the cumulated data from each study – the meta-analysis – and finally the synthesis of the data and the conclusions of the systematic study.

Clinical effectiveness

Research provides midwives and other health care professionals with evidence that ought to add to the individual practitioner's and individual profession's body of knowledge. It is unreasonable to expect practitioners to know everything about any topic, but it is reasonable to expect the professional to be able to explore the literature in order to find the relevant literature and make sense of it. The purpose of these exercises is to improve overall clinical effectiveness.

Clinical effectiveness has been defined by the Department of Health as the extent to which specific clinical interventions, when deployed in the field for a particular patient or population, do what they are intended to do – maintain or improve health and secure the greatest possible health gain from the resources available (DH 1996). This definition clearly identifies clinical interventions for either individuals or populations. Clinical interventions that are deployed to do what they are intended to do include the following:

- For an individual – administration of corticosteroids to a pregnant woman who is going into premature labour, with the intention to reduce neonatal respiratory problems
- For a population – the provision of antenatal services for pregnant women generally

It is important to note that an economic element is included in the definition 'from the resources available'. Health economics are playing a much greater role in the assessment of the provision for health care and this is evident from the recommendations of the National Institute for Health and Clinical Excellence (NICE). Indeed the NICE website now includes the following information:

'NICE is planning to introduce 'recommendation reminders' from December 2006, as part of a new set of products to help the NHS make better use of its resources. The aim is to help the NHS reduce ineffective practice by highlighting recommendations from existing NICE guidance.

Reminders will be issued on current NICE recommendations published as technology appraisals and clinical guidelines between 2000 and the end of 2005. They will appear on the NICE website, along with an electronic tool for estimating the local cost implications (http://www.nice.org.uk/page.aspx?o=404910; accessed 6 February 2007).

The concept of clinical effectiveness is also associated with other terms that are often used interchangeably, even though each of the terms has its own specific definition, e.g. efficacy, efficiency, cost-effectiveness, cost benefit.

Efficacy

Efficacy refers to the ability of a specific treatment to have the intended effect, e.g. syntometrine is efficacious in treating postpartum haemorrhage; aspirin is efficacious in reducing pyrexia.

Efficiency

Efficiency includes an element of measurement between the elements that have to be used in terms of the outcome, e.g. measuring the height of an individual can be done by modelling weight to seating position, clothes size, etc., but the most efficient measure would simply be a tape measure of whatever description, the most reliable being also the most efficient.

Cost-effectiveness

The concept of cost-effectiveness has developed alongside the evidence-based movement; it examines the overall resources that need to be expended to achieve a specific outcome for a specific treatment. Examples of cost-effectiveness include the way access to primary care is organised. The majority of patients visit their GP at a surgery rather than have the GP visit them at home. A single visit at the surgery costs less to the NHS than individual visits to each patient. It is important to note here that the NHS cost is considered here, not the cost to the individual patient. However, even the cost to the individual patient would probably be lower if aspects such as the taxation that would be required to provide such individualised care were considered.

Cost benefit

This considers the costs and benefits of an intervention. Examples abound in obstetrics: e.g. antenatal diagnostic or screening tests are encouraged because the early diagnosis of severe fetal abnormalities can lead to the decision to terminate a pregnancy, with the resulting saving in the cost of supporting a severely disabled child or adult. The calculation of the cost benefit of specific interventions is complicated, but in a system where financial and other resources are limited, as in the NHS, it is important to ensure that resources are carefully allocated so that interventions are not only effective, but also 'good value for money'. These principles can raise important ethical, moral and political questions, but these important aspects are somewhat outside the remit of this chapter.

Systematic literature searching

The information provided so far makes obvious the importance of being able to search the literature effectively and efficiently for all health care professionals, including midwives. It is fair to say that the amount of information presently available is such as to constitute a serious problem for any practitioner who has not developed a systematic approach to data searching and management. Before even starting to search the literature, it is important for all midwives to develop a sound system of data management. Computer software packages are available to help in the retrieval, storage and use of references (e.g. EndNote: http://www.adeptscience.com/products/refman/endnote). Using such a program to collect, organise and use references to support practice is invaluable in our age of information overload.

Once a references management tool has been selected, it remains to find the research evidence. This can be complex, but some fundamental principles and plenty of practice will make the process easier. There are three main areas of evidence:

- Books
- Journals
- Electronic databases

Books are useful but tend to be based on opinions rather than evidence, take a long time to get published and are quickly outdated.

Journals, and in particular peer-reviewed journals (i.e. journals that only publish papers that have gone through the scrutiny of peers before being accepted for publication), are more likely to provide up-to-date research information. However, the manual searching of journals, even through indexes of titles or titles and abstracts, can be extremely tedious and very time-consuming.

Electronic databases provide a much more cost-effective way of searching the literature. Midwives will find the following of particular interest to help them find relevant evidence to support their practice:

- PubMed (http://www.ncbi.nlm.nih.gov/entrez/query.fcgi)
- CINAHL (Cumulative Index for Nursing and Allied Health)
- The Cochrane Library

A systematic approach to data retrieval is important to get the most of the information that is available on numerous databases. It is useful to know that EndNote can be connected to some databases and therefore facilitate the retrieval and storage of selected references directly onto the referencing program – a detail that is not to be neglected! The first step in data retrieval is formulating a sound question and the next is to understand how best to use facilities such as MeSH (Medical Subject Headings). Anyone wishing to explore the literature systematically would be well advised to attend an introductory course led by a specialist health librarian, or to follow the guidelines that health librarians often make available for practitioners who are relatively new to the topic. PubMed also has its own 'Tutorials' material that can be accessed from their home page.

Implementation of evidence-based midwifery

Recent developments in midwifery practice and management have seen the emergence of consultant midwives or research and development midwives, and this demonstrates an eagerness on the part of the NHS to see evidence-based midwifery in practice. This does not mean that individual midwives are no longer responsible for their personal updating. Far from it; it simply demonstrates an additional commitment that ought to support midwives in their continuous professional development. Indeed, engaging in practice development may support individual midwives' professional development (Joyce 1999).

Engagement with evidence-based midwifery can be seen at two levels: the individual practitioner and the clinical set-up. Midwives who are looking after individual women must ensure that the care they provide is based on evidence. No more amazing theories such as the cabbage leaf treatment for breast engorgement that made the rounds in the 1980s! Women should not be advised to follow treatments that are not based on sound evidence, unless they are told that no evidence is currently available and that this is therefore the best suggestion that can be made. At the same time, midwives ought to keep information about the areas of care where they find a lack of evidence to support their practice. This would be an initial step for personal and/or group reflection, literature searching, assessment of the available evidence and the setting up of personal or unit guidelines.

Recent developments by NICE have seen the publication of guidelines for antenatal and postnatal care, as well as the use of electronic fetal monitoring and induction of labour (NICE 2001, 2003, 2006). A draft guideline on intrapartum care was finalised in 2007. Other guidelines have been developed by midwives e.g. (Spiby and Munro 2001), and by international bodies e.g. (World Health Organisation – Regional Office for Europe 1986).

Midwives should not feel that the responsibility for providing evidence-based care rests solely on their shoulders. Networking is important and there are a number of interest lists that midwives can subscribe to in order to meet like-minded people and exchange ideas. One of the most useful Internet sites is www.jiscmail.ac.uk, where midwives can search the many interest lists. A keyword search of 'midwi' or 'birth' will identify a number of lists of potential interest and enable anyone who joins to identify colleagues who have similar interests and thereby foster a community that can develop evidence-based midwifery practices.

Conclusion

Evidence-based practice has evolved from the principles of research-based practice, but has taken into consideration the huge developments in the production of scientific publications, access to electronic facilities such as the Internet, but also and perhaps more importantly, electronic databases and electronic journals.

Midwives are now required to ensure that their practice is based on evidence wherever possible, and where this is not the case, it makes sense that midwives should generate questions that can be answered empirically. This requires them to develop the skills necessary for retrieving relevant material and a sound knowledge of research methods to enable them to appreciate the strengths and limitations of various publications. Midwives, however, do not work in isolation from other practitioners and more and more facilities are becoming available to ensure that they can work in collaboration with other practitioners and develop networks of specialist interest. The situation is becoming more complex but the tools are developing to ensure that all midwives ought to have access to knowledge and to colleagues. The application of sound EBP principles in the maternity services by midwives and other health care professionals should in the long term be in the interest of mothers and babies as this approach should ensure that the care proposed is the best and most cost-effective that can be achieved. This should ensure the promotion of good practice and the relegation of outdated practices to the confines of maternity services history.

References

Committee on Nursing (1972) *Report of the Committee of Nursing* (Briggs Report). London: HMSO.

Department of Health (1996) *Promoting Clinical Effectiveness: A Framework for Action in and through the NHS*. Leeds: NHS Executive.

Donovan, J., Mills, N., Smith, M. et al. (2002) Quality improvement report: Improving design and conduct of randomised trials by embedding them in qualitative research: ProtecT (prostate testing for cancer and treatment) study. Commentary: presenting unbiased information to patients can be difficult. *British Medical Journal* 325(7367): 766–70.

Greenhalgh, T. and Hurwitz, B. (1999) Narrative-based medicine: why study narrative?, *British Medical Journal* 318(7175): 48–50.

Joyce, L. (1999) Development of practice. In S. Hamer and G. Collinson (eds), *Achieving Evidence-based Practice: A Handbook for Practitioners*. London: Bailliere Tindall and RCN.

Mays, N. and Pope, C. (1995) Qualitative research: observational methods in health care settings. *British Medical Journal* 311(6998): 182–4.

NHS Centre for Reviews and Dissemination (2001) *CRD Report 4*, 2nd edition. York: University of York.

National Institute for Health and Clinical Excellence (2001) *NHS*. London: NICE.

National Institute for Health and Clinical Excellence (2003) *Antenatal Care – Routine Care for the Healthy Pregnant Woman*. London: NICE.

National Institute for Health and Clinical Excellence (2006) *Routine Postnatal Care of Women and their Babies*. London: NICE.

Nursing and Midwifery Council (2004) *Midwives Rules and Standards*. London: NMC.

Polit, D. and Hungler, B. (1991) *Nursing Research, Principles and Methods*. London: J. B. Lippincott.

Sackett, D., Strauss, S., Richardson, W. et al. (1997, 2000) *Evidence-based Medicine, How to Practice and Teach EBM.* London: Churchill Livingstone.

Spiby, H. and Munro, J. (2001) Evidence into practice for midwifery-led care. *British Journal of Midwifery* 9(9): 550–2.

UKCC (1991) *Midwives Rules.* London: UKCC.

World Health Organisation – Regional Office for Europe (1986) *Having a Baby in Europe.* Copenhagen: WHO.

Statutory Supervision of Midwives

Kath Mannion

Introduction

The United Kingdom is unique in that it is the only country where midwifery supervision is enshrined in legislation. The Local Supervising Authorities (LSAs) are responsible for the provision of statutory supervision of midwives in their area. They appoint supervisors of midwives to undertake statutory supervision and ensure that every midwife in the LSA area has a named supervisor of midwives. Every midwife who practises in the UK needs to notify her intention to practise to a Supervisor of Midwives. The Supervisors of Midwives pass on the notification of intention to practise to the LSA, which in turn informs the Nursing and Midwifery Council that the midwife is practising within the LSA area. The LSAs also ensure that all midwives have access to a supervisor of midwives for support and guidance at all times. Through this system safe and effective midwifery practice is facilitated. By enabling safe and effective practice supervisors of midwives protect the public and ensure that midwives are supported in their everyday work.

History

In order to understand what statutory supervision of midwifery in the UK is today, it is essential to understand how the midwifery profession and statutory supervision have evolved over time.

Supervision is not a new concept, Towler and Bramall (1986) in their book on the history of midwifery reported that in the 1500s the chief physician of the city of Frankfurt supervised midwives. The earliest records of midwifery show that medicine and men have attempted to control midwifery practice (Donnison 1977; Witz 1992).

The drive to legislate midwifery practice in the UK arose from a desire to reduce the high perinatal and maternal morbidity and mortality evident in Victorian England, and 'protect' the public from untrained midwives. Midwives were characterised as ignorant, drunk and lazy, and ridiculed in the guise of Sairey Gamp in Charles Dickens' *Martin Chuzzlewit* (Heagerty 1996). Heagerty (1996) however notes that most midwives were hard-working and skilled. With the founding of the Midwives' Institute (the forerunner of the Royal College of Midwives) a number of prominent women began to push for legislation which would legalise the practice of midwifery and gain greater recognition for the profession (Towler and Bramall 1986).

Statutory supervision of midwives came into effect when the Midwives Act was enacted in England and Wales in 1902. Scotland followed in 1915 and Ireland in 1918 (Jenkins 1995). Midwives were recognised legally and appropriate training had to take place before registration with the Central Midwives Board (CMB). Registration was not without its opposition as many saw that this was putting midwives under the control of men/doctors (Donnison 1977; Robinson 1990; Witz 1992; Kirkham 1995). Kirkham (1995) notes that men and non-midwives dominated the composition of the CMB. It was not until 1920 that the CMB was required to include midwives, although several notable nurses and members of the Midwives' Institute were already members. LSAs were responsible for enacting statutory supervision of midwives and reporting to the CMB. The CMB was the statutory body that was to rule midwifery for the next 70 years until the formation of the United Kingdom Central Council of Nursing and Midwifery in 1983.

Statutory supervision of midwives, 1902–1937

Supervisors of midwives were known as Inspectors of Midwives until 1937. Inspectors were selected from women in society, for example middle-class and wealthy women, who had undergone nurse training but did not go on to work in nursing (Kirkham 1995). Towler and Bramall (1986) note that the focus was on the social and moral aspect of the midwives being supervised rather than their clinical skills. This finding is supported by Heagerty (1996), who recorded that these inspectors of early midwifery had little or no education in midwifery supervision. Almost all were from the middle or upper class and their knowledge and inspection methods were more concerned with cultural and moral issues than actual clinical practice. With little or no background knowledge apart from what was available to them in largely medical textbooks and the *Midwives Rules* there was no possibility of these inspectors being able to offer constructive comment on clinical issues.

Reports to inspectors from other sources such as doctors were often made without any substantive evidence (e.g. the midwife being drunk at a birth), even though this could result in midwives being struck off the register or severely censured (Heagerty 1996). The midwife had no leave to appeal and Kirkham (1995) reports that many were struck off simply because of 'offences' relating to the poverty of their clients when the rules required the midwife to summon medical aid but the family would not and could not as they had no means pay the doctor's fee. This left the midwife in a dilemma between the rules that governed her practice and the wishes of her clients.

Donnison (1977) regards the *Midwives Act 1902*, along with all subsequent Acts, as a disadvantage for midwifery on several counts compared to other professions. She regards midwives as subjected to supervision and likens it to controls on tradesmen; it therefore did not promote the profession. Investigations of misconduct, which included review of the private life of the midwife, were defined under strict criteria with no recourse to appeal if the midwife was struck off. Leap and Hunter (1993) describe the fear many midwives experienced as unannounced visits from an inspector were common.

Statutory supervision of midwives, 1937–1974

In 1937 the term inspector was dropped in favour of supervisor, and a two-tier system of medical and non-medical supervisors came in. The medical supervisor was usually the Medical Officer for Health for the area, with the non-medical supervisor being a midwife, nurse or health visitor. Strangely, although it was recommended that the non-medical supervisors of midwives should have some experience in midwifery practice, it did not recommend that those who were currently in clinical practice should be supervisors of midwives (Kirkham 1995).

Towler and Bramall (1986) report that the creation of medical and non-medical supervisors was an acknowledgement of unsuitable appointments in the past. As the medical supervisor of midwives was usually the Medical Officer for Health and was therefore aware of the social and public health issues of the area, supervision was more knowledgeable and demonstrated understanding of the everyday issues that midwives encountered in their practice (Allison and Kirkham 1996).

Allison and Kirkham (1996) describe how non-medical supervisors were community-based during the 1940s. These supervisors were practising midwives and worked in the community as part of the domiciliary maternity service. They knew the conditions that the midwives worked in and therefore were much more supportive than the previous inspectors. They formed a valuable resource and were also responsible for recording and passing on to the medical supervisor statistics that enabled information on birth and maternity outcomes to be produced (Allison 1996).

Jenkins (1995) and Kirkham (1995) believe the changes that took place in statutory supervision of midwives in 1937 sowed the seeds for what supervision should be today, i.e. the supervisor being the supporter and friend of the midwife.

Throughout the 1940s and 1950s most women continued to give birth at home. A small number chose to give birth in hospital and midwives were employed to provide care for women who delivered there and also to assist doctors. Supervisors did not have any control over hospital midwives until 1942, when it became mandatory for these 'institutional' midwives to notify their intention to practise to the LSA (Bent 1993). Statutory supervision was provided to hospital midwives by senior community-based supervisors (Robinson 1990).

Kirkham (1995), in a consensus conference report, discussed the 1951 Midwives Act and noted that supervision continued to be linked with issues of control. This Act stipulated that midwives were required to attend a refresher course every five years, and it was in the remit of the Supervisor to check that midwives adhered to this.

Statutory supervision of midwives, 1974–1985

Jenkins (1995) notes that despite major consolidation of midwifery legislation in 1951 there were no changes to the requirements for supervision until 1974. The changes in legislation, when they came, were a result of the reorganisation of the National Health Service. This transferred the powers of the LSAs from local authorities to Regional Health Authorities (England), Area Health Authorities (Wales), Health Boards (Scotland) and Health and Social Services Boards (Northern Ireland).

All midwives were now employed by the NHS and supervision was transferred from community-based supervisors to hospital-based midwives, with the supervisor usually being the head of midwifery services (Jenkins 1995).

Medical Supervisors of Midwives also became obsolete with the reorganisation of the NHS in 1974 and finally ended with an order in 1977 that all supervisors had to be experienced practising midwives and also dropped the criterion that a supervisor required a year's experience of domiciliary practice (Jenkins 1995).

Statutory supervision of midwives, 1985 to the present day

The *Midwives Rules* (UKCC 1993) saw the addition of Rule 45, which detailed how a LSA must discharge its functions. One of the features of this rule was that for the first time each LSA had to make available to all midwives practising in its area a list of all supervisors and how contact could be made with them at any time. This was to facilitate support to midwives whenever they needed it and to heighten awareness of who the supervisors in each LSA were. A more comprehensive definition of the role of the Supervisor was considered by the UKCC for inclusion in the revised *Midwives Rules* of 1998. This, according to Steene (1996), was an effort to improve the understanding and purpose of supervision.

The Association of Radical Midwives held a consensus conference in April 1995 following the publication of *Draft Proposals for Midwifery Supervision* (ARM 1994). The consequences of this conference were far-reaching with the spotlight being firmly placed on supervision and its relationship in supporting changes in midwifery practice, as described in *Changing Childbirth* (DH 1993). The conference proceedings were to become one of the first books on midwifery supervision and were soon followed by Kirkham's (1996).

In 1996 consortia of LSAs were organised in England and Wales as a result of the abolition of Regional Health Authorities. The reason behind the consortium arrangements was that there were technically 127 LSAs in England alone, which hardly fostered equity of supervision standards across the country. The LSAs were amalgamated into eight regions with one or two LSA officers being appointed to each region on a full-time basis. This provided equity of approach in the provision of support and advice to supervisors and midwives alike (Sauter 1997).

The *Nursing and Midwifery Order* (HMSO 2001) led to the establishment of the Nursing and Midwifery Council and the continuing recognition and support for statutory supervision of midwives.

The consortium arrangement of LSAs in England proved to be valuable, with the LSA Midwifery Officers meeting on a regular basis and developing guidelines for supervision across England. With the reorganisation of the NHS in 2006 there are now ten LSAs in England based in Strategic Health Authorities. Each LSA has an appointed Midwifery Officer who is responsible for ensuring that statutory supervision takes place to the required standard as determined by the NMC (2004a). Wales, Scotland and Northern Ireland have now adopted similar consortium arrangements with LSA Midwifery Officers appointed as prescribed by the *Midwives Rules and Standards* (NMC 2004a).

Midwives Rules and Standards

The *Midwives Rules and Standards* (2004a) is the legislation under which every midwife practises in the UK. Supervisors of Midwives use the *Rules* alongside the *Code of Professional Conduct* (NMC 2004b) to guide midwives through the principles of professional, safe and effective midwifery practice.

One criticism of the *Midwives Rules* is that until the latest publication in 2004 they had passed down virtually unchanged since the first *Rules* were issued following the passing of the *Midwives Act 1902*.

The early *Rules* dictated clinical practice in an effort to stop the spread of infection, promote competent practice and safeguard the mother and baby.

The *Midwives Rules and Standards* (NMC 2004a) now provide midwives and Supervisors of Midwives with a framework in which safe and effective midwifery practice can be based. By providing rules, standards and guidance in one document the NMC has combined legislation and practical advice for all midwives.

Role and responsibility of a Supervisor of Midwives

Rule 12 of the *Midwives Rules and Standards* (NMC 2004a) details the minimum role and responsibilities of a supervisor of midwives. However, this does not give a descriptive account of what the Supervisor of Midwives may encounter in her role. This has led the UK Forum of LSA Midwifery Officers to develop role descriptions under three main categories of what is expected of supervisors of midwives (see Table 18.1).

Table 18.1 Advice and guidance

Statutory

1. Receiving and processing Notification of Intention to Practise forms to verify that the statutory requirements for practice have been met
2. Ensuring that midwives practise within the statutory *Midwives Rules and Standards* (NMC 2004a) and that regulations for the supply, storage, administration and destruction of drugs used within the sphere of their role are met
3. Providing guidance on maintenance of registration and identifying updating opportunities in relation to statutory requirements
4. Investigating critical incidents to identify the action required, while seeking to achieve a positive learning experience for the midwives involved, liaising with the LSA as appropriate
5. Reporting to the LSA serious cases involving professional conduct where the NMC Rules and Codes have been contravened and when it is considered that local action would not achieve safe practice, recommending referral to the NMC.
6. Being available for midwives to discuss issues pertaining to their practice and to provide support. This includes those midwives who practise independently. supervisors of midwives must participate in providing 24-hour supervisory cover
7. Arranging regular review meetings with individual midwives at least once a year to help them evaluate their practice and identify areas for development and agree the means by which their midwifery expertise can be maintained and developed
8. Ensuring that effective communication exists, with all stakeholders engaged in determining health services policy, in order that relevant issues are appropriately addressed and resolved

Professional

1. Recognise own accountability to the LSA for all supervisory activities
2. Provide professional leadership to create a practice environment that supports the practitioner role and empowers professional practice through evidence-based decision-making
3. Enhance knowledge of own role and individual professional development needs Attend at least one meeting a year convened by the LSA Midwifery Officer to discuss relevant issues and share information and experience
4. Monitor the integrity of the service to ensure that safe and appropriate care is available to all women and neonates
5. Identify when peer supervisors are not undertaking the role to a satisfactory standard and take appropriate action
6. Audit the standards for statutory supervision (at least) annually. The LSA Midwifery Officer, through visits to practice sites, will validate standards. Validation of standards may also be achieved by external audits performed by other supervisors
7. Maintain records of all supervisory activities for at least seven years. Records may be electronic or manual and must be stored in such a way as to maintain confidentiality. Participate in the safekeeping of all maternity and midwives' records for 25 years

Continued

Table 18.1 *Continued*

Practice issues
1. Ensure that midwives have access to the statutory rules and guidance, evidence and local policies to inform their practice
2. Monitor the standards of midwifery practice through audit of records and assessment of clinical outcomes and take appropriate action
3. Contribute to activities such as Confidential Enquiries into Maternal and Child Deaths, risk management strategies, frameworks for clinical governance or any other relevant enquiry relating to the maternity services
4. Lead activities such as standard-setting, clinical audit and the development of evidence-based guidelines and protocols
5. Contribute to curriculum development of pre-registration and post-registration education programmes for midwives
6. Participate in the preparation and mentorship of new supervisors of midwives
7. Issuing of controlled drug authorities, if required, for midwives undertaking homebirths
8. Be available to guide and support midwives through difficult clinical situations

Source: LSA National Forum 2007

The NMC has issued competencies for supervisors of midwives (NMC 2006) and these are reflected in the role description in Table 18.1. The suggested role description is not exhaustive but for the purpose of this chapter the following key themes have been identified and will be explored briefly.

Named Supervisor of Midwives

The LSA has to ensure that each midwife who submits her intention to practise has a named supervisor of midwives who will offer support on an individual basis (NMC 2004a). The guidance issued within the *Midwives Rules and Standards* (NMC 2004a) also informs the midwife that she should have a choice of supervisor. Hobbs (1997) encourages independent midwives to use supervisors of midwives as a support. She recognises that personality clashes may occur and advises on how to change Supervisor if necessary.

Access to a Supervisor of Midwives

Rule 12 of the *Midwives Rules and Standards* (NMC 2004a) determines that all practising midwives should have 24-hour access to a Supervisor of Midwives in every LSA. This is facilitated in many different ways e.g. on-call rotas ensure that all midwives within an LSA area can speak to a Supervisor of Midwives for help and advice at any time of the day or night. This advice relates to midwifery practice and should not be confused with seeking advice from managers regarding organisational issues.

Intention to practise

Every midwife in the UK has to complete an Intention to Practise (ITP) form and hand this to a supervisor of midwives before she takes up employment or commences practise in an area (NMC 2004a). The period covered by the annual intention to practise coincides with the financial year (April–March). The process continues in that every January all midwives who have notified their intention to practise in the previous year are sent an ITP form by the NMC. These forms are completed and handed to the midwife's named supervisor of midwives. The Supervisor checks on behalf of the LSA that each midwife is eligible to practise and if they are, signs the forms before sending them by the stipulated date to the LSA.

The LSA send the ITP data electronically to the NMC and the information that the midwife has notified her intention to practise is included on the register. Any employer, supervisor of midwives or member of the public can check with the confirmation service at the NMC to see if a midwife is 'live' on the register. Unless a midwife has submitted an ITP she may not practise anywhere in the UK unless in an emergency. In an emergency she may practise providing that she notifies her intention to practise to a supervisor of midwives within the next 48 hours (NMC 2004a).

Choice of Supervisor of Midwives

Rule 12 of the *Midwives Rules and Standards* (NMC 2004a) states that every practising midwife must have a named supervisor of midwives provided by the LSA. The guidance also indicates that midwives must be offered a choice of Supervisor and that if either the midwife or Supervisor finds that the relationship is not beneficial a change can be requested (NMC 2004a). The LSA Midwifery Officer, as part of the annual audit of supervision within the LSA area, checks that all midwives are offered a choice of supervisor and also have the opportunity to change supervisor if necessary (LSANF 2007).

Annual meeting with named Supervisor

Rule 12 of the *Midwives Rules and Standards* (NMC 2004a) informs midwives that they are expected to meet their named supervisor of midwives at least once a year. The purpose of this meeting is to review the midwife's practice and to identify her training needs. The focus of the meeting is on the individual's needs and how both the Supervisor and midwife can work to achieve the midwife's identified goals. Skoberne (2003) notes that statutory supervision of midwives aims to encourage learning by reflection, and all meetings with the named Supervisor should adopt this approach. Yearly (2003) also recognises that a proactive approach to supervision can be facilitated by using guided reflection.

Although the *Midwives Rules and Standards* (NMC 2004a) dictate that the midwife is expected to meet her supervisor of midwives at least once a year, in practice midwives may meet with and work alongside their Supervisors every day. Midwives recognise that such contact provides essential support and guidance in their everyday practice (LSANF 2007). Dimond (2006) also recognises that the best approach to proactive supervision is when the supervisor of midwives adopts an open and accessible approach. She recommends that open contact and freely offered guidance encourages midwives to practise in a safe and effective manner.

Support for student midwives

Within the local supervising authority standard, set out in Rule 12 of the *Midwives Rules and Standards* (NMC 2004a), student midwives must be supported by statutory supervision. This can take many forms, including student midwives being supported by a named supervisor of midwives in their practice placement area. Although there is no requirement for each individual student to have a named supervisor of midwives, the development of this mechanism is seen as supportive of the concept of a proactive supervisory relationship once the midwife has qualified (Mannion 1999).

Statutory supervision and clinical governance

Clinical governance came into being in the NHS with the publication of *A First Class Service* (DH 1998), which described a framework which supported professional self-regulation, clinical standards, evidence-based practice, learning from critical incidents and poor performance. Kirkham (2000) recognises that the aims and dilemmas of clinical governance are the same as those of statutory supervision of midwives.

By meeting all midwives practising in their area every year, supervisors of midwives ensure that not only are the *Midwives Rules and Standards* (NMC 2004a) met but that statutory supervision can be used as a proactive tool which supports clinical governance.

Support for women and promoting normality

It is important that statutory supervision of midwives is recognised as a support mechanism for women accessing maternity services. supervisors of midwives help women achieve their aims and support both women and midwives to meet challenges. Jones (2000) recognises that proactive statutory supervision is an enabling factor in establishing midwifery-led units. Mayes (1995) regards statutory supervision as supporting good practice and sees the supervisor as being the co-ordinator who enables midwives and mothers to achieve their aim – safe childbirth.

The NMC requires that supervisors of midwives promote childbirth as a normal physiological event by being involved in the development of strategies, guidelines and services based on sound evidence (NMC 2006).

Suspension from practice

Although they may recommend it to the LSA, suspension from practice cannot be undertaken by a supervisor of midwives. Suspension from midwifery practice may only be enacted by two organisations within the UK. The LSA may suspend a midwife from practice in accordance with Rule 5 of the *Midwives Rules and Standards* (NMC 2004a); and the NMC can suspend a midwife from practice under the powers of the Nursing and Midwifery Order (HMSO 2001).

Supervisors of midwives investigate serious incidents and allegations that individual midwives' fitness to practise may be impaired. The Supervisors liaise closely with the LSA Midwifery Officer and report any concerns to her/him. Suspension from practice by the LSA is a serious matter and can only be undertaken following an investigation (NMC 2004a). The midwife must be involved in the investigation and informed of the suspension from practice and the reasons why this has been necessary. The suspension must also be notified immediately to the NMC, which will decide if the suspension is warranted and if there are grounds for imposing an interim suspension order.

How to become a Supervisor of Midwives

Rule 11 of the *Midwives Rules and Standards* (NMC 2004a) sets out the minimum requirements for eligibility for appointment as a supervisor of midwives. In addition to these statutory requirements, prospective supervisors must be nominated by their peers before being considered for appointment by the LSA. The current national guidelines issued by the UK Forum of LSA Midwifery Officers advise on the many routes available for midwives seeking nomination to become a supervisor of midwives (LSANF 2007).

This is a considerable change from the 1970s and 1980s when supervisors were mostly heads of midwifery/managers of the midwifery services and were appointed because of their position within maternity services. In the 1990s senior midwives apart from heads of midwifery were nominated. The move to appoint supervisors at all levels of the profession is seen by Walton (1995) as a positive move. McCormick (1996) recognises that the qualities and person specification of people nominated as supervisors are very important. She advises that nominations should be sought by advertising, selecting and recruiting midwives capable of fulfilling the supervisor's entire role. Evidence suggests that where midwives are fully involved in the process of nomination, they nominate those peers who they feel will meet the needs of local midwives (Stapleton, Duerden and Kirkham 1998). Guidance issued by the UK forum of LSA Midwifery Officers reflects this advice (LSANF 2007).

There were no set ratios of supervisor to midwives until the *Midwives Rules* of 1993 stipulated a standard of 1 : 40. The ratio that is now recommended is no more than 1 : 15 (NMC 2004a) and the LSAs are charged with appointing sufficient numbers to ensure that statutory supervision can be effectively provided within the LSA area.

Supervisors of midwives must have credibility with the midwives they supervise and with Trusts' senior management. They should be able to demonstrate ongoing professional development at a minimum of degree level. They must be experienced, academically able, perceived as approachable by their colleagues and able to communicate effectively with senior management so that they can contribute effectively to developments in midwifery practice (ENB 1999).

Education of Supervisors of Midwives

Early supervisors of midwives received little in the way of education on statutory supervision. The first main drive towards modern education for supervisors came about as a result of the English National Board developing the *Preparation of Supervisors of Midwives* (ENB 1992). This invaluable tool formed the basis of many courses in all areas of the UK. Thomas and Mayes (1996) report that supervisors benefited from the structured format of the pack, which was based on a more educational and reflective mode than previous courses of preparation. They conclude that the pack was instrumental in informing both supervisors and midwives of the positive benefits of supervision, but that is should be updated regularly if it is to remain a live resource.

The pack was revised and reissued in 1997 (ENB 1997) and again in 2002 (NMC 2002). The pack was seen as an evolving resource and much valued by students on the preparation for supervisors of midwives course as well as established supervisors of midwives. The pack promoted reflective practice by the supervisor with each section encouraging the reader to examine their own thoughts on the subject covered as well as those of colleagues. The focus of supervisory education is now on supporting and nurturing midwives which improves practice (Steene 1996).

The NMC now sets the requirements of all preparation for supervisors of midwives courses in the UK (NMC 2004a). The publication of the *Standards for the Preparation and Practice of Supervisors of Midwives* (NMC 2006) details the competencies expected of supervisors of midwives. A further update to the *Preparation for Supervisors of Midwives Pack* (NMC 2002) is being commissioned, with the emphasis on the pack as a resource for both midwives and supervisors of midwives.

After appointment, supervisors of midwives have a minimum requirement of six hours' education relating to statutory supervision a year in addition to their PREP requirement (NMC 2006). The NMC requires that the LSAs provide educational opportunities for the supervisors of midwives (NMC 2004a). This can be undertaken in a variety of ways – conferences, study days and local activities around statutory supervision.

Is there a need for statutory supervision of midwives?

Jenkins (1995) questions the need for supervision as midwives are now educated to diploma and degree level and as such should be able to determine their own learning needs. Cross (1996) questions whether supervision is really necessary as the professional accountability of each midwife obviates the need for supervision. However, the Royal College of Midwives, in a position paper on supervision (RCM 1996), saw statutory supervision as a cornerstone of the profession. The College viewed supervision as self-regulation of the profession coupled with the fostering of practice by reflection and development, and concluded that it supports the autonomous practitioner status of the midwife.

Flint (2002) suggests that statutory supervision having being implemented as a means of control by the medical profession now has the additional problem of being influenced by the personality of individual supervisors of midwives. However, Fraser (2002) also suggests that midwives are in the fortunate position of having the system of statutory supervision in place as it offers support, guidance, counselling and friendship.

Wells (2004) found that whilst midwives regard statutory supervision to be necessary, many voiced concerns that it needed reviewing. She reports that conflict was evident as managers within organisations are accountable for systems within their department but statutory supervision of midwives remained within the control of the profession via the LSA Midwifery Officers and supervisors of midwives.

Wells (2004) reports that supervisors perceived that organisational systems and supervision were seen as a duplication of work, rather than a reinforcement of systems. She urged supervisors to focus on statutory supervision as otherwise the supervisory system could be lost, with organisations fighting to take total control to ensure all staff are performing effectively (Wells 2004).

The NMC, by being more explicit about the expected role of the supervisor of midwives and the LSAs (NMC 2004a, 2006), also supports the continuation of statutory supervision in the UK.

Conclusion

Supervision of midwives is evolving to become more supportive of modern midwifery practice. This change requires supervisors to become more proactive in the supervision that they give to midwives on the one hand, and on the other, acceptance by midwives that supervision and supervisors are not there to check up on them, but to enable and support midwifery practice in an ever-changing health environment. Statutory supervision of midwives should enable all midwives to practise safely and therefore protect the public.

References

Allison, J. (1996) *Delivered at Home*. London: Chapman and Hall.

Allison, J. and Kirkham, M. (1996) Supervision of midwives in Nottingham 1948–72. In M. Kirkham (ed.), *Supervision of Midwives*. Hale: Books for Midwives Press.

ARM (1994) First draft proposals for future midwifery supervision. *Midwifery Matters* (Spring): 26–7.

Bent, E. A. (1993) Statutory control of the practice of midwives. In V. R. Bennett and L. K. Brown (eds.), *Myles Textbook for Midwives*, 12th edition. Edinburgh: Churchill Livingstone.

Cross, R. E. (1996) *Midwives and Management: A Handbook*. Hale: Books for Midwives Press.

Department of Health (1993) *Changing Childbirth: The Report of the Expert Maternity Group*. London: HMSO.

Department of Health (1998) *A First Class Service*. London: HMSO.

Dimond, B. (2006) *Legal Aspects of Midwifery*, 3rd edition. Hale: Books for Midwives Press.

Donnison, J. (1977) *Midwives and Medical Men*. London: Heinemann.

English National Board for Nursing, Midwifery and Health Visiting (1992) *Preparation of Supervisors of Midwives Open Learning Pack*. London: ENB. Revised edition, 1997.

English National Board for Nursing, Midwifery and Health Visiting (1999) *Advice and Guidance for Local Supervising Authorities and Supervisors of Midwives*. London: ENB.

Flint, C. (2002) Supervision of midwives. Are we celebrating our shackles? *The Practising Midwife* 5(2): 12–13.

Fraser, J. (2002) Time to celebrate supervision. *The Practising Midwife* 5(2): 13–14.

Heagerty, B. V. (1996) Reassessing the guilty: The Midwives Act and the control of English midwives in the early 20th century. In M. Kirkham (ed.), *Supervision of Midwives*. Hale: Books for Midwives Press.

HMSO (2001) *The Nursing and Midwifery Order*. London: HMSO.

Hobbs, L. (1997) *The Independent Midwife*, 2nd edition. Hale: Books for Midwives Press.

Jenkins, R. (1995) *The Law and the Midwife*. Oxford: Blackwell Science.

Jones, S. R. (2000) *Ethics in Midwifery*, 2nd edition. London: C. V. Mosby.

Kirkham, M. (1995) The history of midwifery supervision. In Association of Radical Midwives, *Super-Vision Consensus Conference Proceedings*. Hale: Books for Midwives.

Kirkham, M. (ed.) (1996) *Supervision of Midwives*. Hale: Books for Midwives Press.

Kirkham, M. (ed.) (2000) *Developments in the Supervision of Midwives*. Hale: Books for Midwives Press.

Leap, N. and Hunter, B. (1993) *The Midwife's Tale*. London: Scarlet Press.

LSA National Forum (2007) *Guidance for Supervisors of Midwives*. Cambridge: East of England LSA.

Mannion, K. (1999) Midwives' Perception of Statutory Supervision and Supervisors of Midwives. Unpublished MSc Dissertation. Queen Margaret University College. Edinburgh.

Mayes, G. (1995) Supervision of midwives. In Association of Radical Midwives, *Super-Vision Consensus Conference Proceedings*. Hale: Books for Midwives.

McCormick, C. (1996) The chosen few. In English National Board for Nursing, Midwifery and Health Visiting, *Midwifery Supervision: A New Perspective*. London: ENB.

Midwives Act (1902) *The Public General Acts England and Wales* Edw VII C17 London.

Nursing and Midwifery Council (2002) *Preparation of Supervisors of Midwives Open Learning Pack*, revised edition. London: NMC.

Nursing and Midwifery Council (2004a) *Midwives Rules and Standards*. London: NMC.

Nursing and Midwifery Council (2004b) *Code of Professional Conduct: Standards for Conduct, Performance and Ethics*. London: NMC.

Nursing and Midwifery Council (2006) *Standards for the Preparation and Practice of Supervisors of Midwives*. London: NMC.

Robinson, S. (1990) Maintaining the independence of the midwifery profession: a continuing struggle. In J. Garcia, R. Kilpatrick and M. Richards (eds), *The Politics of Maternity Care*. Oxford: Clarendon Paperbacks.

Royal College of Midwives (1996) *Supervision of Midwives. The Strength of the Midwifery Profession*. Position Paper 6. London: RCM.

Sauter, S. (1997) Supervision from a LSA officer's perspective. *British Journal of Midwifery* 5(11): 697–9.

Skoberne, M. (2003) Supervision in midwifery practice. *Midwives Journal* 6(2): 66–9.

Stapleton, H., Duerden, J. and Kirkham, M. (1998) *Evaluation of the Impact of the Supervision of Midwives on Professional Practice and the Quality of Midwifery Care*. London: English National Board for Nursing, Midwifery and Health Visiting.

Steene, J. (1996) The Council's perspective and vision. In English National Board for Nursing, Midwifery and Health Visiting, *Midwifery Supervision. A New Perspective. 1996 Conference Report*. London: ENB.

Thomas, M. and Mayes, G. (1996) The ENB perspective: preparation of Supervisors of Midwives for their role. In M. Kirkham (ed.), *Supervision of Midwives*. Hale: Books for Midwives Press.

Towler, J. and Bramall, J. (1986) *Midwives in History and Society*. London: Croom Helm.

United Kingdom Central Council (1993) *Midwives Rules*. London: UKCC.

Walton, I. (1995) Conflicts in supervision of midwives. In ARM, *Super-Vision Consensus Conference Proceedings*. Hale: Books for Midwives Press.

Wells, D. (2004) Identification of the Core Competencies for Supervisors of Midwives within the Northern Consortium. Unpublished dissertation. MALIC Course. York.

Witz, A. (1992) *Professions and Patriarchy*. London: Routledge.

Yearly, C. (2003) Guided reflection as a tool for CPD. *British Journal of Midwifery* 11(4): 223–6.

Clinical Governance Framework and Quality Assurance in Relation to Midwifery Care

Cathy Rogers, Sally Luck and Nada Schiavone

Introduction

This chapter provides an introduction to the systems and processes of clinical governance and their application to maternity care. In particular, it focuses on the following key building blocks of clinical governance:

- Evidence-based practice
- Clinical audit
- Professional development
- Risk management

Although these are presented as discrete systems, the clinical governance framework requires the integration of all these systems to achieve quality in clinical care and high standards of midwifery practice.

Included in this chapter are activities designed to help the reader understand and apply the building blocks of clinical governance. In view of the fact that the aim of clinical governance is to ensure that the care provided is built around the needs of the user, the chapter commences by exploring the needs of maternity service users.

What is clinical governance?

Clinical governance is an umbrella term for systems and processes in NHS organisations to promote excellence in practice (Currie et al.

2004). The report by the Department of Health (DH), *The New NHS: Modern, Dependable*, states that the NHS *'will have quality at its heart . . . and that every part of the NHS . . . should take responsibility for improving quality'* (DH 1997). Clinical governance was promoted as the framework for NHS organisations to focus on the quality of care provided (DH 1997).

Improving the patient's experience is at the heart of the clinical governance framework, and successive directions for the modernisation of the NHS and maternity care have been driven by the need to improve the quality of services offered (DH 1997, 1998, 2000a, 2004a, 2007a, 2007b). National bodies to support the implementation of clinical governance throughout the health service include the National Institute for Health and Clinical Excellence (NICE), the National Patient Safety Agency (NPSA), the Healthcare Commission (HCC) as well as professional bodies such as the Nursing and Midwifery Council (NMC). Statutory supervision of midwives also provides a framework for promoting quality in midwifery practice (NMC 2004) (see Chapter 18) and there are many similarities between the framework for supervision and the framework for clinical governance. The central focus of both is the promotion of quality in maternity care. In their review of maternity services at the North West London Hospital's NHS Trust the NMC concluded that *'the safety of women would be enhanced by cohesive clinical governance systems along with clear lines of reporting that incorporate statutory supervision of midwives'* (NMC 2006a).

What women want and how women feel about maternity services

Improving women's experience and outcomes of maternity care is the guiding principle of clinical governance and NHS policy on maternity services (DH 2004a, 2007a, 2007b). The National Service Framework (NSF) (DH 2004a), which has defined current standards for maternity care, specifies that women should have access to supportive, high quality maternity services, designed around their individual needs and those of their babies. These recommendations mirror the recommendations made in previous policy documents; nevertheless, the evidence indicates that quality of maternity care remains a cause for concern. Whilst overall satisfaction with maternity services is high, concern about the quality of maternity care in many NHS Trusts demonstrates the need to ensure that robust mechanisms to promote clinical governance are embedded in practice (National Perinatal Epidemiology Unit 2007).

Poor standards of clinical care have been cited by successive Confidential Enquiries into Maternal Deaths (CEMACH) and successive Confidential Enquiry into Stillbirths and Deaths in Infancy (CESDI) as a major contributing factor in the deaths reported. The most recent CEMACH, *Why Mothers Die, 2000–2002*, reported that more than half the women who died had some aspect of substandard clinical care (CEMACH 2004). The CEMACH study on women with type 1 and type 2 diabetes found that the majority were poorly prepared for pregnancy and had poor glycaemic control around the time of conception and in early pregnancy. This study also raised serious concerns about the care of these women during pregnancy and labour as well as the care of the baby (CEMACH 2005). The findings of these reports clearly demonstrate the need to strengthen the frameworks for clinical governance in maternity.

The HCC is responsible to the DH for assessing standards in health care, including standards in maternity care. The HCC has highlighted a number of concerns related to standards of maternity care in the United Kingdom (HCC 2005, 2006; Kennedy 2005). The HCC identified a number of common themes that undermined the safety of mothers and babies. (Kennedy 2005). These include:

- Weak risk management structures
- Poor working relationships
- Inadequate training and supervision
- Poor environment, with services isolated geographically or clinically
- Shortages of staff
- Poor management of temporary employees

Another important function of the HCC is the investigation of complaints about the quality of care provided by the NHS. Approximately one in ten complaints relate to the quality of maternity services. Concerns about the quality of maternity care received by HCC include:

- Lack of services for ethnic minority women
- Poor communication between professionals and women
- Lack of staff necessary to give the appropriate advice and time to women
- Standards in cleanliness in maternity units

(Kennedy 2005)

Concern over the safety and quality of maternity services has prompted the HCC to focus on a number of projects relating to maternity services commencing in 2007. There is little doubt that the findings of these projects will provide further impetus to strengthen clinical governance processes within maternity services.

The following activity provides you with the opportunity to reflect on your perceptions of the standards of maternity care within your maternity unit and identify potential gaps in the quality of care. The recommendations in Table 19.1 are drawn from recommendations made in the NICE guidelines for antenatal care (2003), caesarean section (2004) and postnatal care (2006a).

Activity

Reflect on the standards of care in your own unit in relation to the recommendations in Table 19.1.

- In relation to local evidence, identify if each of these standards are met.
- Take one recommendation where you consider the standard is not met, and provide a rationale as to why this standard needs to be met.
- List what you feel should be implemented to support the achievement of this recommendation.

It is likely that you will have identified that these recommendations are based on the recommendations of NICE, and each NHS Trust is required to implement them as part of their quality improvement programme.

Table 19.1 NICE recommendations

Recommendations	Met	Not met
1. All women should be offered a booking visit before 12 weeks		
2. All women should be screened for domestic violence		
3. All women should be offered screening for Down syndrome		
4. The pattern of antenatal visits should be determined by the needs of women		
5. Women should be offered one-to-one care by a midwife in established labour		
6. Elective caesarean section should be performed at 39 weeks		
7. Skin-to-skin contact for a minimum of 30 minutes should be promoted		
8. All women should have an individualised care plan in the postnatal period		

Source: NICE 2003, 2004, 2006a

Developing and implementing action plans to facilitate and monitor the implementation of national standards is an important part of the clinical governance agenda in maternity services. Achieving this involves a range of activities including, evidence-based practice, risk management, clinical audit and continued professional development, which are the fundamental building blocks for clinical governance. Successful implementation of these systems requires strong leadership and the commitment of the entire organisation.

To facilitate the achievement of quality in maternity care, many maternity units have a clinical governance subgroup. The maternity clinical governance subgroup is accountable to each Trust's clinical governance group for overseeing the promotion of quality in maternity care. Membership of the group includes midwifery and obstetric leads for clinical audit, risk management, evidence-based practice and professional development in addition to a Supervisor of Midwives. The frequency of meetings is determined by local requirements, but on average the group meets once a month.

Activity

Find out the local arrangements for clinical governance in your maternity unit.

- Who are the members of this group?
- Discuss with a member of the group, the group's overall purpose – this is often referred as the group's terms of reference.
- How does the group relate to the overall clinical governance framework for the Trust?
- Identify the key challenges currently facing this group.
- Ask to attend one of their meetings.

You may well discover that the function of the group is to bring together the different components of clinical governance, so that each part is working in harmony with the others to facilitate continuous quality improvement in maternity care. You may also discover that the core components of clinical governance are:

- Evidence-based practice
- Clinical audit
- Risk management
- Professional development

The following sections will discuss each of these parts. However, achieving quality in maternity care requires the integration of all of them.

Evidence-based practice

The development and implementation of evidence-based practice for the care of women throughout their maternity is key component of clinical governance. Evidence-based practice can be defined as:

> *'the conscientious, explicit and judicious use of current best evidence in making decisions about the care of individual patients, based on skills which allow [the practitioner] to evaluate both personal experience and external evidence in a systematic and objective manner'* (Sackett et al. 1997).

This definition incorporates knowledge and skills gained from personnel experience as well as evidence derived from research (see Chapter 17). The value of individual practitioners' knowledge and skill is also recognised by NICE, which states that although *'clinical guidelines help health professionals in their work, they do not replace their knowledge and skills'* (2006b). However, clinical guidelines have been developed to assist practitioners to provide care within an evidence-based framework (Field and Lohr 1990). Guidelines for clinical practice can be developed locally or at a national level by NICE.

NICE was established because of concern over disparities in clinical practice between regions and hospitals. Part of the remit of NICE is to develop national clinical guidelines *'on the appropriate treatment and care of people with specific diseases and conditions within the NHS'* (NICE 2006b). The group who have responsibility for the development of NICE guidelines is drawn from members of all relevant professions as well user groups. Guidelines in draft form are available on the NICE website and key stakeholders are invited to submit comments and feedback. This is an important part of the production of the guidelines and it is imperative that midwives and other stakeholders are proactive in ensuring that their voice is heard. The Royal College of Midwives, the Consultant Midwives Group and the Independent Midwives Association, amongst others, are registered stakeholders, and individual midwives can have their views represented through these groups. The NICE website provides information on guidance in development, guidance developed and also guidance to be developed, which impact midwifery practice and the standard of maternity care.

Activity

Visit the NICE website at www.nice.org.uk.

- List the guidelines that the NICE have produced in relation to maternity care.
- List the guidelines that are in the process of development or review relation in to maternity care.

You will see that NICE has produced a range of guidelines, all of which can be downloaded.

NICE also produces implementation advice for all clinical guidelines published after October 2005. These offer suggestions on how to implement specific guidance locally, and key drivers to change, as well as potential barriers and strategies to overcome these. Where NICE guidance exists, local guidleines are required to reflect it.

Activity

- Review two guidelines in your clinical area where NICE guidance is available.
- Review your local guidelines in accordance with the recommendations of the NICE guidelines.
- Consider your responsibilities as a practising midwife if local guidelines do not mirror the recommendations produced by NICE.

The aim of national guidelines and standards is to support equality in clinical standards for all women using maternity services as well as the provision of a cost-effective care.

In additon to national guidelines and standards for maternity care, there must be clear local arrangments for the development and implementation of best practice guidelines. The process of developing and implementing guidelines differs among NHS Trusts, although the principles underpinning the development and implementation of guidelines are similar.

The Clinical Negligence Scheme for Trusts (CNST) requires each maternity provider to have a systematic framework for the development and implementation of guidelines (NHS Litigation Authority 2006). The overall responsibility for this rests with the executive board of each Trust, but each Trust division has a structurally identifed group whose members include midwives, obstetricians, anaesthetists, paediatricians, risk manager as well as user representatives.

The responsibility of this group include some or all of the following:

- Take the lead to promote the development and implementation of evidence-based practice across the maternity services
- Ensure that clinical guidelines are appropriately ratified according to Trust policies
- Ensure that guidelines are reviewed in light of recommendations of NICE, NSF standards, CEMACH and new evidence
- Develop a strategy for the dissemination of the guidelines to all members of the multidisciplinary team
- Ensure that information to be given to women is evidence-based
- Develop an audit strategy to measure compliance with current guidelines

The group is also responsible for ensuring that guidelines are reviewed in a timely manner, and for supporting recommendations made by NICE, CEMACH as well as professional bodies such as the Royal College of Midwives and the Royal College of Obstetricians and Gynaecologists.

Individual practitioners have a duty to practise in accordance with the guidelines, taking into consideration the individual needs of women. Rule 6 of the *Midwives Rules and Standards* specifies that a midwife's practice must be based on '*locally agreed evidence based standards*' (NMC 2004). Reasons for non-compliance must be clearly recorded in the woman's records.

Guidelines alone are of limited value in promoting best practice. Therefore, there should be a clear strategy to facilitate their implementation. According to the evidence, multifaceted intervention as opposed to one-off intervention is more successful in embedding guidelines in practice (NICE 2002). Strategies used to support local implementation of evidence-based guidelines include:

- Mandatory education programmes
- Case study review
- Reminders in clinical practice
- Reminders in maternity records
- Discussion at meetings/handovers
- Newsletters
- Information to women
- Reflective practice forums
- Feedback from audit

As part of the implementation process, barriers to the implementation of evidence-based practice need to be identified, and strategies to overcome these barriers identified (NICE 2002).

Activity

Identify in Table 19.2 possible barriers to implementing best practice alongside suggestions for overcoming these.

Table 19.2 Strategies to overcome barriers

Barrier	Strategies to overcome this

You may identify as barriers to successful implementation of guidelines lack of knowledge, fear, resources and ownership, and that strong leadership in practice is critical to overcome these. You may also identify that providing clinicians with feedback on whether the guidelines have been fully implemented is important in promoting compliance. Clinical audit is an important part of the clinical governance framework which aims to achieve this.

Clinical audit

Clinical audit provides a framework for measuring quality in midwifery practice through the systematic analysis of standards and the subsequent implementation of any recommendations to improve the quality of care (NICE 2002). Clinical audit comprises a number of different components, including the identification of audit topics, measuring compliance against agreed standards, and identifying and implementing changes in practice as a result of the audit findings. Further audit is then performed to ensure the successful implementation of recommendations and to monitor effectiveness of the implementation strategy. This process is often referred to as the audit cycle (NICE 2002) (see Figure 19.1). The overall aim is to improve the quality of care.

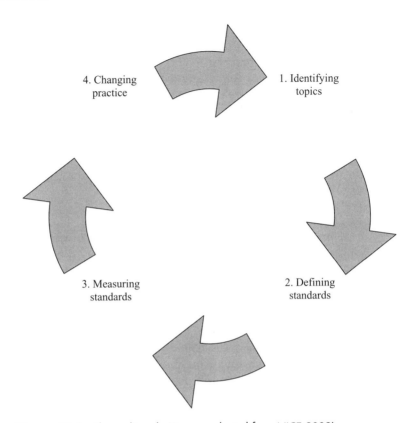

4. Changing
practice

1. Identifying
topics

3. Measuring
standards

2. Defining
standards

Figure 19.1 The audit cycle (Source: adapted from NICE 2002)

Standard 4.3.1 of the Maternity Clinical Risk Management Standards, requires every maternity service to have a systematic approach to the audit of multidisciplinary clinical guidelines (NHSLA 2006). Figure 19.1 shows that clinical audit is concerned not only with reviewing standards of paramount importance, but with implementing the necessary changes to practice resulting from the audit findings (NICE 2002). This ensures that the audit process leads to improvements in practice in line with the aims of clinical governance.

How does audit differ from research?

Many midwives are confused about the differences between research and audit. Although midwifery audit and research have many similarities, the purpose is different. Research is concerned with finding out what we *should be doing*, whereas audit is concerned with what we *are doing*. For example, whilst a midwife researcher might want to find out best practice in the frequency of antenatal visits for women booked for midwifery-led care, the midwife auditor might want to find out if the frequency of visits accords with local guidelines and NICE recommendations.

Activity

Provide an example that shows the difference between midwifery audit and research.

The audit process facilities the achievement of quality in maternity care by providing feedback on current standards, and improves practice through the implementation of action plans. Therefore, each maternity service should have a multidisciplinary audit strategy that is reviewed annually and is communicated to all members of the multidisciplinary team. Audit leads should include representatives from midwifery practice, supervision of midwives and from obstetrics. The role of the audit leads is to ensure that all members of the multidisciplinary team are involved in the development of the audit strategy as well as the audit process.

In order to coordinate and lead the audit process, most NHS Trusts have audit departments and audit lead personnel who are part of the overall clinical governance team for each Trust. Audit facilitators may also be available to provide support for midwives and other clinicians undertaking audit.

Activity

* Identify the audit leads in your Trust for maternity care.
* Discuss the support available to undertake audit with them.
* Identify the audit priorities in your clinical area.
* Find out if there is a local audit strategy for maternity services as well as dates for audit meetings, agendas and minutes for previous meetings.
* Attend an audit meeting.

Doing this will enable you to determine the level of audit activity in your local maternity services.

To reiterate there are a number of components to the audit process, including:

- Identifying of audit topics
- Developing agreeing audit criteria/standards
- Measuring performance against the identified standards
- Analysing results and practice implications

The latter stage should include strategies to ensure that audit recommendations are implemented. This includes a date for re-audit to ascertain progress.

Choosing topics for midwifery audit

Topics for audit projects should reflect national and/or local priorities for improving quality in maternity services, such as recommendations from NICE, CEMACH, National Service Framework as well professional organisations and local guidelines.

Activity

- Write a list of potential topics for audit in midwifery practice.
- Present the rationale for the topics you have suggested.
- Compare your list with the priorities for audit identified in your NHS Trust as you have identified by completing the previous activity.

You may identify a range of midwifery topics covering the care of women in the antenatal, intrapartum and/or the postpartum period. The topics you select may be informed by the recommendations from NICE discussed previously.

Defining standards

In order to measure practice, clearly identified standards are required. Standards for midwifery practice can be identified from a number of sources. Table 19.3 shows sources that can be used to identify appropriate standards for midwifery practice and maternity care.

For the audit to have an impact on the quality of maternity care, standards to be measured must be valid and based on best practice guidance.

Example of valid audit

The NICE Caesarean Section guidelines (2004) recommend that where possible fetal blood sampling (FBS) should be undertaken if

Table 19.3 Useful sources for identifying standards

NICE guidelines
Local guidelines/polices
Literature reviews
CEMACH
Royal College of Midwives
Royal College of Obstetricians and Gynaecologists
National Service Frameworks
Local Supervising Authority
Healthcare Commission

technically possible prior to emergency caesarean section for presumed fetal compromise.

This report highlights that this standard was variably met and that the lack of compliance meant that many women where undergoing unnecessary caesarean sections. Given that this standard is a recommendation of NICE (2004) and an important aspect of the quality of maternity care, an audit to measure local compliance is highly appropriate.

Measuring standards

In order to measure the standards identified, careful attention needs to be given to identify the following:

- What data needs to be collected
- Data collection form
- The methods of data collection
- The amount of data that require collection
- How the data will be analysed

Attention to these areas will ensure the validity of the audit as well as that only necessary information is collected. Getting the support of your audit department to help you choose which tools to use, and the most appropriate methodology to meet the objectives of your audit, is highly recommended.

Take the NICE (2004) recommendation on fetal blood sampling prior to emergency caesarean section for presumed fetal compromise and complete the exercise in Table 19.4.

Doing this exercise will give you a greater understanding of the complexities involved in choosing the methodology. It also clearly demonstrates that for the results of an audit to be meaningful and accepted, the audit requires careful planning and execution. The

Table 19.4 Choosing your methodology

Question	Consider the following
What data do you need to meet the objective of this audit?	• All women who had a caesarean • Women who had an emergency caesarean section only • Women who had an emergency caesarean section only for presumed fetal compromise • Women who had an emergency caesarean section only for presumed fetal compromise and it was technically possible to perform FBS in full • The stage of labour • Status/experience of midwife/obstetrician providing care • Was fetal blood sampling discussed, attempted, performed? • Reason for not performing it/reason for it failing • Results of FBS, number of times performed • The findings of the fetal heart rate trace • Experience of professional in decision-making to perform
Data collection form	• Do you need a pro forma to collect information? • Can it be obtained from your computer database? • What information is essential?
How will you collect your data? Will you collect the data prospectively or retrospectively?	• Patient records • Theatre records • Birth notification • Computer records More than one of these
Sample required	How many samples do you need to make sure that the sample is representative?
How the data are analysed and results presented	• Who will input information? • What system will be used to input data? • Data analysis methods to be used, percentage calculations, statistical methods

final stage in the audit cycle is the dissemination of the results, and the implementation of any identified recommendations.

Moving practice forward

Audits, like clinical guidelines, have limited value on their own in improving the quality of midwifery care (NICE 2002). For an audit to have an effect on the quality of care, strategies to improve practice need to be identified and implemented. Changing practice requires an understanding of change theory, and in particular how both individual and organisational change can be achieved. For further information on changing practice, see *Principles for Best Practice in Clinical Audit* (NICE 2002).

The results of a local caesarean section audit in one NHS Trust showed that FBS was not being offered or performed in accordance with guidelines. Factors identified that contributed to non-compliance included the expertise of staff, lack of knowledge of the benefits of FBS and the fact that the FBS machine was not working.

In order to begin to address the identified barriers, a multifaceted strategy was implemented to change practice with identified leaders in midwifery and obstetrics. This included:

- Dissemination of results in meetings, including multi-professional audit meetings, unit meetings and staff handovers
- Communication of audit findings and recommendations in clinical area
- Regular case reviews held on the labour ward regarding all women who had an emergency caesarean section for presumed fetal compromise
- Clinical guidelines displayed in clinical areas
- Multidisciplinary workshops held to empower midwives and doctors
- Competency assessments of junior doctors, and supportive frameworks to strengthen acquisition of competency in undertaking FBS
- Daily checks on FBS machines

Improving the quality of midwifery practice and sustaining excellence in care is the most challenging and rewarding aspect of the change process and requires strong leadership, constant reminders, and a great deal of motivation.

Professional development

A fundamental component for promoting and sustaining quality in maternity services and midwifery practice is a commitment by the individual practitioner and the organisation to ongoing professional development. The nature of midwifery practice and the challenges facing practitioners requires a commitment to lifelong learning. Continuous professional development (CPD) is mandatory for midwives. The standards for continued eligibility to practise as a midwife are defined in the *Post-registration Education and Practice (PREP)*

Handbook (NMC 2006b). Midwives, like nurses and specialist community public health nurses, are required to renew their registration every three years with the Nursing and Midwifery Council. The *PREP Handbook* details what is required from midwives to renew their registration (NMC 2006b).

Activity

- Read the *PREP Handbook*, which can be found the NMC website: www.nmc-uk.org.
- What are the requirements for midwives regarding renewal of their registration?
- What is the aim of this standard?

Public safety is the overall aim of the NMC, and this is achieved through a number of different mechanisms, including setting standards for entry into the profession, as well as standards for continued eligibility to practise. To meet the PREP standard, midwives are required to demonstrate that they have completed 'at least' 35 hours' learning activity in the three years prior to the renewal of their registration (NMC 2006b). This is the minimum requirement and as a registered midwife you are accountable for your own practice. Part of that accountability is ensuring that you are up to date with the knowledge and skills to provide appropriate standards of care to women and their families. Rule 2 of the *Midwives Rules* requires the practising midwife to have 'the appropriate skills and knowledge to understand interpret and manage as appropriate, the complex physiological, psychological and social changes a woman or her baby may experience' (NMC 2004). Furthermore, Rule 2 requires the midwife to ensure that her practice is up to date and 'tailored to meet the woman's individual needs' (NMC 2004). Continued learning and development is a core requirement for eligibility to practise as a midwife and is an essential part of clinical governance. Your responsibility to meet your learning needs is further highlighted in Rule 6 – Responsibility and sphere of practice.

Neither the *PREP Handbook* (NMC 2006b) nor the *Midwives Rules and Standards* (NMC 2004) specify what learning activities midwives are required to undertake. As autonomous practitioners, midwives are required to identify their own learning needs and take the necessary steps to achieve them. The Supervisor of Midwives is available for discussion and support in order to meet professional development needs.

Activity

- List different activities you could undertake to meet the PREP standard of 35 hours' learning.
- Compare these with the suggestions included in the *PREP Handbook*.

You will no doubt include both structured and unstructured learning opportunities, including reflective practice, reading, participating in workshops and study days and attending courses. The *PREP Handbook* (NMC 2006b) provides excellent guidance to practitioners for recording learning. It is important to demonstrate how that learning has influenced your practice.

Activity

Using the format suggested in the *PREP Handbook* (NMC 2006b), give an example of a learning opportunity you have undertaken recently.

- Describe the learning activity
- How did this learning influence your practice?
- What evidence can you provide to demonstrate its impact on your practice?

Most midwives do not find it difficult to identify and describe a range of learning activities. However, providing the evidence to show how that learning has influenced their practice is more challenging.

The government is committed to promoting ongoing learning as an integral part of the modernisation agenda for health care, and this is reflected in the publication and implementation of the NHS Knowledge and Skills Framework (KSF) (DH 2004c). The NHS KSF (2004c) describes the knowledge and skills that all staff working in the NHS need to deliver quality services. It requires all staff to participate in regular reviews with their manager, and an essential part of that review is the identification of a development plan to support each practitioner's attainment of the knowledge and skills required for each particular role (DH 2004c). Like the *PREP Handbook* (NMC 2006b), it recognises the different ways that practitioners can gain new knowledge and skills, but the most important factor is providing evidence to demonstrate how the learning or experience has influenced ongoing practice.

Continuously improving care provided to women and their families requires a commitment to lifelong learning and development, which is vital part of the clinical governance framework.

Risk management

Risk management is a process that focuses on continuous improvements in the quality of care. This is achieved by taking steps to control actual or potential risks that might adversely affect patient safety or the quality of care (DH 2000a, 2001). There are a number of factors that may adversely affect the quality of care provided to women and their families, including:

- Access to and provision of robust systems for the implementation of evidence in practice
- Lack of a commitment to continuous professional development
- Too few midwives and other staff
- Lack of clinical audit for measuring standards

Risk management is a framework that aims to identify and then control factors both clinical and non-clinical (i.e. lack of beds, poor standards of cleanliness, health and safety hazards) that pose a threat to overall quality of care. The term risk management is used to describe a logical and systematic method of identifying, analysing, evaluating and reducing risks in a way that facilitates continuous improvements in maternity care.

An Organisation with a Memory, a report published in 2000 by the Department of Health (DH 2000b), raised grave concern over the number of potentially avoidable events that resulted in harm to patients. Table 19.5 provides an overview from this report of some of the key findings that occur annually.

The report also identified that there had been little systematic learning from adverse events and service failures in the NHS in the past. The report proposed that a mandatory system should be introduced to identify adverse events in health care, to gather information as to their causes and to synthesise, learn and act to prevent similar events to reduce risk. The process for the identification, investigation, analysis and subsequent action implementation to minimise adverse events recurring forms the basis of the risk management framework (Wilson 2000).

Table 19.5   Key findings of *An Organisation with a Memory* (DH 2000b)

- 400 people die or are seriously injured in adverse events involving medical devices
- 10,000 adverse drug reactions are reported
- 1,150 people in recent contact with mental health services commit suicide
- 28,000 written complaints are received about treatment
- NHS pays out £400 million per year on clinical negligence claims
- Potential liability of £2.4 billion
- Ten per cent of all hospital admissions result in harm to patients due to adverse events
- The cost to the NHS is £2 billion a year in additional hospital stays alone (i.e. excluding wider costs)
- Some specific, relatively infrequent, but very serious adverse events happen time and again over a period of years
- The typical response has been to apportion blame

Risk identification – maternity services

To facilitate the reporting of risks in maternity, many Trusts have developed incident trigger lists to help prompt staff to report certain types of incidents. Any harm, actual or potential, to childbearing women or their newborn babies will comprise an event trigger. Examples include:

- Unexpected poor condition of a baby at birth
- Unexpected intrapartum stillbirth
- Obstetric emergencies
- Third and fourth degree lacerations
- Staffing and workload difficulties
- Equipment shortages and malfunctions
- Major obstetric haemorrhage
- Maternal collapse/admission to an intensive care unit
- Maternal death
- Maternal sepsis

An incident is reported by the member of staff flagging the event, using an incident report form. This is the recognised route within NHS Trusts to report actual or near-miss incidents. Incidents are then assessed and given a rating using the scoring mechanism in operation within each Trust. Incidents are rated according to:

- actual or potential impact severity on the woman or infant
- impact on service delivery
- impact on the reputation of the maternity services
- financial and legal implications

The impact is then considered in conjunction with the likelihood of it occurring again to give an overall incident rating. The scoring mechanism widely used in the UK is the Australian and New Zealand risk assessment tool (Australian and New Zealand Standard on Risk Management 1999).

The process of incident rating discussed above is commonly undertaken by a senior clinician or midwifery manager. Incidents are rated as low, moderate or high depending on the impact and the likelihood of recurrence (Australian and New Zealand Standard on Risk Management 1999).

Incidents that are rated low generally do not require further investigation, but will be recorded and considered as part of trend analysis of maternity services risks. Incidents that are rated moderate to high require investigation. The level of investigation will depend on the severity of the risk or incident, and the actual or potential harm (NPSA 2001). The purpose of the investigation is to identify the contributing factors and to isolate the root cause (NPSA 2005, 2001).

Root cause analysis

All incidents graded high should be the subject of a full root cause analysis (NPSA 2005). Root cause analysis is defined as 'a structured investigation that aims to identify the true cause of the problem, and the actions necessary to eliminate it' (Anderson and Fagerhaug 1999). The purpose is to provide patients and their families with information and explanation of why things went wrong and to prevent similar events occurring in the future. It is also required because of the potential for a serious complaint or legal claim.

There are a number of models used in root cause analysis (NPSA 2005), for example:

- Five why's, a simple questioning technique
- Fishbone diagram for incident analysis
- Gap or change analysis
- Brainshower
- Contributory factors framework

Further information on these models can be found on the NPSA website www.npsa.nhs.uk.

All the models aim to ascertain, and therefore eliminate or mitigate, the factors that may have contributed to the occurrence of the adverse event in maternity.

Activity

- Meet your risk manager for maternity.
- Request a copy of an investigation report into an adverse event occurring in maternity.
- Discuss the process used to identify the root causes.
- Review the subsequent action plan(s) arising from the investigation.

Following root cause identification, recommendations and action planning for improvement should be drawn up. This may involve changes in training policies, clinical guidelines and procedures (NPSA 2001). The effects of the improvement strategies will need to be monitored to evaluate whether they produce the intended results (NPSA 2001). Occasionally, particularly in serious incidents, it is important to start implementing improvement strategies before the root cause analysis has been drawn up, as immediate changes may be necessary to reduce immediate and future risk of a similar incident (NPSA 2001). For example, if the preliminary review of the records of a baby born in poor condition showed that the resuscitaire available at the birth was not functioning correctly, this would need to be rectified or replaced immediately, followed by swift communication of the procedural responsibilities of staff regarding responsibility for checking resuscitaires before deliveries.

Status of the incident report and investigation forms

The Incident Report Form and Investigation Report are confidential and legal documents and so should be kept securely. In the event of legal proceedings they will be required by all relevant parties. Therefore, in line with all professional records, it is essential that they are completed accurately and factually (DH 2006).

Conclusion

Clinical governance can be defined as 'The framework through which NHS organisations are accountable for continuously improving the quality of their services and safeguarding high standards of care by creating an environment in which excellence will flourish' (Scally 1998). Clinical governance therefore provides a framework for all involved in the organisation and provision of maternity care to provide high quality services designed around the individual needs of women and their families in accordance with the recommendations of the National Service Framework for maternity services (DH 2004a).

Providing the best services for women and their families is at the heart of the clinical governance framework and DH policy for the maternity service (DH, 2004, 2007a, 2007b). The most recent national survey of women's experience of maternity reported that overall satisfaction was high and that maternity care has become more individualised and women-centred (NPEU 2007). These findings are encouraging and may reflect the implementation of clinical governance in maternity. Nevertheless there is no scope for complacency given the findings of the NPSA (2007). According to the NPSA Bulletin 2007, over 60,000 patient safety incidents occurred in maternity between 2003 and 2006 and many of these incidents were related to delays in treatment and the failure to recognise complications (NPSA 2007). An article published in the *Independent on Sunday* (2007), based on a report by the NPSA, highlighted the need to strengthen clinical governance frameworks in maternity (Griggs et al. 2007). The report highlighted the fact that many women and their babies are put at unnecessary risk each year, with many suffering both physically and mentally (Griggs et al. 2007).

Moreover, the rise in caesarean section rates (23 per cent in 2006 compared to 3 per cent in the 1950s) clearly demonstrates the need to have robust systems for achieving clinical governance (DH 2007). These trends, alongside the concerns over the quality of maternity care, support the need for robust frameworks for monitoring and addressing standards of practice. Clinical governance provides a framework for this and is of concern to all of us involved in maternity care. The interrelationship between clinical audits, risk management, evidence-based practice and continued professional development to promoting a quality maternity service needs to be widely acknowledged. These processes should be a normative part of midwifery and maternity care practice and are the responsibility of every professional.

References

Anderson, B. and Fagerhaug, T. (1999) *Root Cause Analysis. Simplified Tools and Techniques*. Milwaukee, WI: ASQ Quality Press.

Australian and New Zealand Standard on Risk Management. AS/NZS 4360: 1999.

Confidential Enquiry into Maternal and Child Health (2004) *Why Mothers Die 2000–2002. The sixth report of the confidential enquiries into maternal deaths in the United Kingdom.* CEMACH.

Confidential Enquiry into Maternal and Child Health (2005) *Pregnancy in Women With Type 1 And Type 2 Diabetes 2002–2003.* CEMACH.

Currie, L., Morrell, C. and Scrivener, R. (2004) Clinical governance: quality at centre of services. *British Journal of Midwifery* 12(5): 330–4.

Department of Health (1997) *The New NHS: Modern, Dependable.* London: HMSO.

Department of Health (1998) *A First Class Service. Quality in the New NHS.* London: The Stationery Office.

Department of Health (2000a) *The NHS Plan. A Plan for Investment, a Plan for Reform.* London: HMSO.

Department of Health (2000b) *An Organisation with a Memory.* London: HMSO.

Department of Health (2001) *Building a Safer NHS for Patients: Implementing an Organisation with a Memory.* London: The Stationery Office.

Department of Health (2004a) *National Service Framework for Children, Young People and Maternity Service.* London: HMSO.

Department of Health (2004b) *The NHS Improvement Plan. Putting People at the Heart of Public Services.* London: HMSO.

Department of Health (2004c) *The NHS Knowledge and Skills Framework and the Development Review Process.* London: HMSO.

Department of Health (2006) *Safety First. A Report for Patients, Clinicians and Healthcare Managers.* London: HMSO.

Department of Health (2007a) *Making it Better for Mother and Baby. Clinical Case for Change.* Report by Sheila Shribman, National Clinical Director (Read) for Children, Young People and Maternity Services. London: HMSO.

Department of Health (2007b) *Maternity Matters: Choice, Access and Continuity of Care in a Safe Service.* London: DH.

Field, M. J. and Lohr, K. N. (1990) *Clinical Practice Guidelines: Directions for a New Program.* Washington, DC: National Academy Press.

Griggs, I., Hodgson, M. and Owen, J. (2007) Birth in Britain: too few midwives, too many risks. *The Independent on Sunday*, 4 March.

Healthcare Commission (2005) *Review of Maternity Services Provided by North West London Hospitals NHS Trust.* London: HC.

Healthcare Commission (2006) *Investigation into 10 maternal deaths at, or following delivery at, Northwick Park Hospital, North West London Hospitals NHS Trust, between April 2002 and April 2005.* London: HC.

Kennedy, I. (2005) Kennedy Calls for Improvement in Poor Performing Maternity Services. http://www.healthcarecommission.org.uk/news-andevents/pressreleases.cfm/widCall1/customWidgets.content_view_1/cit_id/2010.

National Health Service Litigation Authority (2006) *CNST Maternity Standards. Clinical Risk Maternity Standards.* London: NHSLA.

National Institute for Health and Clinical Excellence (2002) *Principles for Best Practice in Clinical Audit.* London: NICE.

National Institute for Health and Clinical Excellence (2003) *Routine Care for the Healthy Pregnant Woman.* London: NICE.

National Institute for Health and Clinical Excellence (2004) *Caesarean Section.* London: NICE.

National Institute for Health Clinical Excellence (2006a) *Routine Postnatal Care of Women and Their Babies.* London: NICE.

National Institute for Health and Clinical Excellence (2006b) About clinical guidelines. London: NICE. Available from: http://www.nice.org.uk/page.aspx?o=202669.

National Patient Safety Agency (2001) *Learning from Experience.* London: NPSA.

National Patient Safety Agency (2005) *Root Cause Analysis Training and Toolkit.* London: NPSA.

National Patient Safety Agency (2007) *Patient Safety Bulletin* (January). NPSA.

National Perinatal Epidemiology Unit (2007) *Recorded Delivery: A National Survey of Women's Experience of Maternity Care 2006.* Oxford: NPEU.

Nursing and Midwifery Council (2004) *Midwives Rules and Standards.* London: NMC.

Nursing and Midwifery Council (2006a) *Report on the Nursing and Midwifery Council's Review of the North West London Local Supervising Authority.* London: NMC.

Nursing and Midwifery Council (2006b) *The PREP Handbook.* London: NMC.

Royal College of Obstetricians and Gynaecologists (2001) *The National Sentinel Caesearean Section Audit Report.* London: RCOG.

Sackett, D. L., Rosenberg, W. M. and Haynes, B. R. (1997) *Evidenced-based Medicine: How to Practise and Teach EBM.* London: Churchill Livingstone.

Scally, G. (1998) Clinical governance and the drive for quality improvement in the new NHS in England. *British Medical Journal* 317: 61–5.

Wilson, J. H. (2000) Principles of clinical governance. In J. H. Wilson and A. Symon, *Clinical Risk Management in Midwifery: The Right to a Perfect Baby.* Hale: Books for Midwives.

Cultural Awareness Quiz Answers

1. *When is Ramadan and what must Muslims not do during this period?*
   A. The exact date changes every year. Muslims must abstain from all food, food preparation, drink and tobacco from dawn to dusk for a period of 30 days.

2. *Why do Spanish people have two surnames?*
   A. They take the paternal names of both parents.

3. *Why does the Christian festival of Easter move dates each year?*
   A. It is to do with phases of the moon. Start with the Spring Equinox (usually 20 March) then wait for the first full moon. Easter falls on the following Sunday.

4. *What religious group is defined by the 5 Ks and what are they?*
   A. Sikhs are defined by the 5 Ks. The five ks are:
      Keshas long hair
      Kangha comb – to keep hair tidy
      Kara   steel bangle (wear on left wrist)
      Kirpan dagger or small sword (Sikhs are a warrior race)
      Kachha undergarment, like boxer shorts (worn by both men and women)
   These symbols are important and should never be removed.

5. *What is Halal meat?*
   A. Blood-free meat.

6. *What is the origin of Halloween?*
   A. A pagan festival celebrated on 31 October, marking the end
   ·of summer.

7. *What religion is practised by most Indians?*
   A. Hinduism.

8. *What religion is practised by most Pakistanis?*
   A. Islam.

9. *What is the official language of India?*
   A. There is no official national language, although English and
   Hindi are most often used at the national administrative
   level. The individual states that make up India set their own
   official language(s), which vary from state to state.

10. *What are the main religions of Afro-Caribbeans?*
    A. Christianity, Islam, Rastafarianism.

11. *What is the official language of Pakistan?*
    A. Urdu.

12. *From which West Indian island do most Afro-Caribbean people in the
    UK come?*
    A. Jamaica.

13. *Who is/was St Christopher?*
    A. The patron saint of travellers.

14. *What is a Bar Mitzvah?*
    A. A Jewish ceremony for 13-year-old boys, which marks their
    reaching the age of responsibility.

15. *What is Rastafarianism?*
    A. A religion and culture; Rastafarians are now a protected
    group.

16. *What information about Rastafarianism would enhance medical and
    midwifery care?*
    A. Spirituality is central to Rastafarianism. Recognising the
    dignity of each individual, the assertion of self and the

importance of humility and peace come through strongly in their beliefs and attitude.

Natural food that is as whole and pure as possible is highly valued.

Breastfeeding is highly encouraged. Where bottle-feeding is necessary, women will want to know the brand and will avoid those containing animal products.

17. *How many times each day do Muslims have to pray and what do they have to do beforehand?*
    A. Five times a day, while facing Mecca (east). Beforehand they must wash hands, feet, face, top of head and nose.

18. *What is Nirvana?*
    A. Equivalent to Heaven. A state of bliss. The aim of the Buddhist is to achieve Nirvana.

19. *Where do most Buddhist international students come from?*
    A. South East Asia.

20. *What food is acceptable to most religions?*
    A. Vegetables.

21. *What is the ethnic origin of a person with a white British father and a black Trinidadian mother?*
    A. They can choose for themselves.

Glossary

Abortion Spontaneous miscarriage before the fetus is viable (i.e. before the 24th week of pregnancy); or, the deliberate termination of a pregnancy

Abruptio placenta The partial or complete separation of the placenta from its site after the 24th week of pregnancy

Acrosome A package containing enzymes in the head of a spermatozoon

Acute A term applied to symptoms that occur suddenly and for a short period of time

Aetiology The cause of a disease

Agglutination Clumping together

Alpha-fetoprotein A plasma protein excreted into amniotic fluid by the fetus

Amenorrhoea The absence of menstruation

Amniocentesis The removal of amniotic fluid from the uterus through the abdominal wall

Amniotic fluid *see* Liquor amnii

Anencephaly The congenital absence of the cranium including partial or total absence of the cerebral hemispheres

Anteflexion The bending forwards of the uterus

Antenatal Relating to the pregnancy

Anti-D immunogluobulin An antibody against the Rhesus factor

Antibody A protein produced by lymphatic tissue in response to antigens, which circulates in the plasma to attack antigens and render them harmless

Antigen Any substance which stimulates the production of antibodies

Aortocaval occlusion   Occlusion of the inferior vena cava and aorta by the pregnant uterus. Tends to occur if a heavily pregnant woman lies flat. Avoided by adopting a lateral position or using a wedge under the right hip. Also known as supine hypotension

Apgar score   A system devised to apply a numerical score to the condition of a neonate immediately after birth

Apical   The apex of the heart

Apnoea   Absence of respiration for less than 20 seconds

Attrition   A reduction in the number of those who started a programme of study

Bartholin's glands   Two glands situated in the labia majora which have ducts opening into the vagina just external to the hymen. The secretion lubricates the vulva

Bilirubinuria   The presence of bilirubin in the urine

Bonding   Mother–infant interaction

Bradycardia   A slow heart rate, less than 60 beats per minute for an adult, or 80 beats per minute for a baby

Brown fat   A type of fat present in the newborn that can be metabolised for heat production

Caesarean section   A surgical procedure in which the fetus is delivered through an incision in the lower uterine segment

Canthus   The angle at the inner (medial) and outer (lateral) margins of the eye. Also known as the inner and outer commissure

Caput succedaneum   Oedematous swelling of the fetal head due to prolonged pressure

Cardiotocograph   An electrical device which monitors fetal heart rate and rhythm, and the strength and frequency of uterine contractions

Cephalhaematoma   A swelling of blood under the periosteum of the fetal scalp due to shearing forces

Cervical   Relating to the neck of the cervix

Cervix   The lower third of the uterus

Chorionic villus   A minute projection extending into the decidua

Choroid plexus   Blood vessels in the roof of the ventricles of the brain, which produce cerebrospinal fluid

Chromosome   A linear sequence of genes in the nucleus of a cell, composed mostly of DNA, which transmits genetic information

Chronic   Prolonged

Cleft palate   An opening in the hard palate, caused by incomplete fusion

Coitus   Sexual intercourse

Congenital   Present at and existing from birth

Congenital adrenal hyperplasia (CAH) A condition caused by an enzyme defect which interferes with the synthesis of cortisol in the adrenal glands. Often the first indication of this condition may be the presence of ambiguous genitalia, or dehydration (with 'salt' crisis). There may be a history of CAH or unexplained neonatal death

Constipation Infrequent or difficult defaecation, caused by decreased motility of the intestines in which faeces remain in the colon for prolonged periods. Greater quantities of water are absorbed making the faeces hard and dry

Contraception The prevention of conception or of the implantation of a fertilised egg

Contractility The ability of muscles to shorten

Contraction The shortening of muscle fibres, or narrowing of a diameter of the pelvis

Corpus Body

Crepitus The sound of two fractured bone surfaces rubbing together, or the clicking sometimes caused when moving skeletal joints. Also describes flatulence or the noisy discharge of fetid gas from the intestine through the anus

Cyanosis Bluish appearance of skin and mucous membranes caused by insufficent oxygenation

Decidua The endometrium in pregnancy

Diabetes mellitus A disorder of carbohydrate metabolism caused by a deficiency of insulin from the islets of Langerhans, required to control blood glucose levels

Diarrhoea Frequent defaecation of liquid faeces caused by increased motility of the intenstines

Diastole Relaxation of the heart between contractions

Diploid Containing two of each chromosome. All body cells, except gametes, are diploid.

Dislocation The displacement of a bone from its joint

Dysplasia An abnormal development of the tissues or organs

Dysmenorrhoea Painful menstruation

Eclampsia Condition progressing from pre-eclampsia in which convulsions occur

Ectopic pregnancy Pregnancy in which the fertilised egg embeds outside the uterus

Effacement (also called ripening) Shortening of the cervix, resulting in the loss of the cervical canal

Embryo The product of conception from implantation until eight weeks' gestation

Endometriosis The presence of tissue resembling endometrium outside the uterus, which undergoes cyclical change in response to reproductive hormones

Endometrium The lining of the uterus

Engagement Movement of the widest presenting part of the fetus through the pelvic brim

Epidural anaesthesia The introduction of a local anaesthetic into the epidural space to block selected spinal nerves

Epidural space The potential space between the dura mater and the vertebral column

Episiotomy Surgical incision of the perineum during delivery

Epispadias When the urethral opening is found on the dorsal (upper) surface of the penis

Fetus The product of conception from the 8th week of gestation until delivery

Fistula An abnormal opening between two cavities such as the rectum and vagina, or between a cavity and the skin surface

Fontanelle An area of membrane between the bones of the fetal skull

Forewaters The bag of amniotic fluid formed in front of the presenting part of the fetus

Fornix One of the four recesses formed by the protrusion of the cervix to the vagina

Fourchette The fold of skin where the labia minora join posteriorly

Frenulum A longitudinal fold of mucous membrane that connects the underside of the tongue to the floor of the mouth

Fundus The base of a hollow organ situated furthest from the opening

Gestation The normal period required for the fetus to mature sufficiently to live independently of the mother

Gravid Pregnant

Guthrie test A test carried out on neonates on the sixth or seventh day after delivery to screen for phenylketonuria and other metabolic disorders

Gynaecoid (Pelvis): the type of pelvis most suited to childbirth

Haemorrhage Excessive blood loss

Hereditary Genetically transmitted from parents to offspring

Homeostasis The physiological process which maintains the body systems in constant balance

Hormone   A chemical secreted by an endocrine cell or gland, which has its effect on another part of the body

Hydrocephalus   An extremely serious pathological condition characterised by an abnormal collection of cerebrospinal fluid. Usually this causes an increase in cerebrospinal fluid pressure with related dilation of the ventricles within the cranial vault. The congenital condition is usually demonstrated by a rapid increase in the size of the occipital frontal diameter. Signs and symptoms directly relate to the amount of pressure and trauma caused to the brain and brainstem

Hymen   The membrane covering the vagina, which either perforates spontaneously before puberty or ruptures on first sexual intercourse

Hyperemesis   Excessive vomiting

Hyperglycaemia   High blood glucose levels

Hyperplasia   The increased production and growth of normal cells

Hypertension   High blood pressure

Hypertonic   Describes frequent strong contractions

Hypertrophy   The enlargement of muscle fibres due to cells increasing in size, rather than dividing

Hypospadias   When the urethral opening is located on the ventral (underside) surface of the penis

Hypotonic   Describes deficient muscle tone during labour

Hypoxia   Decreased level of oxygen in body tissues

Immunity   The body's resistance to infections

Induction of labour   Initiating labour by amniotomy or the use of hormones

Infertility   The inability of a woman to conceive, or of a man to induce conception

Instrumental delivery   Delivery of the fetus with the use of forceps or ventouse

Introitus   The entrance into a cavity or space, e.g. the vaginal orifice

Ischaemia   A deficiency of blood flowing to a particular part of the body, caused by constriction or blockage of blood vessels

Isthmus   A narrowed part of an organ or tissue

Jaundice   The yellow discolouration of the skin or the whites of the eyes caused by an excess of fat-soluble bilirubin in the blood

Ketonuria   The presence of ketones in the urine

Labour   The process of childbirth

Lactation   The production of colostrum then milk by the mammary glands of the breast

Lanugo   Fine hair present on the fetus, shed at about 40 weeks

Linea nigra   Pigmented line running from the umbilicus to the mons pubis, which women develop during pregnancy

Liquor amnii (also called amniotic fluid)   The fluid produced by the amniotic membrane in which the fetus is contained

Lochia   Discharges from the uterus during involution

Meconium   Waste material formed in the gut of the fetus in utero, excreted as the first stools of the newborn baby

Meiosis   The type of cell division by which gametes are formed, with the haploid number of chromosomes in each cell

Menarche   The start of menstruation at puberty

Microcephaly   A congenital anomaly characterised by an abnormally small head in relation to the rest of the body. Resulting mental retardation is caused by underdevelopment of the brain

Morning sickness   Nausea and vomiting related to early pregnancy

Mortality rate   The number of deaths in a population in a defined period

Moulding   The overlapping of the fetal skull bones

Multigravidous   A woman who is pregnant for the second or subsequent time

Nausea   Sensation of being about to vomit

Neonate   A newborn, up to four weeks after birth

Neural tube defect   A congenital abnormality of the spinal column

Noxious   Poisonous, harmful

Occiput   The back of the head

Oedema   An excessive amount of interstitial fluid

Osteogenesis imperfecta   Also know as brittle bones An autosomal dominant genetic disorder caused by a defective development of the connective tissue. May be suspected on late ultrasound scans. At birth the condition is known as osteogenesis imperfecta type II, with the newborn baby suffering multiple fractures that have occurred in utero. The baby's appearance will be deformed due to imperfect formation and mineralisation after bone fractures. Duration of life may be limited if head trauma has occurred

Oxytocin   A hormone released by the posterior pituitary gland, which is involved in the contraction of the uterus and the myo-epithelial cells around the alveoli of the breast

Palate   The roof of the mouth, separating the mouth from the nasal cavity

Palpation   Examination by touch

Palsy   An abnormal condition characterised by paralysis, such as Erb's palsy

Perimetrium   The outermost layer of the uterus

Perinatal   The period around the time of birth, defined as being from the 24th week of pregnancy until one week postpartum

Perineum   The pelvic floor and associated structures

Peristalsis   Spasmodic muscular contractions that create a wave-like movement along some hollow tubes of the body, e.g. the intestines

Phenylketonuria   An inherited condition in which excessive amounts of the amino acid phenylalanine accumulates in the blood, damaging the nervous system and leading to mental retardation

Phimosis   Constriction of the orifice of the prepuce so that it cannot be drawn back over the glans penis.

Physiology   The study of the functioning of the living organisms

Placenta   The structure in the uterus responsible for the developing fetus's respiration, excretion and nutrition

Polydactyly   Extra fingers or toes

Postnatal   After childbirth

Postpartum   After delivery

Postural hypotension   Lowering of blood pressure occurring during a change of position from sitting to standing, or lying to upright. Frequently accompanied by dizziness and light-headedness, and sometimes syncope (fainting)

Pre-eclampsia (also called pregnancy-induced hypertension)   A condition that can occur in pregnancy, characterised by hypertension, proteinuria and oedema

Precipitate delivery   Rapid labour and delivery

Preconception   Before conception

Pregnancy   The period of time between conception and delivery

Pregnancy-induced hypertension   *see* Pre-eclampsia

Prenatal   Before delivery

Preauricular sinus   A sinus located anterior to the auricle (external ear or pinna) of the ear

Pre-pregnancy   Before pregnancy

Presentation   That part of the fetus entering the pelvis first

Primigravida A woman who is pregnant for the first time

Progesterone A female sex hormone

Prolactin A hormone involved in milk production

Prostaglandin A hormone involved in the initiation of labour and in the inflammatory response

Proteinuria The presence of protein in the urine

Pruritus gravidarum Itching during pregnancy

Psychosis Severe mental illness, whose symptoms include loss of contact with reality

Puerperium The period of up to about six weeks after childbirth, when the reproductive organs return to their non-pregnant state

Relaxin A hormone that loosens the joints of the pelvis during pregnancy

Reproduction The formation of new cells or organisms

Retroperitoneal External to the peritoneal lining of the abdominal cavity

Retroplacental Behind the placenta

Rhesus factor A group of antigens found on the surface of red blood cells, forming the basis of the rhesus blood group system

Rubella German measles

Sacrococcygeal joint The hinge joint between the sacral vertebrae and coccyx

Shoulder dystocia Occurs when the normal mechanism of labour stops as the shoulders attempt but fail to enter the pelvic brim. Occurs with pelvic abnormalities reducing the pelvic diameters or increased bisacromial diameter (distance between the shoulders). This may be due to one (unilateral dystocia) or both (bilateral dystocia) shoulders becoming impacted at the brim or, with a large baby, delay occurs because of the right fit

Sinciput Forehead

Spasticity Hypertonic muscle tone with abnormal reflexes

Special measures Activities/actions designed to generate improvement where other methods have failed or are considered likely to do so

Spina bifida A congenital malformation of the vertebral column

Sternal recession Occurs when the alveoli fail to remain inflated and the compliant chest wall begins to collapse around the stiff lungs. The sternum is seen to recess, rather than expand, with breathing movements

Stillbirth Delivery of a fetus that has shown no signs of life

Striae gravidarum   Marks that may appear on the abdomen, breast and thighs during pregnancy, and seem to result from over-stretching of the elastic fibres of the skin

Subinvolution   The uterus is involuting (contracting) at a slower rate than expected or remains at the same size for several days. This may be due to the presence of retained products of conception, blood clots within the uterus, uterine fibroids or infection. It predisposes to postpartum haemorrhage and is considered a deviation from the normal

Sulcus A   A groove or furrow, e.g. the groove between the cotyledons of the placenta

Supine hypotension   Low blood pressure when lying on one's back caused by the pregnant uterus compressing the vena cava

Surfactant   A phospholipid present in the alveoli of the lungs which decreases surface tension, so preventing the alveoli from collapsing

Symphysis pubis   The cartilage between the public bones

Symptom   Any evidence of disordered physiology perceived by the patient

Syndactyly   Webbing between the fingers or toes

Synergy   Enhanced action resulting from the combined effect of two or more substances

Synthesis   The production of more complex molecules from simple molecules/atoms

Syntocinon   A synthetic form of oxytocin

Tachycardia   A rapid heart rate, above 100 beats per minute for an adult, 160 beats per minute for a baby

Tachypnoea   In babies under six months of age, a respiratory rate persistently above 55 breaths per minute

Torsion   Twisting of the spermatic cord that can cut off the blood supply to structures such as the testes and epididymis. Partial loss of circulation may result in atrophy and a complete ischaemia for approximately six hours may result in gangrene of the testes.

Trauma   A physical wound or injury; or a psychologically painful event

Trimester   A three-month period of pregnancy

Trisomy 21   A condition where an extra chromosome 21 is present, resulting in three chromosome 21s in each cell. Also referred to as Down syndrome

Ultrasound   Sound waves which can be transmitted through tissue to indicate changes in density

Umbilical cord   The temporary structure that carries blood from the placenta to the body of the fetus

Urinalysis   Analysis of the constituents of urine

Uterus (also called the womb)   The hollow muscular organ in the female in which the embryo embeds and is nourished

Ventouse   A method of aiding a vaginal delivery of a baby by attaching a cap to the presenting head to create a vacuum and then applying traction to expedite (in conjunction with the mother pushing) delivery of the baby

Ventricular septal defect   An abnormal opening in the septum between the ventricles of the heart

Vernix caseosa   The greasy covering of the skin of the fetus

Vertex (of skull)   The area of the fetal skull surrounding the posterior fontanelle that presents first in a fully flexed fetus

Villus   Root-like structure of the placenta, which lies in the material sinuses under the placenta

Vulva   External genitalia of the female

Index